Praise for *The Yoga Engineer's Manual*

"A must for your yoga library! *The Yoga Engineer's Manual* is the next step in the evolution of our understanding of yoga anatomy. A yoga teacher, anatomy teacher, and massage therapist, Richelle brings her vast experience to the table to turn conventional yoga alignment on its head and empower students to more deeply understand their bodies and their practices. Practical and insightful (with a dash of humor), this book is a must-read for students and teachers who want to create a sustainable yoga practice that can last a lifetime."

—RACHEL SCOTT, MSc Online Education, MFA, ERYT 500, YACEP, author of *Living Yoga*

"Richelle has a unique gift for translating functional anatomy into a language everyone can hear and for sparking the understanding of one's own body that motivates action and growth. She keeps it real and relevant, always connecting the dots of how what we do on the mat affects the engineering of our body well beyond asana. Richelle has been a steady mentor and guide for me in my work coaching elite athletes for more than a decade. This is a truly important book for all yoga practitioners—an essential guide for inspiring and deepening a sustainable, lifelong yoga practice."

—ERIN TAYLOR, RYT, founder of Athletes for Yoga and author of *Work IN* and *Hit Reset*

"Richelle Ricard will challenge you to question asana cues you've either heard 1,000 times or uttered yourself. She boldly disrupts our assumptions and asks that we open our minds and pay exquisite attention to what is arising in our bodies as we practice. She guides us to a clearer understanding of what we are asking of students and ourselves. You will be a more skillful yoga teacher if you read this book!"

—KAREN SCHWISOW, ERYT 500, founder and codirector of Three Trees Yoga Teacher Training

"This book is a must-read for anyone who practices yoga and absolutely essential information for every yoga teacher. Richelle brings to light the many ways that one single cue for the alignment of a pose cannot serve everybody. She tackles the important information on how anatomical difference needs to be considered in every pose and how to adjust each pose for those differences. *The Yoga Engineer's Manual* allows for a deep dive into the understanding of your own body mechanics and the variation of what functional movement can look like in other bodies.

   This book offers empowering knowledge that the only perfect pose is the one that honors and supports your body and its own unique configuration, while also shining a light for yoga teachers on the important differences in the bodies of their students. With the content of this book, I know my students will practice in a safe and supported way, and we will all be practicing yoga into our nineties!"

—SUZY GREEN, RYT E500, C-IAYT 500 Yoga Therapy Certified, owner of Three Trees Yoga Teacher Training

"*The Yoga Engineer's Manual* is a remarkable resource for conveying the complex subjects of anatomy, biomechanics, and special conditions in a way that is simple to read due to its smart organization and excellent images and visuals. Richelle has created a truly great yoga book for teachers, students, therapists, schools, and trainers! A must-have for every practitioner who loves their body and practices yoga."

—STEPHANIE ADAMS, ERYT 500, YACEP, OES, ACE PT, author of
Cancer Exercise Specialist Yoga

"Are you a yoga instructor? Have you had students develop pain during or after class? Do you wonder if there's something wrong with what you're teaching? There might be, but it's not your fault and there is help!

The yoga industry is not supposed to replace physical medicine, and yet many people will try yoga before they seek medical help—hoping to 'fix' themselves in your class. Thanks to yoga's impact on the nervous system, people often do find relief from various problems without extra guidance. But I can tell you from my experience as a chiropractic physician that just as many people get hurt and quit yoga forever.

Let this anatomy-informed yoga field guide, *The Yoga Engineer's Manual*, serve as the remedy. Richelle Ricard's extensive experience with massage therapy, yoga, and teaching informs her deep understanding of functional anatomy in this wonderful resource for teachers and students alike."

—YA-LING J. LIOU, DC, author of *The Everyday Pain Guide* and founder
of Stop Everyday Pain

THE YOGA ENGINEER'S MANUAL

THE
YOGA
ENGINEER'S
MANUAL

*The Anatomy and Mechanics
of a Sustainable Practice*

RICHELLE RICARD

North Atlantic Books
Berkeley, California

Illustrations on the following pages are original works by Rachel Schneider with digital annotation by Kathryn Stevens and the author: 14, 15, 25, 27 (lower image), 28, 29, 32, 33, 35, 38, 62, 78, 159, and 162. Copyrights reserved.

All photography is the original work of Kathryn Stevens. Editing, labeling, and annotations have been completed by Kathryn Stevens and the author. Copyrights reserved.

Published by
North Atlantic Books
Berkeley, California

Cover art © gettyimages.com/Benjavisa
Cover design by Mimi Bark
Book design by Happenstance Type-O-Rama

Printed in the United States of America

The Yoga Engineer's Manual: The Anatomy and Mechanics of a Sustainable Practice is sponsored and published by North Atlantic Books, an educational nonprofit based in Berkeley, California, that collaborates with partners to develop cross-cultural perspectives, nurture holistic views of art, science, the humanities, and healing, and seed personal and global transformation by publishing work on the relationship of body, spirit, and nature.

North Atlantic Books' publications are distributed to the US trade and internationally by Penguin Random House Publishers Services. For further information, visit our website at www.northatlantic books.com.

MEDICAL DISCLAIMER: The following information is intended for general information purposes only. Individuals should always see their health care provider before administering any suggestions made in this book. Any application of the material set forth in the following pages is at the reader's discretion and is their sole responsibility.

Library of Congress Cataloging-in-Publication Data

Names: Ricard, Richelle, 1979– author.
Title: The yoga engineer's manual : the anatomy and mechanics of a
    sustainable practice / by Richelle Ricard.
Description: Berkeley, California : North Atlantic Books, [2021] | Includes
    index.
Identifiers: LCCN 2020052124 (print) | LCCN 2020052125 (ebook) | ISBN
    9781623176334 (trade paperback) | ISBN 9781623176341 (ebook)
Subjects: LCSH: Hatha yoga—Study and teaching. | Human anatomy. |
    Biomechanics. | Exercise—Physiological aspects.
Classification: LCC RA781.7 .R498 2021 (print) | LCC RA781.7 (ebook) |
    DDC 613.7/046—dc23
LC record available at https://lccn.loc.gov/2020052124
LC ebook record available at https://lccn.loc.gov/2020052125

1 2 3 4 5 6 7 8 9 KPC 26 25 24 23 22 21

This book includes recycled material and material from well-managed forests. North Atlantic Books is committed to the protection of our environment. We print on recycled paper whenever possible and partner with printers who strive to use environmentally responsible practices.

Contents

*This book is dedicated to those curious ones
who seek to peel back the layers
of their own skin to see
the soul of their bones*

Preface

It's hard to believe that I've already been studying and working in the world of movement, bodywork, and healthcare for over twenty-five years. That is a sobering number. I was lucky to stumble into my life's calling at a young age. A somewhat random detour to get out of a high school PE class became the inception of a decades-long professional journey through physiology, physical therapies, fitness, and movement science. That path wound its way through terrain as varied as the US itself: high school athletic teams, high-end day spas, massage clinics and bodywork schools, chiropractic offices, gyms, yoga studios, Olympic-training teams, yoga teacher trainings around the world, retreats in India ...

I am a student, a practitioner, a teacher. I am both a healer and a guide. I endeavor to help each individual connect to their deepest self-awareness. I want to help teachers *see with clearer vision* and *speak with their most authentic voice*. I want to be present when practitioners find their solid foundation and grow from that place. I want to help them build that foundation.

I also want to laugh! I want to energize your intellect and pique your curiosity. I want to offer up a buffet of delicious tidbits that will deepen your understanding of your inner spaces, while keeping you engaged with functional applications that you can go to class and use *today*. On your mat or at the front of a class, you'll be able to use this information in real time.

I am the Yoga Engineer.

I am not a researcher recording data. I am a clinician. I am a practitioner. This isn't just an instructional manual or guide to better teaching but a memoir of my working life as a massage therapist and a yoga teacher. This is my memoir of healing touch in both of those fields, a recitation of how one can witness the sense of movement in our anatomy, observe the relevant actions, and take the time to know a body in the present moment, instead of just what it was and what it could be.

Regardless of your yoga style or lineage, there is a body that shows up on the mat, yours or your student's. That body is made up of tissues with very specific designs and functions. Those tissues and those functions have rules that apply to them, ways they interact with the world around them, their relationship with gravity and the physics of our environment. Every one of us is subject to the same set of rules, but each of us has an individual blueprint, our personal expression of those tissues, and individual needs for alignment and posture in the gravitational field. How do those rules apply to you and your students? This is what the Yoga Engineer aims to translate for every yoga student and teacher.

1

Perspectives on Practice and Teaching

The Yoga Engineer's perspective on practice and teaching differs from that of many mainstream yoga systems. I am interested in unifying your body's truths with the movements of yoga instead of imposing the form of yoga on your body. The following chapters outline how and why the Yoga Engineer philosophy is important to your practice and your teaching.

Why Study Anatomy as Part of Your Yoga Practice?

In yoga we examine and work with the places where the body, brain, and mind intersect and overlap. They are separate parts that can work independently or in concert. It seems we spend our childhood trying to build these connections and diligently learn about our world by touching, tasting, listening, making a ruckus, and "feeling all the feels" at sometimes excruciating extremes. We figure out what works and what hurts, and what hurts but seems worth the

fun. Many of us in adulthood, however, through various physical and psycho-emotional mechanisms, have detached ourselves from our self-awareness so effectively that we must learn it all again: how to observe, how to feel, and how to judge. After all, feeling takes an abundance of energy, and our busy lives tend to be lacking in extra energy these days.

This reconnection, this reawakening to our inner awareness, takes time and practice. Patience with the process and the blocks that arise is what the practice of yoga is all about. Anatomy is a perfect place to begin this journey. By building a base knowledge of the gross aspects of our structure, an understanding of our nature begins to emerge. Over time, this understanding evolves to a finer and finer sense of our experience of the external world, our mind's interpretation of experience, our heart's feeling about our experience, the energetic mechanisms that allow us to take part in the world, and, eventually, the purest knowledge of our existence at the very center of the Self.

In my career as a physiologist, massage and yoga therapist, and teacher of bodywork and movement, I've worked to encourage a sharper and more defined perspective on the body's engineering.

- How does the body's structure serve its functions?
- How do we define those functions?
- How does this relate to our yoga practice?

This training manual answers those questions and encourages more dialogue, exploration, study, and excitement. It dispels much of the rhetoric that is not biomechanically sound but is pervasive in our asana culture. To that end, we'll examine the physical body from the perspective of both structure and function.

This information is meant as a primer on the fundamental concepts of physiology and kinesiology. Even with this sleek approach, you'll be able to observe your anatomy and movement in a more thoughtful way. Like anything, the more informed you are about this subject, the harder it is to take the little things for granted.

Teaching Yoga: Science or Art?

I believe teaching yoga is *both* an art and a science. Perhaps teaching yoga asana is more like architecture than anything. As an architect, one must employ a great deal of technical knowledge within an incredibly creative endeavor. If you aren't artistic, your buildings will not be looked at with admiration or wonder or curiosity … they will not inspire. If you do not use the proper mathematics in your design

and work within the (presumably finite) limits of physics, your building will never stand the test of time, and it will likely present a significant safety hazard—just ask the factory workers in Bangladesh whose building collapsed on top of them.

A lovely new house in India, built to look modern and chic on the outside with beautiful lines and a posh paint job, will still melt and fall to pieces in its first monsoon because it was built of sticks and mud instead of rebar and concrete. Conversely, a state-built flat complex in Moscow will likely never, ever fall down, though it's certainly the last place you'd peg as a monument to the human potential for grace and beauty … it is purely and utterly efficient utilitarianism.

So, as yoga teachers we must observe that we are in a similar boat. We must ride a line between science and art, because like it or not, certain rules actually do apply to the working of the human body in this world. Therefore, we must prepare ourselves with a clear, linear understanding of the mechanics of the body and its relationship with gravity, all while calling upon a beautiful creativity and motivational tone. Neither knowing the mechanics of the body nor creativity alone will make a great teacher.

What Sets the Yoga Engineer Functional Anatomy Apart from Other Muscle-Focused Programs?

This is certainly not the only anatomy book written with yoga practitioners in mind. Most of them focus on the muscles at play in individual postures, offering beautiful images that light up what is stretched and what ought to be working. Some others talk in a dry tone about the technicalities that may or may not be applicable to your personal yoga practice. On one hand, I believe that the more information you have about your body, the better off you are. On another, I wonder if this particular information offers you any actual improvement or refinement to your practice.

This book takes a different approach. I'm more interested in telling you how your body works while it's moving on and off the mat. I think that if you have an understanding of how your tissues function and how your joints are designed, you are more likely to pay attention to how you move through space and time, not just where you feel a stretch. (I'm also sure you know exactly where you are feeling a stretch in any pose, not just because a picture showed you.) If you understand the relationship between your body and gravity, you are more likely to stack your joints precisely and use your muscles in the most efficient way to support those joints. This approach may sound stifling and clunky at first, but I assure you, when you learn to be strong and mobile at the same time, grace appears, and you are able to move with a controlled fluidity that is remarkably safer than simply flinging your body around on your mat in time to your playlist.

Most of the time, a technical anatomy class is *dry as hell*.

There, I said it.

This is boring stuff in the wrong hands. If you took any anatomy and physiology courses in college, even if you were fascinated by the subject, it's still not very exciting in class. Unless you had an exceptional teacher, you were probably bored stiff. That does not make

for good, solid, long-term absorption. My expertise in workshops has been in translating some very boring information into useful, actionable lessons that get you excited about learning some otherwise mundane data—and doing it in an entertaining way. I dance around like a monkey and act out the most crazy stories ... in person, it's pretty involved. I've tried to embody that sensibility here in writing as well. This book is ideal for those who retain details by reading and just soaking it up, but also included are experiential learning exercises for those who prefer a more interactive learning experience. In addition, online resources are available at YogaEngineer.com to supplement the written content here before you.

It is my intention with this book to offer you a clear look into the inner workings of the body that make direct impacts on your yoga practice. If you are a teacher, it will go a step further, offering you insights on how to bring this information effectively to your classes without boring your students with overwhelming technicalities. It is written as a manual, a step-by-step, layer-by-layer examination of the physical body. Connections are made between the physical and the subtle energies activated and engaged in asana practice. We'll discuss the mechanisms of breathing and the direct/indirect impacts on the nervous system as well as the energetic body. This information is formatted in such a way that you can easily use it as a home practitioner, or it can be inserted into any existing yoga teacher training.

A Note on Individual Differences

I am loath to try to define my particular style of yoga, though students often ask. (It's funny how attached we are to labels!) I understand that many people already have a basic knowledge of the different styles that are out there, and they are merely curious if attending my class would be appropriate for what they are looking for. On the other hand, I wonder what would happen if we all just walked into random classes and tried them out, owning our limitations in real time and trying something on for size just because it's there. Now, I admit I am actually the first one to be judgey and avoid things that don't immediately sound like the thing I'm seeking out, but I guess that's exactly my point: we could *all* use a little more experience outside of our comfort zones to know what possibilities even exist. After all, we don't know what we don't know.

I bring all this up because in my classes we move very precisely. In many ways I envy the teachers who just let their students run willy-nilly all over their mat and flow freely through the movements as their body and instincts dictate. Unfortunately, I labor under the burden of knowledge that many of the movements that "feel good in the body" are deleterious over time and lead to injury, dysfunction, and eventual disability—if we're not careful. At best we may suffer from neck pain, low back pain, or joint stiffness due to mechanisms that we simply aren't aware of triggering. At worst we can create lifelong injury and distortion. It's my belief that since this body is the vehicle in which we have to move around in this world, no matter your beliefs of the purpose thereof, we should keep it running as smoothly as possible.

The fact is, we are like snowflakes—each one a marvelous individual, one that is unlike any other in all of existence. And yet we are all snow! Very precise atmospheric conditions must be present for us to be snow instead of rain or sleet or hail. If the pressure or temperature or wind patterns are not just right, snow ceases to exist as a cohesive crystalline structure. So too the human body. Our bodies are made of similar tissues and arranged in very similar patterns, yet we are individuals. We all have bones, but our bones are shaped in infinite ways. We all have ligaments, though those ligaments may be long or short depending on our genes and development. We all have muscles, but they are shaped particularly for us, and our own personal brain has a particular way of interacting with that tissue. These individual differences, though, do not preclude us from abiding by the general rules of how each of those tissues works or how each of our joints is engineered. There are fundamental rules that we all must follow if we intend to keep these structures safe and sound long into our late lives.

Unifying the Practice

While the physical body in asana is not in any way the end-all and be-all of our yoga practice, it is in fact the *gateway practice* for a vast number of people. Sometimes I think that my detailed teaching style runs the risk of being pigeonholed as a physical-body practice alone, and honestly, that couldn't be further from the truth.

I believe this is one of the primary reasons we practice asana: to cultivate a sense of connection to our inner Self. Physical movement promotes a baseline conversation with this Self as you get to know it, probing deeper and more profound subject matter. But to be able to understand what the Self is saying to you, you must first establish a common language, and our physical body is the best reference most of us have to start learning that language. Consider how babies learn language; we start pointing out their own body parts ("here is your nose! here is your finger!"), and then how those parts interact with each other ("touch your nose!"), and then how those parts interact with the world ("don't touch the hot coffee!"). The eight traditional limbs of yoga laid out in the Yoga Sutras of Patanjali (Ashtanga Yoga) begin with the external ethics and morals (Yamas and Niyamas), then address the physical body, and only then tread into the depths of the energetic and esoteric body.

My hope is that through the work of refining our awareness in the physical realm, we gain the tools necessary to grow our awareness of the deeper layers of existence and develop a sense of containment of our energies in order to facilitate the deeper work. To that end, I believe there is a tangible reason to learn more about the human body in its physical sense.

So, if we can come to a deep understanding of the safest movements for our particular body, beginning with precision and strict adherence to the rules, building strength and genuine awareness of our finer points, we then can begin to move with more freedom and spontaneity. We may even, eventually, begin to bend the rules a bit, but only to the extent that we remain fully aware of the adaptations and compensations we may be employing along the way. We must always ask if the risk is worth the reward. We must have an ongoing conversation with the physical body to constantly reassess not only the "how" of the progress but also the "why."

Because so many of us are so profoundly detached from even our most basic self-awareness, the physical body is the ideal doorway to a deeper path. Not to mention that we can keep our bodies healthier and prevent debilitating breakdowns if we pay close attention to how we move in time and space. My hope is that this manual will be an ideal tool to reacquaint you with the body you think you know.

2

How to Use This Book

The Yoga Engineer's Manual is written to be relevant to a wide range of readers. Perhaps you are new to yoga and are concerned about how to approach the practice. This manual offers insight to your own body, how it functions, and how it moves in yoga. Are you a practitioner with experience on the mat? This book reveals some of the misconceptions that abound in the common yoga practices, and it shows how to make personal connections to your alignment and action. Since yoga teacher trainings (YTTs) abound these days, this book provides yoga teacher trainees with an in-depth curriculum that applies principles of physiology directly to your practice and future teaching. Maybe you have been teaching yoga for a while but recognize that your understanding of anatomy and physiology isn't adequate to keep your students safe and challenged simultaneously. This manual brings clarity to the how and the why we need to teach specifically to protect certain at-risk joints and tissues.

For the Curious Yoga Student

When you step on the yoga mat, whether it is at home or in class, for the first time or the four-hundredth, you bring your own personal body to the practice of yoga. If your understanding of the body is limited to the health classes you had in high school, or even anatomy and physiology classes in college, there is a large gap in your knowledge of how this body works at the connective-tissue and joint levels, and what that means as you move through your postures. This manual offers you a deep but functional look at the physical reasons your body moves the way it does, and why your asana practice is uniquely yours.

For the Teacher in Training

The path toward being a teacher is a long one and requires years of practice and study, long beyond the range of your 200–500 hour trainings. *The Yoga Engineer's Manual* will act as a textbook for anatomy and physiology but also as a well-rounded guide to teaching from your authentic voice. My interest is not in replacing the old rhetorics with a new script; my interest is in shifting all teachers into a new paradigm of using the body's integral rules as the blueprint for your sequencing and cueing. Within these pages you will be challenged to discard things you may have heard in every single yoga class you've ever attended, exchanging them for a teaching approach based on the actual bodies you see before you.

For the Current Yoga Teacher

When you shift into the seat of Teacher, you take on a certain responsibility for those to whom you offer instruction. You cannot feel their sensations and you cannot make choices for them about how deeply they engage, but you can use a language that ignites their critical thinking as well as their physical feeling. As Teacher, you have an opportunity to help make deeper connections between the physical body, its movements, the breath, and the questioning mind that takes one past a physical practice and into a spiritual one. This manual offers you the detailed threads of that connection. Through the lens of functional physiology and physics, you will see the body more clearly and all its myriad permutations. By building a better understanding of the limits of joints and tissues, the differences that change an individual's personal alignment, and the language that helps foster mobility and stability, you will develop safer, more powerful classes.

For Every Yogi

Whichever camp you are in, one thing is certain: this book is not here to make your job easier. It is here to help you find a deeper wisdom within. It is here to bring you into greater intimacy with your own physical nature, a place from which you will advance your practice through and beyond the physical, and with fewer risks of injury.

There is much work to be done. There are challenges to the common order. *The Yoga Engineer's Manual* will guide you through the technical to the nuanced and into the flowing Nature of your physiology as it pertains directly to your yoga practice. It is meant to be read as a narrative, with concepts building on each other to form a cohesive integration at the end. But it can certainly act as a reference for looking up specific information. If you choose, you can skip through to chapters that directly address your curiosity.

Throughout the manual, you will find stories that offer more detailed observations about particular muscles, joints, movements, and postures—some will debunk long-held beliefs, while others simply offer the Yoga Engineer perspective on particular subjects. All of these will be relevant to you, no matter if you are reading them from the perspective of teacher or student.

In addition, you will find opportunities in the Experiential Learning sections that ask you to develop skills of observation, vocabulary, and cueing. There are also sections dedicated to Adjustment and Modification. Though these may at first seem directed to teachers, students will find them useful too. For example: a line describing how I would make the adjustment may be taken as literal instruction for a teacher, while a student can imagine those adjustments being made directly on their own body.

A Note on Language

Depending on your training, your lineage, your teacher, you will have been offered various perspectives (or perhaps only one) on the use of Sanskrit within your yoga practice and class. The Ashtangis are Sanskrit heavy. I have a colleague who is only a couple degrees separated from Guruji himself, and he really doesn't know many of the English translations for the poses because he learned and practiced them in Sanskrit from the beginning, and that's how he teaches them in turn. Iyengar practitioners also tend toward the exclusive use of the original language of the practice.

Outside of these direct lines, space has been made for the use of English in daily classes. In part this is a form of inclusion, as many students feel intimidated by the long words they don't understand, and they get frustrated at an inability to follow the flow. Personally, my initial immersion into practice happened to be in a gym, but since my teachers had all been trained in both Sanskrit and English, that is how they taught. Gradually, I was able to link the names in my head and proceed with a pretty healthy knowledge of translations back and forth. My YTTs reinforced this knowledge for sure, but admittedly, many trainings have only a slight focus on Sanskrit.

A whole other book could be written (and probably has, but I'm not paying good enough attention) to the hows and whys and whether we should be using the original names or not. There are seemingly valid arguments on both sides of the cultural appropriation discussion: that using Sanskrit when you don't understand its underlying culture and meaning is disrespectful, or that using the original language is a primary form of honoring the non-Western origins of the yoga practice. I believe arguments could be made either way, so I will not dive down that particular path here.

In this book, I have chosen to use both Sanskrit and the common English translations as I've learned and practiced them. There are specific yoga styles that have created their own vernacular for the postures in English, which are different at times from what is presented here. So my apologies to those practitioners who find confusion in that regard; hopefully the pictures will help in clarification.

I try to introduce postures in both English and Sanskrit the first time they arise in the text. After that, to keep the text less cluttered and to ease the reading for those who have English as their primary understanding, which I believe at this point is the vast majority, pose names will be in English only. Where style and formatting dictate, I include both again, for consistency in keeping things looking good. What can I say, I like it to look good too.

So, if Sanskrit is not your first language of yoga, hopefully this book will help make those connections, since outside of YTT or yoga magazines, seeing the Sanskrit written out is not common. I'd love it if this piqued curiosity for more study. If Sanskrit is fascinating to you, I encourage you to dive deeper into the learning. Local teachers in many areas are trained by the American Sanskrit Institute and are likely to offer in-person workshops, or you can go right to the source (www.americansanskrit.com). I'm sure the Institute folks are not the only ones in the game; they are simply the ones I'm most familiar with. They are the go-to for many of the YTTs I've been a part of.

Additional Resources

Depending on how you'd like to utilize this book, I'd like to offer some other tools to help you on your yoga journey. Throughout the book you will be offered online resources, noted by this symbol:⚙. These are references to pages at YogaEngineer.com/resources/readers, accessible only to you, the reader. The resources include images and videos to further or deepen your experience of the written material in the print version. You can access these resources using the password *Engineers2021*.

Since the website will continue to evolve long past the printing of this first edition, you'll have access to ongoing updates to support material online. So even if there isn't a symbol directing you there, check in anyway to see what has been added recently—you may find answers there. Or you can use the contact form or any of the Yoga Engineer social media platforms to submit questions directly. Your curiosity may spur an addition to the support pages for everyone's benefit.

Asana Journal

If an asana journal is not already part of your practice, this self-guided project may be worthwhile for you as you dive deeper into your yoga experience. It is a lifelong practice like any other journal. It can look any way you want it to: a three-ring binder, a nice hardcover book, a series of composition notebooks ... the possibilities are endless and dependent only on your own style and aesthetic. My own asana journal is a set of two soft-cover journals outfitted with sticky tabs to help me organize my postures into groups.

The purpose of this project is to create a compendium of knowledge about the asanas themselves. I start with the name of a pose in both English and Sanskrit. On that page I draw a picture of the pose (or cut and paste an image from the internet!). Next I list the actions needed to refine this posture; this could be a bullet list or arrows drawn directly on the image. I go back and forth on which works best for me. From there, I start writing what I know about the pose—or wish I knew about the pose. Things like:

- What are words I can use to describe the energy or affect of this posture?
- What are related poses for preparing or countering this posture?
- Is there a mythology associated with this pose?
- What are the contraindications of this posture?
- Are there any specific risk factors to be aware of?
- Common misalignments?
- Is it in the traditional Ashtanga sequences, or has it developed in the "modern" yoga practice?

There are no hard rules for this process and no particular end point. This project offers you the chance to dig a bit deeper and do some research across intellect and experience. If you are a teacher or trainee, you might make notes after each class based on observations you made in your students' bodies. It gives you the opportunity to study the minutiae of a pose and its refinement, without the pressure of students hanging on your every word. This practice of journaling offers a chance to develop your own language around each posture and different ways of coming at it in class, whether purely physical or more energetic. If you use this for your own asana practice, you may write down new cues you heard or breakthroughs you made in class, or note a new teacher's perspective on something you've otherwise done the same way for years. It becomes a reinforcing/

questioning mental practice after the physical work is done for the day.

Over your lifetime, this journal will expand and morph. Your intentions for it may change over time, and as long as it continues to serve your practice, it can become an integral part of your evolution as a person and as a yogi. You may be surprised by what aspects begin to interest you most as you take notes. It may guide you down a path you never knew spoke to you before.

Here are the groups I've separated my own journal into:

- Backbends
- Forward Folds
- Twists
- Warrior I Standing Poses (neutral hips)
- Warrior II Standing Poses (open hips)
- Balance
- Side Bends
- Inversions
- Arm Balances
- Binds
- Sun Salutations
- Restoratives

These are by no means the only categories, nor are they the "right" way to organize the postures. These are simply what make sense to me. Perhaps yours are more simple: Seated, Standing, Lying Down. It only matters what works for you. Period.

I'd love to hear your feedback on this asana journal practice once you've been at it for a little while. Please send me your comments on the Yoga Engineer Facebook page, so I and others may learn from all of your experiences with it.

3

Terminology and Reference Points

In order to understand anything better, you must become accustomed to the language of that subject. In the case of yoga, learning even the most basic Sanskrit adds to the experience by bringing you closer to the origin of the postures, the mythology, the context in which these movements were developed. These shapes tell a story of their origins, and our English translations can not only miss the mark but can be so adulterated by our own cultural sensitivities that they convolute the intention completely. *Balasana* becomes *Short Prostration*, becomes *Prayer Pose*, becomes *Child's Pose* because "prayer" may be too triggering to the religious or anti-religious in kind. But the root of the pose is actually bowing in supplication. That was the point.

You are certainly not less-than if you prefer your classes to be taught in English, or any other mother tongue for that matter, but the brain really does engage in a different way when the postures are communicated in their native Sanskrit. (Chanting is another example, but that's a whole book of its own.)

The same holds true for the science of anatomy. We can use lay terms all day long, and perhaps that is the most appropriate language to actively use in class, but I believe it's important to learn the technical language first, so you can be as specific as possible in your translations. You do not want to communicate half-truths because you lack the fundamental understanding of the original terminology. It is our goal to communicate as clearly as possible with our students, and that means starting with a clear and consistent, accurate vocabulary.

In addition, you'll learn the Yoga Engineer's Principles of Physiology. These outline some primary concepts that support how and why we approach practice as we do.

Basic Terminology

Technical language isn't always appropriate to teaching in class, but it enhances the context of the material as you gain knowledge of the structure and function of the human body.

Reference Words

- **Anatomical Position** = Mountain pose (Tadasana), essentially; all reference terms are defined from this shape. Even if you change positions relative to the floor, actions are defined precisely as if you were still in Mountain pose.
- **Medial** (also **Internal**) = toward the midline (the breastbone is medial to the ribs)
- **Lateral** (also **External**) = away from the midline (the hip joint is lateral to the pubic bone)
- **Superior** = above the current reference point (the ribs are superior to the pelvis)
- **Inferior** = below the current reference point (the ribs are inferior to the skull)
- **Distal** = specific to the limbs, away from the torso (the hand is distal to the elbow)
- **Proximal** = specific to the limbs, toward the torso (the shoulder is proximal to the elbow)
- **Deep** = level under the skin, toward the bone/central channel
- **Superficial** = opposite of deep, toward the skin and away from the bone/central channel
- **Anterior** = the front of the body or toward the front
- **Posterior** = the back of the body or toward the back

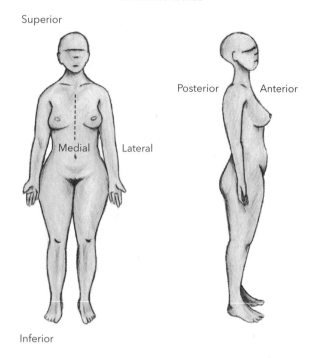

Reference Words

Superior

Posterior   Anterior

Medial   Lateral

Inferior

Range of Motion

Form follows function. I forget where I first heard this adage, but I suspect it was in my middle school biology class. Everything in Nature has a purpose, and that purpose defines how a thing is built, because energy is seldom wasted on building things that have no purpose to begin with. In our bodies, this plays out in every cell and every tissue. It is perhaps most noticeable in how our joints are shaped. Each joint has a specific job to do and therefore has a particular shape. That shape defines its total range of motion. The shoulder, for example, is differentiated from the hip in that the hip is built to bear weight as we walk on two legs, while the shoulder is built for reaching around in our world. While both of these joints are considered *ball and socket* joints, they are free-moving or restricted in different ways in order to achieve their purpose with the greatest efficiency.

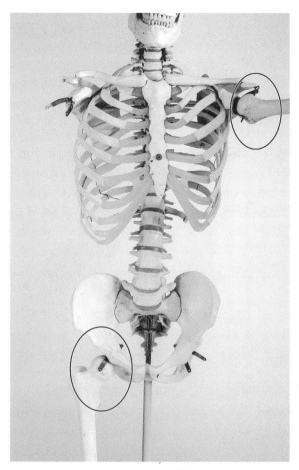

The two major ball and socket joints have different structural design, therefore different functions.

Planes of Movement

In kinesiology (the study of joints and their movement) we isolate movements onto very specific planes before we integrate them back together as full range of motion. While we can swing our arms around in all sorts of directions, it's easier to understand the healthy limitations of the shoulder joint if we break down its range into individual movements first. We do this by dividing each joint along **planes of movement**.

Consider a pane of glass, flat, hard, unbending. Now imagine that the pane of glass cuts your body in two. There are many different directions with which you could split the body, and we have named a few of these specifically:

- The **sagittal** plane cuts the body left from right.
- The **coronal** (or **frontal**) plane cuts the body back from front.
- The **transverse** plane cuts the body top from bottom.

Every joint is bisected by these various planes; the diagram offered here illustrates the joints of the spine as they are intersected by the planes of movement. You would also have a sagittal plane for your shoulder joint, one for your hip, knee, elbow, wrist, etc.

Planes of Movement

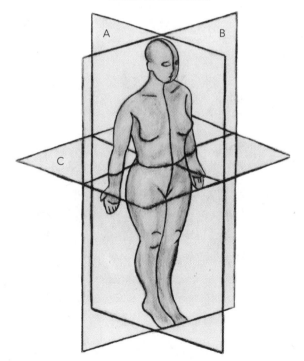

(A) Sagittal plane, (B) Coronal plane, (C) Transverse plane

Defining Range of Motion

Consider this model: the wheels of your car spin on an axle. The axle is perpendicular to the wheel, allowing the wheel to spin in only two directions (forward and backward), *on one plane*. The only way that wheel may go a different direction is if the axle itself is moved to intersect another plane.

If you think of the spine lined up on a sagittal plane (the wheel), intersected by a perpendicular axis (the axle), the spine should only be able to move forward and back on that plane. Those are the only two actions available on that plane—forward and back (we call this *flexion* when we bend forward and *extension* when we bend back). The same is true on the sagittal plane of the shoulder, knee, hip, elbow, wrist, etc. The *only* movements available on the sagittal plane are flexion and extension.

The same is true for every defined plane of movement: only certain movements are available on each one.

- **Sagittal** = flexion/extension = movement forward and back

- **Coronal** = lateral flexion (side bending at the spine); abduction/adduction = reaching out to the side, and returning back toward the centerline

- **Transverse** = rotation = twisting left and right at the spine; internal/external or medial/lateral = turning the arm or thigh in toward the midline or away from the midline; supination/pronation = turning the forearm in toward or away from the midline

For our purposes going forward, it's important to note that movements and actions will differ slightly in reference to specific alignment in postures. **Movement** will refer to the gross movement through space to make the general shape of an asana. **Actions** will refer to fine motor contractions once in the pose in order to support your joints efficiently and safely in gravity.

Principles of Physiology

These principles are the backbone, so to speak, of the Yoga Engineer approach to asana practice. They represent the most fundamental aspects of physiology as it is relevant to yoga. *Kinesiology* is the study of the movement of joints, and we integrate that important perspective here as well. Since I believe in an education grounded in concept and principle and not only of rote memorization, you will be well served to commit to understanding these fully over time. These principles are all immediately applicable to every single posture, so by learning them you can more easily assess the technical characteristics of any body in any pose. While each individual is unique, these are the things that we all share.

Sensation is not always the best barometer of effective movement. Our brain has impressions of where we are in place and time, but these impressions may not be accurate. Our proprioception may be altered by recurrent postural misalignments … so what feels "normal" may not actually be "straight."

Our brain can have a hard time discerning the difference between stretch and compression. These sensations may at first feel the same. Going further into this sensation may cause damage to soft tissues and joint structures.

Just because you can go there doesn't mean you should. A lack of sensation does not always mean "go further to get in it." Some of us have long, supple muscle tissue, in which case reaching the sensation of stretch can be difficult. In fact, there is the possibility you'll stretch too far. If your muscles are at their longest, you'll start stretching into your tendons and ligaments. This is not good. Over time, it will lead to instability and degeneration of the joint tissues.

Muscles are their strongest when in their midrange. In essence, any muscle that is too long or too short is not as strong as it can be. From 75 to 110 percent of its resting length is where every muscle belly is strongest. Shorter or longer than this range, the muscle loses integrity and power. Note that you have way more play in the "short" category than in the "long" category—an active muscle can only lengthen by 10 percent before it loses integrity.

The shape of your bones is as individual as your fingerprints, and it defines your movement. Some traditional alignments are not beneficial for some joints, and they can even cause damage over time. Once you observe and understand your own bony shape, it is in your best interest to tailor your practice to the shape of your bones, not the pictures in a book.

Habits are hard to break, but you can do it. Your brain has worked hard to observe patterns in your world and in your actions ... you'll have to work ten times as hard to change those patterns. You'll need to strengthen new muscles, relearn how to use old muscles, and reinterpret sensations. It won't be easy, it will likely be unpleasant, but you can do it.

Counteraction: the way we stabilize our skeletal system. When opposing muscles work against each other to reach equilibrium, they effectively stabilize a joint through isometric contraction (a muscle contracting without changing length). True counteraction cannot take place in a locked joint.

The Law of Compensation. A restriction of movement in one place transfers force to the next available mobile point.

Over time, repeated movement at the compensation points results in *hypermobility*—a joint moving beyond its normal range—and instability. This isn't good. Hypermobility is a common factor in joint degeneration. When a joint is too sloppy, the tissues sustain far greater impacts in regular movement than when those two surfaces are closely articulated and can translate force cleanly from one bone to the next.

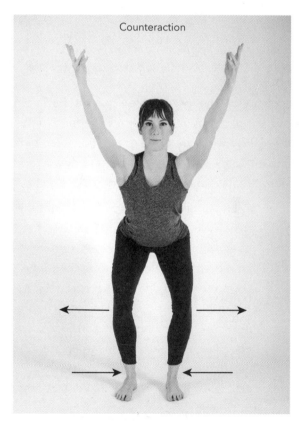

Counteraction

The counteracting abduction and adduction actions of the legs stabilize the hip joints and activate the entire length of the leg, creating support for the upper body.

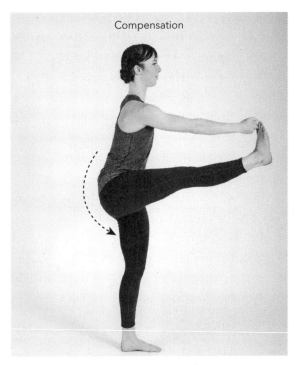

Compensation

Without sufficient mobility in hip flexion, the spine will compensate with flexion of its own.

Gravity. The force of gravity is a constant in our world, so our body is always adapting to this force. How we move in the gravitational field will impact which muscles engage and how ... and vice versa. We must acknowledge two things:

*   First, our orientation in space will determine which muscles need to fire to hold us up. Consider this: when in a side plank, with your left hand on the mat, your left side-body must contract to lift the ribs and hips up away from the floor (essentially creating a left side bend). If you make that same shape when standing upright, however, it will be the right side-body that contracts to control your movement and hold you up in gravity.

*   Second, we can engage gravity actively and make it our ally instead of our enemy. To that end, we will be well served to understand a particular law of physics ...

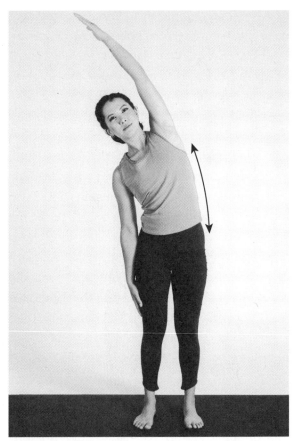

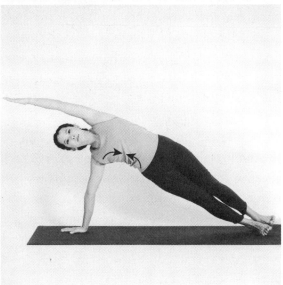

In the side bend, Elena's long side is using eccentric contractions to control her movement, getting longer. In side plank, the exact same shape uses the opposite side in concentric contraction to create movement, getting shorter.

Newton's Third Law. "For every action, there is an equal and opposite reaction."

This distilled version of Newton's law is the linchpin to a successful yoga practice, both within the body and in our relationship to Earth's gravity. When we engage opposing muscle groups (counteraction), we employ Newton's law. When we root our feet down in order to feel rebound upward, we employ Newton's law. If we acknowledge that Earth is actually pushing on us with the same amount of force that we apply to it, we can feel a productive levity. Think to yourself, "I only need to do half of the work, because the ground is doing the other half." You will feel more buoyant, and your postures will seem to float instead of drag you down.

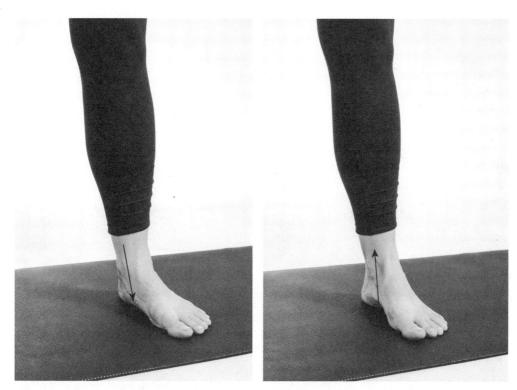

On the left, the foot is inactive so the arches fall. On the right, Richelle is actively pressing the edges of her feet through the mat, so the arches rise.

4

Relevant Human Systems

If this were a generic Anatomy and Physiology class, we'd cover all the systems of the body, but it's not a generic class, so we won't waste your time. Instead, you should be informed in the basics of just a couple of those systems. You should understand the fundamental functions of each and a bit about how they interact. These systems cannot act in isolation; they are fundamentally integrated, one action creating a reaction elsewhere, one serving the other in an intricate circuitry. For purposes of simplicity, we'll isolate them in theory only, in order to try to grasp their most basic functions as relevant to our practice and teaching.

The primary systems of interest to us are:

- Nervous
- Endocrine
- Respiratory
- Skeletal
- Integumentary
- Muscular

The Nervous System

The nervous system can be broken down two ways: the physical division and functional division. Of course, since this is science, these two categories can be broken down as well. The physical division becomes the *central nervous system* (CNS) and the *peripheral nervous system* (PNS). The CNS = brain + spinal cord. This is "central command," where all the processing of data happens. The PNS = all the nerves outside the spinal column. These nerves connect the CNS to all the sensory and motor structures throughout the body. The functional division breaks down to the somatic and the autonomic. The *somatic nervous system* = conscious action and motor control. We use this to consciously move our body through space. The *autonomic nervous system* = unconscious sensory/motor control: organs, glands, etc. The autonomic then splits into *sympathetic* and *parasympathetic*: stress vs. relaxation.

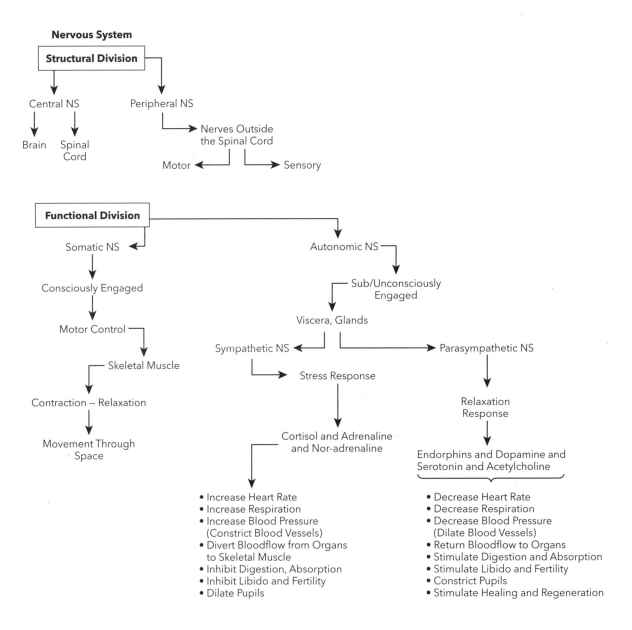

It seems obvious, but the brain is the end-all, be-all of our experience in time and place. From infancy the brain is making and recording observations. It gathers data through its sensory organs—eyes, ears, skin, taste buds, and proprioceptors in our muscles. (*Proprioceptors* are biosensors throughout our muscles that tell the brain where we are in place and time; the brain bases many assumptions about our reality on the data gathered here.)

It creates a hierarchy of processing based on the things it sees most often and begins organizing itself based on observed patterns. This process is called *neural networking*.

The peripheral nerves that leave the spinal cord to enervate our organs, muscles, and skin have both sensory and motor pathways. We use the sensory information to create motor actions. If either path is damaged or impaired, we lose acuity in our interaction with the world. Moving our body through space-time helps keep these pathways clear and the brain's perceptions pliable and fine-tuned. Impairment of this system can be the result of reduced circulation due to impingement by bones or soft tissue, stretching, or, of course, trauma that severs the nerve completely.

As we continue to grow, the brain reacts to stimuli based on these patterns and, for efficiency, begins to filter out much of the information around us, paying attention to only about one-third of the available data in our environment. Typically, we see mostly what is already familiar to us until some significant distraction moves our attention to the new and surprising. Our mind begins to add judgment to this process, and the details of our perception are refined further. Our perception literally becomes our reality. Once a neural net is in place, it is there for good. New networks may be established with new patterns, but flipping the switch to the new network is tough. Habituation is real and is difficult to change because there is literally a physical brain component to those habits. It takes work to instill new patterns without reverting to old ones. It can be done though.

The Endocrine System

The endocrine system is where we produce and distribute hormones. Hormones are chemical messengers, like little bio-instruction manuals that trigger our organs to function in specific ways. We may often think of them working solely in the area of sex, but they are responsible for ensuring nearly all the functions within our cell walls, organs, and body as a whole.

Because of this total-body necessity, the endocrine system is deeply linked to the nervous system. Most primally, the hormones associated with how we respond to stressors in our environment affect the fundamental functions of respiration, heartbeat, and blood flow. This is our link between our survival instincts and the actions that will keep us alive when faced with danger.

For our purposes, it's sufficient to be familiar with the autonomic division of the functional nervous system that breaks down to the sympathetic nervous system (SNS) and the parasympathetic nervous system (PNS).

The SNS is our stress response, the "fight-or-flight" reaction to stressors in our environment. The hormones adrenalin, noradrenaline, and cortisol flood our system, so we have the immediate capacity to face our foe or run from them, fast. These chemicals dull pain, increase capacity for muscular contraction, and help us focus our attention to a very sharp point. There are obvious responses such as increased heart rate to move more blood to the muscles that will require more oxygen, and also increased respiration to provide that oxygen. But there are more subtle responses as well: blood vessel dilation to the muscles to accommodate the increased blood flow, the cessation of nonessential organ functions such as digestion and peristalsis (movement of the intestine), diversion of blood away from these organs to better serve the muscle tissue, the dilation of the pupils to take in more light and therefore more information in every moment, and perhaps the most fascinating aspect: the increased processing of that information in the brain. If you've ever been in a highly stressful situation—a car wreck or an assault or witnessing something traumatic like a fight—then you may have experienced "the slow down." It's that moment when time seems to literally creep by, and you're witnessing your environment as if in slow motion, the details of which may be razor sharp and brilliant compared to normal. This is your brain taking the time to process much more data than its typical 30 percent. Time is relative, it turns out … especially in the brain.

The PNS is our relaxation response. Once we fight or flee, burning through our stress hormones in the process, our PNS kicks in to offer endorphins, serotonin, and dopamine to our overworked body, chemicals that calm us down, help us heal, and begin regeneration processes. Our heart slows and blood pressure drops, sometimes very quickly, and we call this *shock*. It can be a dangerous condition if not addressed, as the brain and other organs can run short of blood and oxygen. Under normal circumstances, however, the blood pressure regulates, the respiration returns to normal, digestion turns back on, and the metabolism increases as tissues assess and begin repair processes for any injured parts from the fight or the flight.

This particular process is important to understand with regard to our yoga practice, because we typically stimulate both systems in the course of a class. Most people in modern society experience a whole different kind of stress environment than our distant, primal ancestors did. Survival was on their minds: shelter, food, safety from predators and enemies; but they encountered major stressors infrequently and had a life span that topped out around thirty years. But in our world now, we are on a constant drip-line of stressful stimulation. We rarely actually fight or flee … we just keep up, get the work done, and pay our psychotherapist and cardiologist. Yoga—and frankly any kind of exercise—can break this

cycle of adrenal overload and reset our systems for healthier episodic stress responses, while also providing the relaxation response through quiet sitting, concentration, and meditation. More active styles of yoga can physically burn through our stress hormones and bring us down to the quiet place for Corpse pose (Savasana). We should take care, though, because if we do not give careful thought to our nervous system and stress response, our sequencing could actually serve to turn up our stress chemicals and not effectively turn them back down. We'll discuss this soon.

The Respiratory System

The respiratory system serves all our cells by oxygenating the blood circulating throughout our body, and removing the waste gases produced in that system. The lungs dissolve oxygen out of the air into our bloodstream, and then the cells pull that oxygen out of the blood for use in their own operations. This system also works hand in hand with the nervous system, since our stress/relaxation responses rely heavily on the oxygenation of tissues to react accordingly to various stimuli.

Mechanics of Breathing

The organs of breath are, obviously, the lungs. But the lungs themselves are not muscular and therefore require external forces to fill them with air and empty them again. The primary muscle of breath is the diaphragm.

The *diaphragm* is a muscle shaped like an overturned bowl or the dome of an opened umbrella. Its edges attach to the bottom rim of the ribs and the front of the spinal column, around the levels T10–L3 (see p. 59 for an explanation of vertebrae numbering). Its muscle

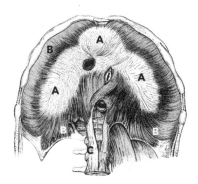

(A) Central tendon, (B) Attachments to inner surface of lowest ribs, (C) Attachments to anterior spine

fibers start at these edges and go up to the top of the dome where they insert into a patch of connective tissue called the *central tendon*. This is the diaphragm in its relaxed state.

- **Inhale**: When the diaphragm contracts, the volume of the rib cage—and thereby the lungs—increases, creating a vacuum. Air comes in through the nose and mouth to fill this newly created space.

- **Exhale**: As the muscle relaxes, it returns to its original shape, re-shrinking the chest cavity and pushing air out through the mouth or nose.

The ribs themselves are mobile, connecting to the spine at hinge-like joints. Notice in the illustration that the rib cage widens as the ribs lift up when the diaphragm contracts and flattens out. This too increases the overall volume of the chest cavity, allowing for deeper breath. While there are intercostal muscles (between the ribs) that are the prime movers for the rib-lift, every single muscle that attaches to the ribs has an effect on the depth or intensity of the breath. They will impact either the inhale or the exhale. We have a lot of potential to intentionally alter the rhythm and depth of our

Inhale

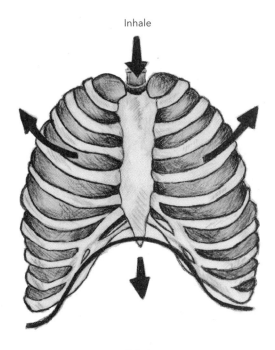

Exhale

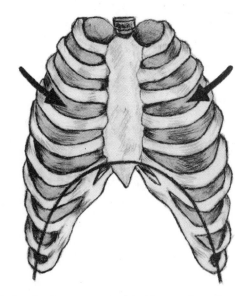

Inhale: diaphragm contracts/descends + ribs rise/widen = increased chest volume = air pulled in. Exhale: diaphragm relaxes/ascends + ribs fall/narrow = decreased chest volume = air pushed out.

breath; it is not at the whim of the stressors around us. We have control.

Also consider the spinal attachments of the diaphragm. These muscular threads attach just at the transition point in the spine where nervous control changes from sympathetic to parasympathetic. Why might this be significant? As the diaphragm contracts those long fingers of muscle, the peripheral nerves can be directly stimulated. When the diaphragm engages in hard, fast contractions, the sympathetic nerve roots are affected, while slower, longer contractions will stimulate the parasympathetic nerve roots. So, the control of our breath can act as a proactive switch on our nervous system. The ancient sages may have had some really good ideas about using Pranayama practice to elicit certain states of being, even without any technical knowledge of the nervous system as we know it.

The Skeletal System

A friend of mine once said that my lectures on anatomy can really be broken down into just a few parts: hard, pokey bits; soft, squishy bits; and all the movey bits. The hard, pokey bits are of course the bones. So let's talk about bones. You know what they are … but we should know some specifics about their structure and function in relationship to kinesiology instead of just basic anatomy and physiology.

Our bones are hard but light, made of a matrix of crystalline salts: calcium, magnesium, phosphorus, etc. The calcium especially is stored here for use elsewhere when needed, as in muscular contractions. We take calcium from our food, place it in our bones for safekeeping, and then draw it out again when we need a shot. This means that the bones are actually constantly changing—they are plastic and not fixed. We will keep more calcium in the bones if the bones require more strength and less if they aren't working very hard. Hence, the adage that impact keeps our bones strong and dense.

Density is not the only adaptation the bones make over time—they can change shape as well, at least to a certain extent. The bones will build up where muscles attach if those muscles are used often and place stress on those attachments. If you look closely at a "naked" skeleton, you'll notice that anywhere there should be a number of big muscular attachments, the bone is bumpy and rough. This is illustrative of forces that those muscles apply to the bones in action in gravity.

If we continue to consider that "form follows function," then looking at the shape of our bones will tell us a ton about what they are made to do. While some bones are long for leverage, some are small puzzle pieces arranged to accommodate forces from many angles, and some are totally irregular in order to provide lots of surface area for large muscles to attach and serve a very specific purpose. One thing you can be assured of: if a bone has a lot of pokey-outy bits, many muscles attach to it; if it has large, flat surfaces, then big bulky muscles are likely to make a home there.

Bones may also build up extra bone in places where compression or friction occurs on a regular basis, and we call these *spurs*. Some people, depending on their genetics, are more prone to this phenomenon than others. Bone spurs themselves can be painful because they increase friction at the point of contact, but they can also cause soft tissue pain or nerve impingement, depending on where they are located.

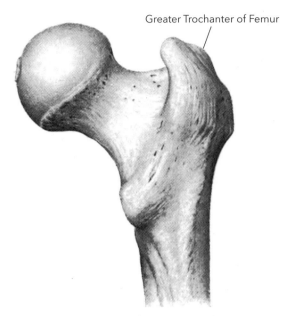

Greater Trochanter of Femur

The bone grows knobby and textured where muscles stress the attachment points, such as on the greater trochanter of the femur where the hip muscles attach.

Every bone is encased in a form-fitting sheath of connective tissue called the *periosteum*. This tissue assists with circulation in and out of the bone marrow, and it provides a connective medium so tendons and ligaments can firmly attach to form joints.

The Integumentary System

This is the fancy word we use to describe the system of connective tissues that hold our body together. It consists of fascia, tendons, ligaments, linings, vessels, and skin. Pretty much any tissue that holds other stuff together falls into this category. Our specific interest lies in just a few:

- Fascia (Deep Fascia in particular)
- Tendons
- Ligaments
- Scar Tissue

Fascia

Fascia is the integral tissue that holds all of our cells together. Without fascia, we would literally be a puddle of goop on the floor. It consists of a matrix of fibers—mostly collagen, but also some fibrinogen, elastin, and a few other bits—arranged in varying densities depending on the tissue's purpose. These fibers are molecular, not cellular, so they are not "alive." They are suspended in a special fluid-like, liquid-crystal substrate that varies in viscosity, again depending on the specific role to be played. There are live cells interspersed within the matrix as well, some of which are believed to be contractile. Recently, it has been observed that nerve endings terminate within fascial layers, suggesting that fascia itself may be sensory. A ton of basic research is still being done to understand the roles that fascia plays, and clinical research is happening in the medical and rehab fields as well. There is so much left to learn.

The collagen offers the tissue a great amount of tensile strength, and the more densely packed those fibers are, the more stress or tension the fascia is capable of withstanding. The alignment of the collagen has a

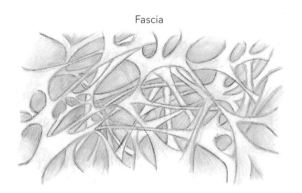

Fascia

The collagen fibers connect in a fluid manner, clinging together in thicker bands or thinner, depending on the forces applied to them. ✿

direct effect on how the tissue moves and in what directions it will withstand stress; tension is best absorbed along the lines of the collagen, not across them. Elastin fibers allow for the tissue to stretch beyond its original shape and then return to that shape. We call this *elasticity*. Some fascia is equipped with a lot of elastin, while other connective tissues have little to none.

The texture, health, and functionality of fascia depend upon three factors: hydration, heat, and movement. When the tissue lacks any of these three conditions, it will become hard, sticky, and stiff. When this happens, the layers of fascia can bind together instead of sliding freely past one another; we call this *adhesion*. This can and will impair the efficient movement of individual muscles and impact the range of motion of the nearby joints. Pain can occur at or around the adhesions, creating altered movement patterns that can have farther-reaching postural effects, resulting in a vicious cycle of dysfunction that is very difficult to undo.

Keeping your fascia hydrated is essential to preventing the aforementioned issues. Without water, fascia cannot move with fluidity. Once the tissue is dehydrated, the collagen fibers stick together and, over time, become increasingly difficult to separate. It also makes it more and more difficult to rehydrate. Consider this model: A kitchen sponge that you haven't used in a while will not only dry out but kind of crinkle up and shrink a bit, almost folding in on itself. Then, when you want to use the sponge again and you run it under water, what happens to the water at first? It doesn't just soak into the sponge right away; it beads up and rolls off for a while. You need to squeeze and manipulate the sponge a bit before it can absorb the water. Fascia works in a similar way. Once the collagen fibers are adhered together, it is tough for fluid to flow in between them. You need to move and warm up and maybe even mechanically separate those fibers … massage is a good option.

Adhesion of Fascia

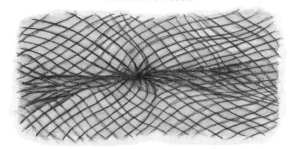

Even a small point of stickiness will pull on fascia from all directions.

Not drinking enough water is one way to dehydrate your tissue, but there are other ways too. Compression is the biggest culprit— sitting too much (the weight on your hamstrings) or sleeping in one posture (lying on one shoulder for hours at a time). You can also dehydrate fascia by overstretching a muscle … like wringing out a wet washcloth.

As yoga practitioners we are interested mainly in the **deep fascia** (the tissue that holds our muscles together) and the tendons and ligaments. Deep fascia wraps around each and every muscle fiber, like a long sleeve. The sleeve extends past the end of the fiber itself to make a little tendril or tail. Muscle fibers within their fascia sleeves get bound together in bundles and are wrapped in another layer of deep fascia, extending past the end of the bundle to envelop the tendril/tail of each individual fiber. A few of these bundles may then be bundled together and wrapped in another layer of fascia, and so on until sufficient fibers/bundles are there to do a specific job. We call this a *muscle belly*.

There are layers of deep fascia that create continuity from one muscle belly to another, building long chains of myofascia that add stability to our form and grace to our movement. If there are dysfunctions at any point upon the chain, the entire chain will be affected. These patterns have been dubbed "anatomy trains" by a pioneer in the field, Thomas Myers. I highly recommend reading his book of the same name for a better understanding of these connections and relationships. It will inform your practice and teaching in some fascinating ways, especially if you plan to go into private or therapeutic yoga at any point.

that muscle to a bone via the periosteum. Simply put, tendons attach our muscles to our bones. They are thicker and more densely packed with collagen than the deep fascia, and they have less vigorous blood supply. This fact leaves them lacking in the healing-up department.

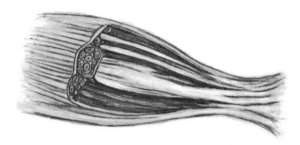

Muscle bellies comprise bundles of muscle fibers wrapped in fascial layers. Tendons are the extension of those fascia layers beyond the muscle fibers.

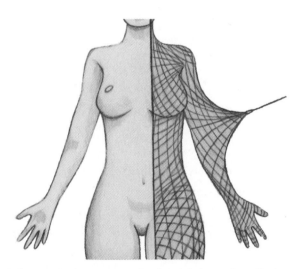

When a single point on the fascial sleeve is pulled, the entire system responds.

Tendons

The deep fascia layers that extend beyond the end of the muscle fibers, bundle upon bundle, make the *tendon*, the tissue that will attach

TendonTissue

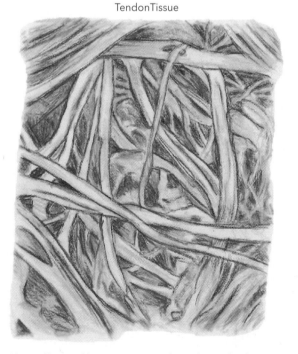

The collagen fibers are more densely packed in tendon tissue than in other connective tissues.

It's important to note that because the tendon is made directly from the layers of deep fascia, it is integrated fully into and through the muscle belly, and therefore all forces applied to the system will be distributed much more evenly than if the tissues lacked such continuity. It is this continuity that gives our muscular system its tensile strength and the potential for such sublime support as a *tensegrity* system.

Ligaments

Ligaments are the tissues that connect bone to bone, creating and reinforcing joints. Often they are an external component of a complex synovial joint (we'll talk in detail about this in chapter 5), but sometimes they are the only structures keeping two bones together (a *ligamentous joint*).

Like fascia and tendons, ligaments are made of densely packed collagen fibers, but they lack the other more elastic components of those tissues. Without elastin to give rebound, a ligament, once stretched, will not return to its original shape or size.

Note that ligaments will not bounce back from being stretched.

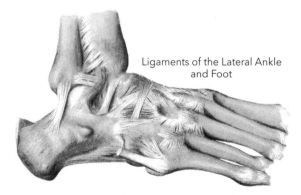

Ligaments of the Lateral Ankle and Foot

Ligaments connect bones to bones, reinforcing joints. They lack the elasticity of deep fascia and tendons in order to keep joints secure and stable.

Most of the time, a stretched ligament is not a choice, occurring because of an external trauma like twisting an ankle. It is possible, however, to stretch these tissues under slower, more innocuous circumstances—namely, holding yoga postures in poor alignment with no muscular support. I would ask: If this tissue's primary function is to keep bones connected to one another, why would anyone want it to be any longer to begin with?

Some styles of yoga claim that the health of this tissue relies directly on methodical stretching. I will argue against this 'til the day I die, or at least until there are repeated, large-scale, very well-designed studies to prove me wrong. These styles use direct joint capsule stretching techniques to access the tendons and ligaments because they believe that the tissues will otherwise contract over time and lead to shrinking joint capsules and compressive decreases in range of motion. I would argue that there is a big difference between the "contraction" they describe and the natural drying and hardening of all the connective tissues as we age. If you mobilize these joints, thereby mobilizing, heating, and hydrating the muscles, tendons, *and* ligaments, these tissues will remain both pliable and resilient long past their prime. Stretching them is likely to create too much space and mobility in any given joint, rendering it more susceptible to degeneration instead of the opposite.

(That said, I fully support the work of these styles of yoga to work directly on the deep fascia and muscle fibers, just not on tendons and ligaments.)

Scar Tissue

Ahhh, scar tissue. So misunderstood. It has really good intentions in our body, and mainly it accomplishes its duties quickly and well. Sometimes it does its job too well.

When you push a tissue beyond its limits, it will fail. In the case of a muscle belly, it will tear; the fascia and muscle fibers will pull apart from one another, oftentimes across their fibers, as shown in the visual model on the next page.

The tears themselves may be very small or very large. We may not even feel them happening, they are so small. But they are there nonetheless, and the body knows it. When a tear is detected, the body injects into the torn space a special fiber called *fibrinogen*. This fiber goes in much like silly string being sprayed from a can, all willy-nilly and in a fantastic mess of coils and bends. It is very sticky and binds to the walls of the torn tissue and to itself. Once laid in, it starts to shrink, all the twisted bits pulling closer in on themselves and drawing the torn sides back together. Well, almost together, because all that fibrinogen is in the way of them completing the union. This is what we feel as

TENSEGRITY ⊙

Such a funny word, *tensegrity*. This term originates in the construction industry and is the combination of *tension* and *integrity*. It describes a structure that relies on tension cables to apply compression forces to rigid members, holding them in space though the rigid pieces never meet. In this system if you change the length of one tension cable, all the other cables must also change length to maintain tension; otherwise it will collapse.

In the case of the body, we can say that the bony system of the skeleton is kept supported and upright by a system of tendons and deep fascia that are under tension. If the length or tone of one muscle or one section of deep fascia changes, the entire system must adjust. Many of us may have heard the old wives' tale about losing a pinky toe, and how a person can't walk without it … I assure you that this is an overstatement, but at its heart is a simple truth: you will never walk exactly the same as you did with that pinky toe intact, because now there is a missing link to how your feet touch Earth, and how the ankles respond to that base, and the hips respond to the shifted balance, and so forth. They may be only small shifts, perhaps unnoticeable at first, but they still make an impact on the entire form. On the surface it seems absurd to think that a "knot" in our shoulder (technically an adhesion in the fascia layers near your shoulder blade) could change everything about our posture, but consider the adjustments you might make in response: how you hold your arm, or move your head, or hunch your spine.

The human body will adapt almost too readily to these subtle anomalies, and sometimes those shifts have lasting and detrimental effects themselves.

a tight knot of thickened tissue anywhere we scar—like on our skin after a bad cut, or under the skin after a surgery.

This scar tissue is there for good. You can't get rid of it. You can sometimes change the texture of it if you apply certain massage techniques in the stage where it is shrinking and before it totally hardens, but you'll never change it completely or remove it.

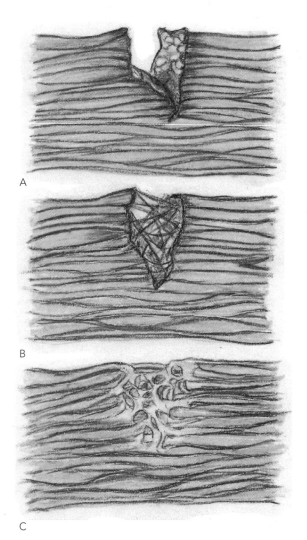

When a muscle is torn (A), fibrinogen rushes to fill the space and stick to the sides of the wound (B) then shrinks upon itself to pull the sides back together (C).

The Muscular System

Although muscles are considered a tissue, they have even deeper levels of classification (remember, science!). More importantly for yoga teachers, muscles are absolutely fundamental to building poses; as such, we need to have a thorough understanding of not just their what, but their how and why.

There are three kinds of muscle: skeletal, smooth, and cardiac. Cardiac cells are found only in the heart, whereas smooth muscle builds our organs and arteries. These two types of muscle cells are controlled unconsciously: we don't have to think about them in order for them to contract. However, skeletal muscle—the muscle that attaches to our bones and moves us through space—does require conscious effort to control.

For our purposes, the skeletal muscle is of most interest.

Structure

Muscle Cells. Also known as *sarcomeres*, muscle cells are complex machines (so complex that we are really simplifying them here) that use a lot of energy to function and in turn produce a lot of heat and waste. Perhaps because of this complexity, they are not very good at regeneration. Therefore, once a muscle cell is injured, it doesn't regain its proper function and isn't readily replaced—in other words, it's a good idea to take care of our muscle tissue. Since these cells don't regenerate well, scar tissue will be the first fix, and that comes with some trouble down the road.

Each cell should be able to do three things: contract its ends toward its center (*contractility*), relax back to its original shape and size (*relaxation*), and stretch beyond its normal length AND return again to normal (*extensibility/elasticity*). To contract, a chemical reaction incites the ends of the muscle to be pulled toward its center. It's important to note that a single cell can only turn on (contract) and off (relax)—there is no proverbial dimmer switch. It may also interest you to know that a muscle cell requires energy to relax. In fact, it takes just as much chemical energy to relax that cell as it did to contract it. This metabolic imperative can cause some issues—when a muscle cell (or group of cells) is stuck in a contracted state, we call this a *spasm*.

There is a fallacy out there that is popular and rhetorical: you must tear muscle to build it. Well, friends, I'm here to dash that notion out of existence. Tear muscles and you get scar tissue, that's all. So, how about the real scoop?

Muscle cells depend on energy to contract, and that energy is metabolized in the engines of the cell: the mitochondria. The more work you ask a muscle cell to perform, the more energy it will need, and the more mitochondria will be built into the cell over time. So as you increase your weight bearing, or extend the time doing work, the body will respond by building up the necessary tools to do that extra work. Those tools take up space and expand the size of the cell. If you decrease the workload for an extended time, the mitochondria will die off so as not to waste energy, and your cells will shrink down once more (*atrophy*). Getting stronger isn't a matter of adding muscle cells, it's those mitochondria bulking up the cells you already have.

Muscle Fibers. A series of skeletal muscle cells strung together in a long, thin fibril (*myofibril*) makes a muscle fiber. There are no typical cell walls but instead overlapping molecules, leaving you with a long, multi-nucleated string. Each muscle fiber will exhibit the three qualities listed earlier (contractility, relaxation, elasticity).

When a muscle fiber contracts, it contracts all the way; it is either "on" or "off." Each fiber has a somatic nerve ending to signal it to contract or relax, which affects every cell in that fiber. The cells will each pull their ends toward their own middle, effectively shortening the entire fiber in a balanced way.

Muscle Bellies. As pictured in the illustration, a muscle belly is composed of a series of bundles of muscle fibers. Each fiber has a thin layer of deep fascia surrounding it. A group of these fibers is bundled together by another layer of deep fascia. A group of these bundles is then held together by another sleeve of deep fascia. All of these layers of connective tissue extend past the end of the muscle fibers to form the thick tendon, as described earlier. Muscle bellies are reliant on this fascia to hold them together and attach them to bones.

Each belly's fibers are visible to the naked eye, like the striations you see on a beef roast,

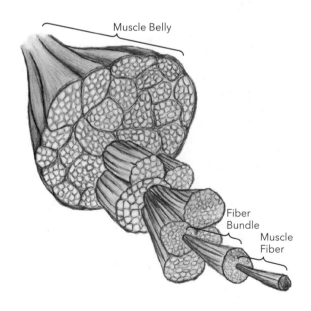

Muscle Belly

Fiber Bundle

Muscle Fiber

and the direction of these fibers tells us precisely what action any given muscle will perform. It is this information that we will use as we learn about types of contractions and range of motion.

Proprioceptors. These are special cells that measure actions of the muscle belly. They tell the brain what the muscle is doing and assess where it is in space. *Proprioception* is defined as the brain's impression of when and where your body is at any time. These little sensors help gather the data to make those calculations. The muscle spindle cells are spaced out within the muscle bellies and measure how long a muscle is and how quickly it is lengthening or shortening. The Golgi tendon organs are situated at the ends of the muscle fibers where the tendon begins, and they measure the tension on the system. Together they help the brain determine if the muscle is safe doing whatever it is doing.

Each proprioceptor has its own reflexive response if the signals it's receiving exceed certain thresholds. If the spindles determine that a muscle is getting too long too fast, its reflex is to trigger full contraction. The muscle is trying to prevent itself getting so long that the tendons pull off the bone or tears occur within the belly. In contrast, the Golgi tendon organ's reflex will relax a muscle when too much tension on the belly threatens to tear it. By relaxing, the hope is that a little extra length will prevent such injury.

Both of these precautionary actions can be effective, but both have the potential to get over- or under-done, still resulting in injury. The more you move through space and gravity, however, the more you will program these receptors to your norms, and the more prepared they are to react only in your extreme need.

Strength

Strength is a bit more complicated than it first seems. Here are the basics:

- **Contractile Strength** = the number of fibers contracting at once and their capacity to contract against force
- **Stamina** = how long the muscle can hold a contraction before it fatigues
- **Tensile Strength** = how well the fibers hold together under stress (density and strength of its fascia)

Since a muscle fiber is either "on" or "off," the body has set up an ingenious system of neural units. A *neural unit* is a small group of muscle fibers that receive information from a single nerve ending and contract together as a team. Each belly has a number of these neural units that fire sequentially depending on the current needs of the desired action. After all, it takes much more power to lift a brick than it does a pencil. The more work needed, the more units will fire for a longer time. The more efficient this system gets, the better stamina can be.

Midrange is where we find the most efficient and safe contractile strength—and the least likelihood of straining the muscle. If a muscle is shortened or lengthened too much, it loses strength and increases the risk of injury. It is strongest between 75 and 110 percent of its resting length. When translated to our practice, this means that if we are overstretched while trying to do work, we're very likely to do damage. Even a little damage can build up over time, so we need to consider working diligently in the midrange of our muscles and keep them subtly engaged even as we stretch. There is a sense of yin/yang here: even in restorative postures, we can engage to a slight degree to help keep from going too far too fast; and in active postures, we need to maintain just the slightest bit of room in the joints, not working at our absolute deepest point.

If a muscle doesn't have the tensile strength to hold its fibers together or remain attached to the bone, it will tear—no matter how powerful the muscle fibers are. The more we stress a muscle, the more collagen fibers the deep fascial system will lay down in order to build resistance to that stress. This results in stringy, sinewy muscle texture and eventually leads to decreased pliability.

Contractions

Skeletal muscle contracts in a variety of ways depending on the action required:

- **Isometric** = static; the muscle contracts but doesn't change length
- **Isotonic** = dynamic; the muscle contracts and changes length

Isometric would be holding a weight at shoulder height and keeping it there—no lengthening, no shortening; static contraction.

Isotonic would be lifting the weight to shoulder height and then lowering it again—shortening, then lengthening; dynamic contraction.

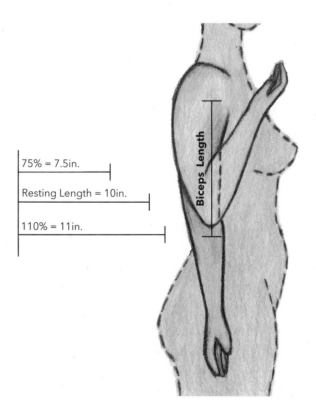

75% = 7.5in.

Resting Length = 10in.

110% = 11in.

Biceps Length

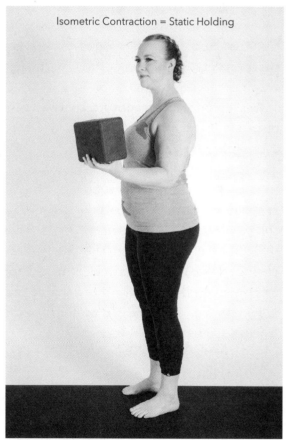

Isometric Contraction = Static Holding

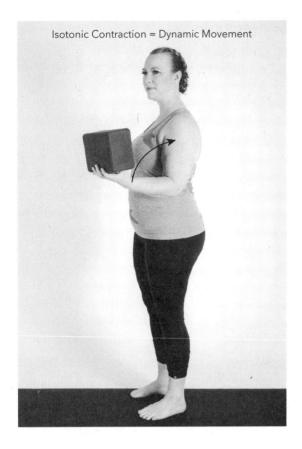

Isotonic Contraction = Dynamic Movement

This isotonic contraction can take two forms:

- **Concentric** = shortening
- **Eccentric** = lengthening

When you bend your elbow to lift the weight, your biceps is getting shorter (concentric contraction). As you lower the weight, you are not relaxing the biceps—it remains contracted as it lengthens (eccentric contraction). If you were to simply relax the biceps, you would just drop the weight quickly according to gravity. Instead, we are equipped to control the lengthening of the muscle through the eccentric contraction. It is said that eccentric contractions have the most strengthening potential, though injuries are also more common with this type of contraction.

Consider your yoga practice for a moment. As you flow from Warrior II to a Triangle pose, your front knee goes from bent to straight. The quads on the front of the thigh get short while the hamstrings on the back get long. Being active in gravity is a constant dance of concentric and eccentric contractions working in a balance. Make sure they remain balanced throughout your movements, and you will control your flow with grace and safety.

Creating Movement

Movement depends on:

- **Leverage** = the relationship of muscles to bones
- **Mechanical advantages** and power differentials = the relationship of muscles to other muscles
- **Gravity** = specifically, *our relationship* to gravity

Each muscle belly connects to two or more bones across a joint. In the case of the biceps, for example, one end of the muscle attaches to a point at the shoulder and the other end attaches to the forearm, crossing the front of the elbow joint. If we place a dot at each attachment point, and we see that the fiber direction of the biceps runs straight between one dot and the other, we can see that a concentric contraction will pull the two dots closer together, bending the elbow. Even if you don't know what that movement is called, you can tell how the body will move when the muscle contracts. This will be your key to understanding the roles muscles play without having to memorize each one off the bat. Fundamentally, the muscle fiber direction defines the action that muscle performs.

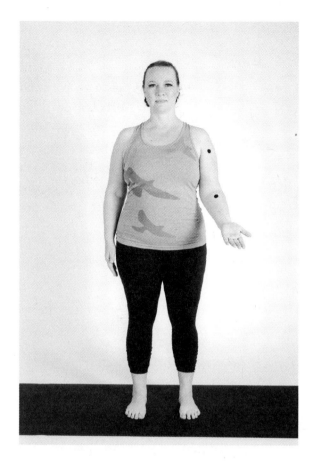

You will always know the primary action of any muscle if you ask yourself these questions:

1. **Which joint does it cross?** This is the joint it will move.

2. **Where does it attach?** This shows you the ends of the muscle in question.

3. **If the two ends are brought closer together, which bone will move, and in which direction?** This answer essentially defines the action it creates.

Once we see this clearly, we can begin to define the roles muscles play in moving our joints:

- **Agonist** = primary muscle creating the movement

- **Synergist** = muscles assisting this action

- **Antagonist** = muscle opposing the movement (usually on the opposite side of the joint)

The body couldn't move fluidly without these relationships—we would move in very robotic and clunky ways without the constant shifting and balancing of these roles. The brain is making constant assessments and adjustments as we move through our world. These adjustments are based on the calibrations of our proprioceptors.

You can tell even more about a muscle just by looking at it. When looking at a diagram, you can make some pretty solid assumptions about the muscle's function by assessing its shape and relative size. Short, squat muscles attaching close to a joint are fundamentally *stabilizers*. Long or broad muscles that attach at a point farther from their joints are fundamentally *mobilizers*. Some muscles play both roles, but for our purposes, these principles usually hold true.

Regions of the Musculoskeletal System

In science and medicine, we typically talk about the body region by region ... scientists love to categorize everything! This is how we end up with finer and finer specialties, but I digress. Later, when we start talking specifics, we'll break it down into three primary regions: the spine/core, the lower extremity, and the upper extremity. There are smaller bits within these regions that we'll define and explore with more specificity over time. In the beginning though, we'll peel away all the complicated layers of muscle and connective tissue and start with the bare bones.

The skeleton is hopefully something we are at least basically familiar with. I think it's important to recognize the regions of the body in both technical and lay terms. The lay terms, though, should become very specific. The arm, for example, is different from the forearm and only a small part of the upper extremity. Let's list them out:

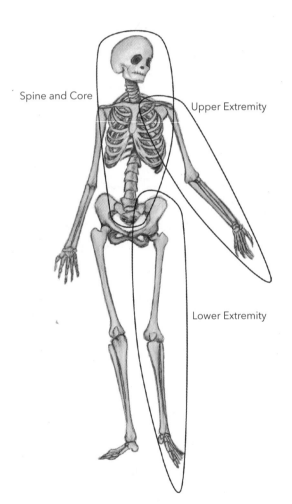

Spine and Core

Upper Extremity

Lower Extremity

Axial Skeleton = Spine + Core

- Skull = head
- Spinal Column, Vertebrae = backbone(s)
- Costals = ribs
- Sternum = breast bone

Upper Appendicular Skeleton = Upper Extremity

- Scapula = shoulder blade
- Clavicle = collarbone
- Humerus = arm
- Ulna + Radius = forearm
- Carpals = wrist
- Metacarpals = hand
- Phalanges = fingers

Lower Appendicular Skeleton = Lower Extremity

- Ilia + Pubis + Ischia = pelvis
- Femur = thigh
- Patella = kneecap
- Tibia + Fibula = leg
- Talus = ankle
- Calcaneus = heel
- Tarsals = midfoot
- Metatarsals = forefoot
- Phalanges = toes (yep, same as the fingers)

5

Fundamentals of Physiology and Kinesiology

Bones

Bones are a rigid framework of hard, nonliving minerals. They have live cellular components that break down and build up your bone tissue according to the forces applied to them. If muscles pull hard on their attachments, the bone will build up there in order to accommodate the stress. If bones start rubbing against each other in unnatural ways, the bone may build up in that spot to "make space" as it were. We call this a *bone spur*. The more impact you apply to long bones in gravity, the more dense their structure becomes to withstand that stress. If you don't apply stress to the bones in some way, they will become less dense and more weak as the body leaches minerals for cellular functions elsewhere. This is referred to as *osteoporosis*. The bones, therefore, are constantly changing according to how we use them. Form follows function.

This holds true in other ways as well. The shape of our bones is the first thing we look at to determine the range of motion of any joint. The articulating surfaces fit together in precise ways and determine if the joint will work in flexion/extension, rotation, or adduction/abduction. Some bones will allow more direction one way than the other, as in the elbow. Ideally the elbow can flex fully, bringing the hand toward the front of the shoulder, but it will only extend back to neutral. If it goes further than that, we'd refer to it as *hyperextension*; any time a joint moves beyond its normal range, it's considered *hypermobile*.

Hypermobility is not good. When a joint has extra movement, the tissues that hold it together undergo more stress, strain, and friction than they are designed for. Over time, these tissues degrade more rapidly and lead to dysfunction, disability, and disease.

Joints: Structure and Function

There are different kinds of joints, defined by what tissues form them. Some joints are two bones held together with a squishy bit of fibrocartilage, conveniently called *cartilaginous joints*. Some joints are simply two bones held to one another with ligaments and no cartilage. These are *ligamentous joints*. (You coulda called that one, I bet.) Neither type of joint is meant to move much, though cartilaginous joints can flex at the cartilage, offering just a little give in the system. The bones of the skull are held together with *suture joints*, where the two bones have tiny serrated edges that fit together like puzzle pieces and have only a millimeter of movement at the most.

Synovial joints, however, are built for movement and are the primary focus of our study. We will encounter cartilaginous joints in the spine, but mostly we are concerned with the freely moving joints like the shoulder, hip, and knee.

Synovial Joint Tissues

Hyaline Cartilage (A). This cartilage protects the ends of the bones by absorbing shock and reducing friction. It can also be found in the rib cage, joining the sternum to the ribs.

Joint Capsule (B). This thick connective tissue creates a sack around the articulated bones. The capsular membrane is similar to ligament in texture, but it has slack to allow the joint full movement in all its prescribed ranges

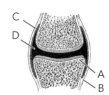

(A) Hyaline cartilage, (B) Capsular membrane (joint capsule), (C) Synovial membrane, (D) Synovial fluid

of motion. Under the wrong circumstances, the slack in this membrane can fold on itself and get impinged or adhered, causing pain patterns and reducing range of motion. Frozen shoulder is one such version of this phenomenon.

Synovial Membrane and Fluid (C, D). Lining the capsular membrane is the synovial membrane, a thin secretory layer that produces synovial fluid. This fluid helps keep the joint lubricated and hydrated. Movement stimulates the production of this fluid, which explains why joints can feel stiff when they've been at rest for too long. It's also the cause of osteoarthritis, the inflammation of a joint due to not enough synovial fluid production. As much as the pain keeps you from wanting to move the joint, it is movement that will help re-lubricate the joint and reduce the inflammation over time.

Ligaments. Ligaments usually exist outside the actual joint capsule but are an integral part of the joint structure. Some joints are built with tons of ligaments surrounding them, and these ligaments are the primary limiters of movement. The joint where your finger meets your hand is actually a ball and socket joint, meaning that at the bony level the finger should move in any direction without restriction. But since there are ligaments built specifically to limit this range, we get much more flexion than extension, and adduction/abduction are also limited. This makes these joints much more stable overall and helps us focus energy on the movements that are useful to us in life instead of wasting muscular energy trying to stabilize the other directions.

This functional aspect is one reason we should never focus on stretching the ligaments—and in fact should avoid it whenever possible. Remember, once a ligament has been stretched, it will not return to its original shape. They have no elasticity. If the ligaments get stretched, that will lead to hypermobility, and as discussed earlier, this leads to degeneration, dysfunction, disability, and disease. Not. Awesome. Save your ligaments! Your older self will thank you.

Menisci/Labrum. Some joints have an additional component. The knee, for example, has two fibrocartilage rims on the top of the tibia. These crescent moons are called *menisci* (or a *meniscus*, singular), which assist in keeping the movement of the femur in line. The shoulder and hip have a *labrum*, or hyaline cartilage lip, which helps extend the reach of the socket around the ball of the limb bone. In any case, these are cartilage structures that do not have a good blood supply and are therefore vulnerable when injured; they cannot heal. Visuals of these will be provided when we detail specific joints.

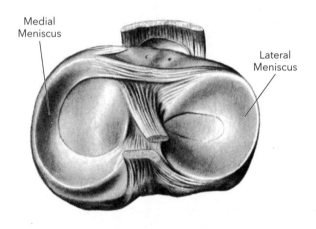

Medial Meniscus

Lateral Meniscus

Types of Synovial Joints

Because the shape of the bones defines range of motion in our synovial joints, we categorize the joints by their shape and structure. The shape of the joint will define which planes it can move on. Remember, there are three planes: sagittal, coronal, and transverse. All of the movements will be defined from a Mountain pose.

Hinge. Pretty much like it sounds, two long bones open and close around a pivot point. The designs vary greatly, but all hinge joints move only in flexion and extension on the sagittal plane.

Examples: Elbow, ankle (talocrural), middle and distal fingers (interphalangeal)

Modified Hinge. This joint works on two planes, sagittal and transverse, allowing for rotation only when the joint is flexed.

Example: Knee

Ball and Socket. Simple, a ball fits in a round socket. These joints work on all three planes, freely moving in any direction, including the combination of the fundamental movements. This combo is called *circumduction* and can only truly be done at ball and socket joints.

Examples: Hip, shoulder (glenohumeral), proximal finger (metacarpophalangeal)

Ellipsoid. Also referred to as a *condyloid* joint, it is an oval dish hosting an oval bone. Because it isn't round, these joints only allow movement on two planes, sagittal and coronal. You can flex, extend, abduct, or adduct here.

Examples: Wrist, subcranial (C1-skull), subtalar

Pivot. Where one bone pivots around another bone, or where the end of one bone pivots in a still-point formed by connective tissue. Rotation is the name of this game, working only on the transverse plane.

Examples: C1–C2, elbow/wrist (humeroradial/radioulnar)

Gliding. When two flat bones articulate, they can essentially slide across each other in any direction. These joints have no defined range of motion and are limited only by the connective tissue and the shape of surrounding structures, as in the spine. These joints are also called *facet* joints, like the facets of a cut gemstone.

Examples: Spinal facets, wrist (carpals), midfoot (tarsals)

Hinge

Ball&Socket

Ellipsoid

Saddle

Pivot

Gliding

Risk Factors

By now you have probably heard plenty about the risks of a yoga practice. Undoubtedly you know someone with pain in their shoulder, wrist, or knee from one posture or another. Sometimes they know exactly when and how it happened, but sometimes it seems to creep up on them, even after they've practiced for a while. There are books written specifically about the nature of injury in yoga, though many practitioners don't want to read them out of fear that they may inadvertently be convinced not to practice yoga anymore. There are whole styles of yoga where famous teachers undergo secret surgeries on their hips and knees, without ever acknowledging to anyone that their yoga practice was the likely culprit. In some lineages, the yoga injury is deemed to be a sacred rite of the practice—that you cannot possibly learn how to be a good human without hurting yourself in the process. Well, I'm calling "Bullshit!" on all of that.

Of course there is risk involved. There is not a moment in your life in this world that is absent of risk. Some of us hurt ourselves in our sleep, for cryin' out loud! You think moving through the world is gonna be void of opportunity to injure yourself, much less while moving in odd and otherwise not-normal ranges of motion while Gravity maintains its eternal grip on you? Funny.

I believe it's integral to be aware of the trouble before it arises. Not that I'd like you to wrap yourself in pillows and only leave your house when the coast seems clear, because frankly that's just no way to live. We cannot let fear of the truth be the thing that turns us away from our highest practices. What I ask is that you learn about your own individual body in a way that enables a healthy respect for the possibility of injury, know the mechanisms by which they are most likely to occur, and then willfully strengthen and stabilize to minimize those risks.

So, what can happen? The joints are the place most of our troubles arise. Sometimes we can push a muscle belly beyond its limits, but many of us will experience a joint injury long before we get to that point.

- **Sprain**: A stretch or tear of a ligament.

- **Strain**: A tear (micro or macro) of a tendon or muscle belly.

- **Tendinitis**: Inflammation of a tendon, sometimes due to overuse (repetitive stress, not necessarily a tear).

- **Tenosynovitis**: Inflammation of the sheath that encases some tendons. They may adhere together or be irritated by the nature of the friction between them when dehydrated.

- **Bursitis**: Inflammation of a bursa (synovial fluid–filled sac).

- **Impingement**: A pinch or compression of a tendon, ligament, nerve, or fat pad. May occur between any combination of hard and soft tissues.

- **Subluxation**: A joint leaves its ideal alignment and then returns to its original place.

- **Dislocation**: A joint leaves its ideal alignment and cannot return to its original place.

- **Torn Labrum**: In the shoulder or hip, the cartilage ring that helps form the joint socket can be sheared or compressed to the point of fracture or tearing.

- **Arthritis**: A generic term for all sorts of joint mishaps that include inflammation of joint tissues, though most often it's referring to the degeneration of cartilage, inflammation of the synovial membrane, and a lack of lubricating synovial fluid. It comes in many forms, some brought on by poor form, some due to autoimmune dysfunction.

Each and every joint has its own story to tell about what is ideal and what limits it will express. Through the following chapters, we will explore these specifics and how they apply directly to your yoga practice. You may be surprised by what you find. Some things you have been told about certain parts of your body, and how to best protect them, are just plain wrong. I endeavor to tell you what's really going on in those parts, how to begin to listen to your own internal truth, and even how to observe other bodies with a finer eye to their own limits. From here on, an open mind and a curious heart are necessary. Are you ready?

6

Integrating Anatomy into Practice and Teaching

For most teachers, their first hurdle is finding their own teaching voice. Not only have new YTT graduates just absorbed a ton of new information and been exposed to unexpected perspectives, they have also heard their own yoga teachers cue in particular ways—usually for years—and assimilated that language into their understanding of postures and sequencing. We often revert back to the rhetoric of our original teachers instead of automatically integrating the new data from training. In order to find a better way to apply the Yoga Engineer information, whether you are a newbie or a veteran, it will be important to explore the way you communicate, the way you see your students, and the manner in which you extricate yourself from old habits and commit to your new vision.

This chapter will offer tools and commentary on how to build a new and familiar language that is true to your voice while addressing the very real differences between the individuals in your classes. Our goal here is not to just insert a new rhetoric, but rather to insist that you use your critical thinking skills to assess the needs of your students in real time. To do that, you'll need to develop a system to really SEE your students' bodies. You'll need to notice their misalignments with relation to THEIR OWN body, not a glossy-magazine standard. So, we'll also discuss the ways that old cues have gone wrong and offer a new perspective on teaching to those bodies actually in your classroom.

Principles of Observation and Practice

Probably the most valuable skill a teacher can develop over time is their ability to see what is in front of them and make assessments about the safety, functionality, and pranic flow within a particular body. It is only from there that effective adjustments can be made with either the words or the hands. Please be clear: this has nothing to do with fixing a pose to look like the "ultimate expression" picture in some book. This is instead about helping a student find *the most effective version of alignment for their own body.*

Observation Skills: Clothing, Bony Landmarks, Prana

When I was in the fourth grade, my teacher had us write out the instructions for making a peanut butter and jelly sandwich. She brought a jar of peanut butter, and a jar of jelly, and a loaf of bread, and she tried to make a sandwich using our directions. This left an indelible impression on me, because only one person gave her the information she actually needed … TO OPEN THE JARS OF PEANUT BUTTER AND JELLY. If you miss this step, nothing else works. So I invite you as teachers to *open the jar.* Start at the foundation of the pose, choosing what needs to be stable and what needs to move. Then, teach. Teach each part in its stability or movement: where to place your parts and how to get them there. That is the most fundamental definition of teaching yoga. All the other philosophical, metaphorical, esoteric, and mythological parts will flow naturally into your vernacular once you gain confidence in simply telling people how to move.

Clothing. It sounds crazy, but I'm telling you, the clothes a person wears often mimic the lines and folds of the bones and fascia underneath the skin. A frame that is out of balance will stretch on one side and bunch up on the other. Your shirt will do the same thing. Learning to first look at the clothing will help you to build finer observation skills over time.

For example, in Triangle pose (Trikonasana), both side-waist lines should be long and even, with no side bending apparent. Look at your student's shirt; does it bunch up on the bottom waist line and stretch on the top waist? If so, you know you need to instruct them to adjust either the ribs or the hips in order to balance out the two sides.

Bony Landmarks. Next you'll want to pay attention to bony landmarks. Any bony bits that are visible under the skin are valuable to you in assessing alignment. The tips of the shoulders, the crease of the elbow, the thumbs, the crease of the wrist, the pubic bone, the sacrum, the edges of the shoulder blades … see where I'm going with this?? You'll want to get familiar with what solid, average alignment should look like, observe variations from this in the individuals in your class, adjust accordingly, and finally determine whether further tweaking is needed due to individual differences. That will take time to learn, so start small and practice, practice, practice.

Prana. Well, this is a tough one. Some of us are blessed with the ability to readily see the flow of energy in other individuals. Some of us need to practice. A lot. This is a skill that can surely be developed by anyone who dedicates the time and effort, but it may be much more difficult for some of us. So, what are we looking for, exactly? Imagine looking at a drum—a drum with a skin stretched over a wood frame. If that drum skin is taut, tuned up, and ready to play, it has a visible tension to it. Without even touching it you get a sense that it is positively thrumming with the potential of vibration ready to burst forth once it is struck. Now imagine that same drum with the skin yet to be fully stretched, fully engaged. It is less taut and has a softness, a slackness, to it. Before you even reach out to touch it, you *know* there will be dullness—no reverberations, no satisfying sound. This is your sense of prana. This is akin to your ability to see the pranic "thrum" in a yoga student.

When you observe your student, you first look at the activity in their joints—locking out, collapse, hyperextension—then address the tone of the muscles working. Assess the balanced use of the entire body. Are they lacking tone in their feet? Their hands? Are they engaging the continuum from their limbs to their core, or vice versa? The more you practice this view, the finer your awareness will become. You'll get a sense of their connection to or through the earth and their expansion upward or outward. You'll start to see lines of force through their bones when they are aligned properly, or the lack thereof when they aren't engaged. It's a painstaking process to get to that point, but once it clicks, you'll know it *and* feel it. You'll immediately be able to see if they are letting go to gravity or engaging to press the earth away.

"Getting the Feel" for Observing While Teaching, Then Teaching to Those Observations

Along with just getting your eyeballs dialed-in to seeing these things in the first place, you'll also need to develop the ability to catch patterns you see coming up in multiple bodies and adjusting your teaching in real time. For example, I constantly notice that the majority of students thrust their hips forward when coming up from a forward fold and reaching overhead. Not only is this a pet peeve of mine because it is so hard on the low back over time, but it also strikes me as something that

virtually no one is aware that they are even doing. That means I am responsible for pointing it out to them *while they are doing it*. So I can't just keep to my typical rhetoric for how to come to standing, I have to add stuff in about those pesky hips ... which means I may have to skip some things I normally say in order to get this new cue in within that one inhale. I may need to say it three or four different ways in order for it to click with everybody. This could lead to repeating this movement more times than I originally anticipated, or I may actually stop class to workshop this one particular tiny movement, just to bring awareness to the fact that it's happening *all the time*.

This is one really good reason to consider teaching on the fly, with only a loose script instead of a hard-set sequence in place—sometimes the best-laid plans are thwarted by the people actually doing yoga in your class today. That said, even in a totally scripted class, you need to be able to adapt to the immediate needs of those before you. This means slowing down your rhythm to the point that you can see the bodies in the pose before they are moving on through a transition. You need to have them hold a posture long enough that the cues you offer can be tried on, felt out, and then repeated. Repetition is key because it's very likely that you'll be working hard to unwind years and years of postural patterning here. That definitely doesn't happen the first time around.

You'll also benefit greatly from *not* demonstrating your entire sequence, or even part of it. Unless you are showing a new variation, or it's apparent that people aren't comprehending your words, I strongly suggest walking around the class the entire time. If you are on your mat at the top of the class and never venture out into the fray, you have a very limited perspective on how those bodies are really moving. It truly helps to see them from all angles. Every body is different, so seeing them only from the front can be very deceptive. Two people may look like they are lifting their tail, but from the side or back it becomes apparent that they are not. The reverse is often true as well. I constantly have to check myself from not putting someone into hyperlordosis (overly arched low back) because from the front they look like they are tucking their tail, but from a lateral viewpoint their spine is in a lovely neutrality.

Vocabulary

Terminology Relevant to Physiology and to Class

There is a distinct difference between technical terms and specific terms. To be effective, we must be fluent in the concepts and language of physiology and kinesiology, but this language is not always appropriate in the classroom. We need to be able to fluidly translate this anatomical information into lay terms that can be understood and absorbed in the real-time asana class. This takes practice—lots and lots of practice.

Let's start with an example. In Mountain, I'd ask people to stand with their feet hip-width. What is "hip-width," though? The first few times I teach students, I need to help them define this in their own body, because no two pelvises have the same proportions. There is, however, a kind of shorthand or blueprint that each body has: our two fists aligned side by side are nearly exactly as wide as the space between our coxal joints. The actual joints, not the greater trochanters or the outer width of our fleshy thighs. So I need to be able to tell

them about this miraculous personal proportion until it becomes ingrained. I take my time about it too, partly a stylistic preference on my part, but also because this learning stuff takes time to sink in, and I want to offer them that time. It may seem tedious at first, but eventually it makes more and more sense and they become so familiar with it that it becomes second nature.

Here is how I'd cue it:

"Your two fists, real fists, hard fists, equal your personal hips' width. Place these two fists in between your ankle bones ... not your big toes, not your inner arches ... make the knuckles of your hands span the space just between your ankles— those pokey bits that stick out."

Yes, it sounds wordy, but you are a teacher. Use your words. It's okay, it's your job. And make sure they do it—they're likely to try to half-ass it. Be specific and hold them to it.

Other simple examples include referring to specific body parts, functions, or tissues by both technical and lay terms interchangeably.

- Sympathetic nervous system = stress response

- Respiration = breathing = pranayama

- Circulation = blood supply = nutritional infusion = blood flow

Lastly, we should be able to describe qualities of our tissues in easy-to-understand terms and short statements.

"Ligaments hold your joints together. Don't stretch them. Your joints will fall apart."

"Ligaments have no elasticity. Don't stretch them. They will remain stretched forever ... and your joints will fall apart."

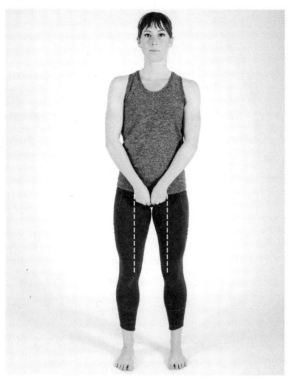

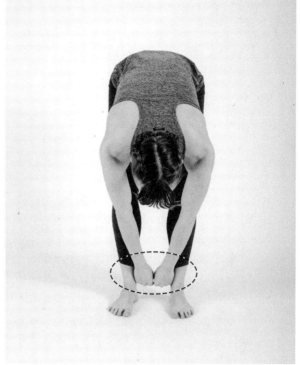

The tone you choose is up to you, but it's important that students learn the how and the why in order to take your specific instructions to heart; otherwise you may just sound like a drill sergeant, and no one really wants one of those in class.

Experiential Learning: Vocabulary

So now it's your turn. Make a list of technical terms from our earlier chapters. These could be names, movements, or functions that seem important in the scope of teaching. Then brainstorm less-technical terms that are still specific. Keep in mind that there isn't always a single-word translation; some of these will require explanation. How would you tell a student about Newton's Third Law? You'd have to make it relevant to them and their practice. Word clouds, outlines, lists—these are all

fabulous ways to approach this exercise. Here are a few to get you started:

- Extension
- Parasympathetic Nervous System
- Compensation
- Tendon

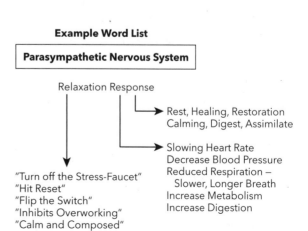

Example Word List

Parasympathetic Nervous System

Relaxation Response

Rest, Healing, Restoration Calming, Digest, Assimilate

Slowing Heart Rate
Decrease Blood Pressure
Reduced Respiration –
Slower, Longer Breath
Increase Metabolism
Increase Digestion

"Turn off the Stress-Faucet"
"Hit Reset"
"Flip the Switch"
"Inhibits Overworking"
"Calm and Composed"

Cueing Principles

So now we get to the nitty-gritty. This is where we take some of our newfound vocab words and put them into use. But how? This is where the principle of **specificity** comes to the forefront. It does no one any good to hear a bunch of words they don't know bandied about like it's Latin 101, but very specific instructions on how to move will sink in eventually.

Here's my list of principles that will help support the idea of specificity:

Eliminate extra words. You are trying to get a ton of information crammed into a very short breath-space. Say more with fewer words. "Place your hands on the mat" becomes "Hands root into mat." "Send your right foot to the back of the mat" becomes "Right foot floats to back of mat" or even "Right foot to back of mat."

Don't name the pose until you've told them how to get there. If you name the posture first, students' habitual movements will take over for sure. By offering precise instructions on how to build this shape, you will ensure that they are engaged from the base up and are less likely to fall into old habits. Take the things they think they know and deconstruct them. They will build better strength, eliminate momentum, and become more precise in their movements.

Stop class to workshop new ideas or concepts. Learning is hard. Many people are resistant to it at first. Only if you knock them out of their rhythm can you ensure that they are hearing what you need them to hear. This is the ideal time to demonstrate a new approach to a familiar posture or transition. It is also how you can emphasize the importance of the how and why! Don't be scared—you know it's good for them.

Use a slightly different phrasing through each repetition. Word variation offers people a chance to absorb the information in different ways. It will click a little differently for each person, so offering multiple expressions can help get everyone on board. This is your critical thinking in action. You've got to get nimble enough to not fall into your own rhetorical cage.

Choose one or two principal themes to teach throughout class. No matter which pose you teach, stick to just a couple primary ideas instead of giving all the detailed cues. You don't need to be an encyclopedia of alignment in each class. Teach to the feet or the knees or the hips or the ribs ... connect the dots from one pose to the next. This will help inform them of particular muscle groups working in diverse ways, no matter where you are in space. Over many classes these principles will integrate nicely, but at first, isolation is key to building awareness.

Describe specific actions. Tell them what part you want them to move, where you want them to put it, and how to get it there. Break down transition movements into component parts before putting them back together as a single fluid movement. The first time you move from a three-legged dog to lunge, it is helpful to do it in four breath-parts: inhale to three-legged dog, exhale knee to chest (stay in the dog shape), inhale, shift forward to three-legged plank keeping knee at chest (keep hips high), exhale, place foot at front of mat directly under knee. The more these actions are practiced as separate parts, the less momentum we use to get the foot to the top of the mat, the more we engage and rely on our core, the stronger and more fluid the full movement becomes over time.

Shifting the Common Rhetoric

Consider for a moment the nature of classical yoga education: A student is essentially apprenticed to a particular teacher for many years, a single teacher with a vast and deep yogic knowledge and perspective. A single voice passes on huge amounts of knowledge over a long period of time. Particular views and practices are indoctrinated and held sacred. The message is clear and crystallized through physical practice and dedicated devotional work. The student eventually becomes the teacher. The system repeats and expands, sharing the work and the words, with slight personal variations, but essentially remaining consistent over centuries. Within this oral tradition lies one potentially fatal flaw: there is very little room for the critical thoughts of the student, and no effective means of questioning the teacher or their perspective. In this system, there is little space for new information to enter the stream of consciousness, and very little opportunity for the student to learn about anything or anyone other than themselves. This can narrow a teaching viewpoint to a concerning degree.

At this point in our yoga culture, while so much has managed to change in the way yoga is practiced and shared, there are still remnants of the traditional ideologies that have been passed down the lineages and remain deeply rooted in daily practice and teaching. Common cues in the yoga vernacular have been used so often and for so long that they are taken as a kind of alignment-gospel. Unfortunately, many of these phrases and instructions are not in any way biomechanically sound. Throughout this manual, we'll address these specifically and offer the how and why these cues should be put out to pasture and replaced with updated information.

For now, we will discuss the nature of shifting out of these old cues and introducing new perspectives. This information isn't just for teachers in training; it's valuable for each of us as practitioners to remember that there is room for adjustment and advancement, that experts in their field are making potent observations that warrant our attention, and that we need to engage our critical thinking skills whenever being offered instruction that will have direct effects on our health. In some ways this is revolutionary, and in some ways it is simply a next step in the constantly evolving nature of personal practice and growth.

Oftentimes in YTT, I am asked some version of this question:

> "How do you get people to listen to this new way of approaching alignment when they've been told thousands of times to do it this other way?"

My answer:

> "It's not always easy. Habits are hard to break, and you're often battling a deeply ingrained message placed there by people they trust."

In order to shift a perspective from a habituated one to an open-hearted one, you'll need to establish a few things with your students. I suggest approaching this with candor and humor. Remind them that yoga is an evolving practice, that there are advancements in knowledge about movement and health that weren't available to our elder teachers, and that yoga has been an oral tradition from master-teacher to student—not an ideal model for incorporating critical questioning. To do that effectively you must:

- **Be kind.** There are times to be a drill sergeant, and there are times to give thoughtful advice. This is the time for thoughtfulness. Remember that you are working with a person who has distinct beliefs about their body and maybe their practice. They may feel vulnerable about trusting you with both.

- **Be humble, but assertive.** You and your message are coming up against a potentially long history with their other teachers. Make it clear that you understand you are asking them to buck a system, but not with disrespect to their prior learning. Focus on the concept that this new way of approaching alignment is based on emergent study—information that wasn't available to the classicists is now available to us, and we have an opportunity to grow our practice in safer ways

- **Hold space for independent, critical thought.** Invite the challenge. Encourage them to ask questions, and then be willing to clarify your position or give it up. Trust your knowledge and translate it as best you can to them, but be open to changing your mind too. You are a teacher but also a student. That's part of what this life is for, questioning, going deeper, following the curious path of the white rabbit ... perhaps you'll see the bottom of the hole ... but only if we all ask the questions.

The "Dirty Dozen" Cues

So ... just to kick things off with a bang, we'll list here some specific cueing that makes my skin prickle (and soon yours too, as you become a master of these Yoga Engineering principles). If the principles of physiology are ideals we want to ingrain into our understanding, the Dirty Dozen are the bits you should immediately remove from your vernacular. They are traditional (or at least rhetorical) but don't correspond with what we now know to be biomechanical facts. The how and why these ought to be eliminated from your classes will become more clear in the following chapters, but considering the information that you've just read, I figure I should give you some particulars to chew on as you proceed. I assure you, you will have more than enough evidence by the time we're through!

One last thing: I fully acknowledge that there are more than a dozen items on the following list, but "Dirty Dozen" sounds way better than "Dirty Fourteen" or "Please Forget These F'ing Fifteen." Okay, perhaps I stand corrected ... that last one could work.

1. Tucking the tail. The lumbar curve is integral to our core's stability in gravity; curves are stronger and more stable than straight lines. When we tuck the tail, we flatten out the lumbar lordosis and engage mostly the "six-pack muscles" in front. This disrupts our ability to engage the deeper abdominal wall, which is our intended tool for stabilizing the core. When the six-pack fires hard, we can't compress the organs, we can't engage the deep fascia that lifts the pelvic floor and Mula Bandha, and we tend to clench the glutes ... oy. I could literally talk about this specific point for a year, so I'll leave it at this for now.

1.1. Press low back into mat for support. This is a fallacy (see the arguments in number 1). That curve is important, especially if you are working with your legs stretched out while on your back. You need the whole core to be active to sustain that leverage in a healthy way. Maintain the lumbar curve! The only time it should disappear is when you are rolling into a ball intentionally like Balasana or Cat pose.

2. Drawing down the shoulders. The shoulder blade is built to rotate upward and downward. The full range of motion of the upper extremity is only available when the shoulder blade + collarbone (shoulder girdle) move freely and fully. When reaching overhead, the shoulder girdle must upwardly rotate, or else the humerus compresses soft tissues in their small bony gap. Turning the arms outward makes a bit more space there, but it is eliminated the moment you depress the shoulder girdle. Over time this impingement leads to pain, weakness, degeneration, and disability. Once overhead, if you instruct the turn-out strongly enough, the shoulder girdle finds its perfect happy place and there is more than enough room between shoulder and neck. A soft face and throat will greatly improve the feeling of this new alignment.

3. Rolling up from forward fold. The muscles of the low back essentially "tap out" when the spine is in deep forward bends; they're just too small to take on such a great task as pulling the entire weight of the upper torso to upright. So the thick connective tissue kicks in and does about 75 percent of the work. Rolling up not only puts the lumbar musculature at risk of strain but also puts the discs at maximum anterior compression with NO core activation or support. It's essential that the spinal muscles work only to align the vertebrae into the neutral curves, stabilizing them so the hips can do the heavy lifting.

4. Press into "L" of the hand. The saddle joint that attaches the thumb to the wrist is a vulnerable joint. It is not on the same plane as the rest of the palm or fingers, so if we bear weight there, the joint tends to twist in an unnatural way, stressing the ligaments and wearing on the cartilage. Hello, arthritis!! If we instead focus our effort on transferring gravity/energy in the most efficient line from the fingers to the shoulder, we can still engage the palm but save the saddle joint in the process.

5. Twisting in low back, especially in supine twists. The lumbar spine is built to rotate a very small amount, but many of us put all of our twisting energy there. This repeated action leads to hypermobility and degeneration of some already fragile bits. In fact, most lower back pain I've encountered (in myself and others) is remedied by reducing this rotational range and restrengthening the low back muscles.

6. Feet together. Most bodies don't accommodate this foundation in standing poses without a fair amount of compensation through the knees and hips and eventually low back. Most bodies out there will feel better in the long run with feet hip-width in all poses … yes, even in Chair. Because of physics, placing the feet on the midline disrupts the natural supportive flow from foot to spine, putting undue torsions on the arches, ankles, knees, hips, and sacroiliac joints. Allowing the natural architecture of your base support you makes better sense.

7. As in doing a Kegel, squeeze your perineum to engage the pelvic floor. Here's the deal: the perineum and the pelvic floor are totally different muscle groups responsible for different things. The perineal muscles are small linear muscles associated with the external genitalia and the pelvic outlet, while the pelvic floor muscles are thin sheets of circular muscles at the pelvic inlet that infiltrate the deep abdominal and anterior sacral fascia. We activate these in subtle ways, pulling the deep abdominal wall straight back toward the sacrum, not by clenching the perineal muscles as in deep Kegels. Clenching can lead to the lack of strength in the deep core instead of stabilizing.

8. Inner thighs roll back in forward folds. Oh goodness. This action increases the torsion on the knees in profoundly unsettling ways. This action rotates the hips too far and puts added stresses on the knee ligaments, contributing to hyperextension and instability. There are very efficient ways to activate the legs to support you better in forward folds, but this is the opposite of that.

9. Thigh parallel to ground in standing postures/knee 90 degrees. This position requires the feet to be very far apart, taking most effort out of the back leg and transferring it directly to the front hip. For most bodies, this "ideal" shape puts the deep structures of the hip at risk, as well as strains the hip and thigh muscles. As you'll learn later, muscles at the extremes of their length (short or long) are not stable or strong. The hip joint is not constructed to hold up your body weight in this position for long; doing so leads to imbalances in the short and long muscles that leave you vulnerable to subluxation. (That would be the femur falling out of the pelvis, which actually happened to a friend of mine—and she was strong as hell—so I mean it when I say that this is not ideal at all.)

10. Hips "square" in Warrior (Virabhadrasana) I. Because of the shape of the hip joints, the back leg in Warrior I has limited extension, pulling that side of the pelvis back (usually looks like rotation toward Warrior II). This is even more marked when the feet are at traditional heel-heel alignment rather than hip-width. Overstretching the front of that hip will lead to hypermobility and joint degenerations. Don't do that. As long as your effort is true from your roots to your core, you're all good.

Some slight adjustments to your feet alignment could make all the difference here.

11. Hips "open fully"/parallel to edge of mat in Warrior (Virabhadrasana) II. Conversely, we ought not to force the pelvis all the way open in Warrior II poses for similar reasons. The shape of the hip joints themselves resists this, not just the length of muscles. To force it is to compress the joint tissues, which usually leads to misalignment and injury further up the chain in the sacroiliac and low back. Instead, allow the pelvis to open only to the point of resistance, making sure the thigh bone and knee aren't pulled along for the ride.

12. Flex foot to protect the knee. This one is complex, and we'll dive deep in later chapters. For now, I'll say this: flexing the foot does not in any way protect the knee. There ya go. In some cases, in Pigeon variations for instance, flexing the foot can actually lead to injury. The foot is more complex than we give it credit for, especially regarding its relationship to the knee and hip. This oversimplified instruction blurs too many lines.

13. Lift kneecap to protect the knee. This is ubiquitous in many hot yoga environs and used in the balance postures. Unfortunately, when standing, lifting the kneecap is a movement that usually sends the knee joint into hyperextension. This is a dangerous place, so again, it does not protect the knee. In fact, it can lead to real harm.

14. Hands under shoulders. Oh boy. Do you know where your shoulder joints are? I swear to you they are not in your armpits, or under your collarbone, which is where most people actually put them on the mat. This alignment collapses the chest, impinges shoulder joint tissues, compromises the strength and stability of the wrist, and sets up your core for weakness. It's no wonder so many people hate Plank (Phalakasana) and Low Plank (Chaturanga Dandasana). The shape of your own individual arms will tell you precisely where to place your hands on the mat. I swear it'll make sense soon!

15. Lift your sternum. This cue is intended to remove a hunching upper back, but instead it tends to create a distinct breaking point in the mid-back, sometimes referred to as *rib shear*. We need to be able to lift the entire rib cage off the pelvis in a balanced way, not just tip the front side upward. We also need to be able to move the shoulder blades separately from the rib-spine to achieve the sense of open heart and chest that this cue is really trying to elicit.

It will take time and practice to ensure that these items are dispelled from your mind and body. For many of us, they have been ingrained over many years with many different teachers. What we know for certain is this: your brain can change its ways, and so can your body. You will only achieve this through mindful practice, by turning off your autopilot and actively eliminating them from your rhetoric. The following chapters add supporting evidence that these cues are not in keeping with the body's imperatives, so the deeper you dive, the easier it will be to make these shifts in perspective and speech.

7

The Spine and Core: Structure and Nature

Did you know that we are the only mammals who generally move around on just two feet? We are the only truly upright beings, walking, running, even sitting with our head stacked over our hips ... actually, not many of us truly manage that one! Many of us move through the world without any awareness of our spinal body until it hurts. Mostly, it starts hurting because we haven't been paying attention to our posture. Those of us who *have* been paying attention have unfortunately been given some bad information about that posture and are supporting habits that will end up hurting us down the line.

When you start to look closely at the spine, at its individual bones and how they fit together, how the layers of connective tissue overlap, and how muscles layer and connect to wrap around our abdominal organs, a distinct story unfolds. This story is detailed and intricate, subtle and strong. This is the story of how we ought to support ourselves in gravity. It is not so simple as the front body and back

body working together or against each other. It is a complex system that involves multi-range counteractions, strategic compensations, and hydraulic pressurization. This is the engine that drives this machine of ours.

The spine is at the center of our ability to stand upright, to move through space. It is the axis from which our appendages move. In fact, they are defined specifically as the *axial skeleton* (skull, spine, ribs, and sternum) and the *appendicular skeleton* (all the other bones). Understanding the nuances of this system, how it works, and how to isolate or integrate these disparate parts is integral to being able to teach an integrated, safe, and logical yoga sequence.

When we can see clearly how the spine can support us in gravity, we can teach a detailed blueprint posture like Cow/Cat (Bitilasana/Marjaryasana) and then apply these principles throughout class as they are reflected elsewhere (or everywhere!)—in our standing postures, backbends and twists, inversions, and arm balances.

There are two fundamental questions for every posture in your sequence:

- Is the spine mobile or stable?
- Does the spine support the limbs, or are the limbs supporting the spine?

These questions become the heart of your sequencing and teaching, and in the long run they serve to support a safe and confident yoga practice.

Throughout the following pages, I will allude to and sometimes state directly what NOT TO SAY. We want to eliminate the flow of that bad information and insert new models and practice in its place. I want to assure you that in future chapters, I will offer you the new models in excruciating detail. We will practice within new alignment paradigms, and you will develop new language to support those. So don't freak out now! In this chapter, try to focus on understanding how and why things work the way they do, and recognizing the risk factors that require us to refigure our approach to cueing and alignment; that way, when you get to chapter 8 all our new models make sense.

Bones

The genius of the spine is in its funky-shaped bones and how they fit together. The combination of both cartilaginous and synovial joints makes for a versatile system that provides structural stability while still allowing a remarkably wide range of motion. The spine is made up of a series of stacked bones called *vertebrae*, separated by fibrocartilage *discs* and bound together by layers of ligament. Their purpose is manyfold: to protect the spinal cord, which runs through the tube that is formed by their stacking; to give us height and range of motion

Vertebrae

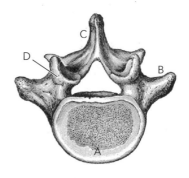

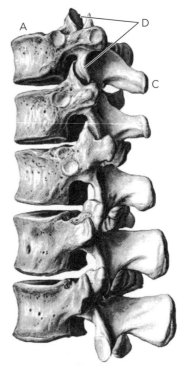

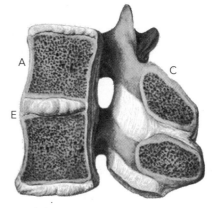

(A) Body, (B) Transverse process, (C) Spinous process, (D) Facets, (E) Intervertebral disc

to increase our reaching ability; and to afford better visual range. Since form follows function, the vertebrae are shaped precisely for the level they inhabit and are designed to allow or limit movement accordingly.

When you look at the skeleton, notice how each bone is shaped. What do you see? What is the difference between the top and the bottom bones? Are the shapes different? Are the angles of the pokey bits consistent or different? The more closely you observe these details, the more you'll be able to deduce about how those bones will move relative to one another.

You'll notice that each vertebra has a *body*, thick and dense, which stacks on the bone below it. This is the weight-bearing portion of the spine. Two bony bridges called *lamina* sweep out laterally and around the spinal cord creating the pokey bits on each side (*transverse processes*), then they meet up on the back to create the pokey bits we can feel beneath the skin on our back (*spinous processes*). We can tell from all this surface area that tons of muscle will be attaching through this area. Consider how all of those pokey bits relate to each other. Are they close together? Would they compress against each other in range of motion? How could they limit or allow movements?

Lastly, you have to look quite closely to see this in the skeleton model, but there are a set of bony shelves that extend from both the bottom and top of the vertebra near the spinous process. These shelves are called *facets*, and we'll discuss those in just a moment when we talk about the spinal joints.

The spine is divided into the following regions, from top to bottom:

- **Cervical** = neck; seven bones, numbered (from the top) C1 to C7: The cervical vertebrae are built mostly for mobility. The first and second levels are specialized to work together for

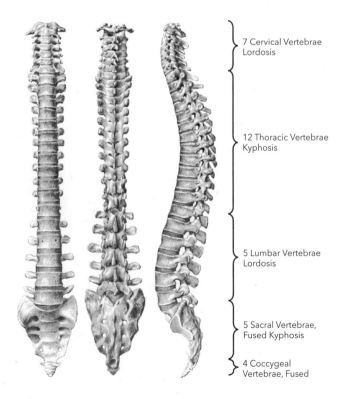

7 Cervical Vertebrae
Lordosis

12 Thoracic Vertebrae
Kyphosis

5 Lumbar Vertebrae
Lordosis

5 Sacral Vertebrae,
Fused Kyphosis

4 Coccygeal
Vertebrae, Fused

ample rotation of the head. Short lateral processes mean ample space for side bending. Some of the spinous processes stick out quite far and stack very closely to one another, indicating that range of motion will be limited in some fashion at those levels; they are very stable in extension. Notice too that there is a hole present in each transverse process that an artery can travel through. While it's very difficult to injure these blood vessels in normal range of motion, it's important to acknowledge that some risk does exist there.

- **Thoracic** = rib spine; twelve bones, T1–T12: Upon inspection, the thoracic vertebrae have some distinct differentiation from the neck bones. The spinous processes angle sharply downward in some cases, cascading over one another. This shape allows the bones to glide over each other instead of stopping each other in their tracks. One thing to observe is that the ribs themselves anchor to multiple vertebral levels at once, creating a great deal of stability in this section, regardless of the shape of the spinal bones. The mobility in the ribs, therefore, will have a direct impact on the mobility of the thoracic spine.

- **Lumbar** = low back; five bones, L1–L5: The lumbar vertebrae have oversized bodies compared to the cervical and thoracic, because these bones bear the majority of our weight. They are also more noticeably wedge-shaped instead of columnar. This shape defines the lumbar curvature so it doesn't stack straight up and down in a column. The processes are thicker and larger to offer large muscles and thick connective tissue a place to take hold. Take a close look at the facets of the lumbar levels in comparison to the upper sections; they face a totally different direction! This is pertinent information as we begin to talk about facet joints and range of motion.

- **Sacrum** = triangle-shaped base of the spine that fits into the pelvis; five fused bones, S1–S5: The sacrum is a hollow, curved bone that begins as five separate vertebrae in utero that then fuse into a single unit. It is hollow to accommodate the end of the spinal cord and has holes in it that the nerve roots can pass through. The curvature of the sacrum varies between men and women, as does its angle relative to the lumbar spine. This is pertinent because as we look at bodies in class, the pitch of the sacrum may cause some optical illusions, making it appear that someone has a much more curved lumbar spine than they actually do!

- **Coccyx** = tailbone, may or may not be fused to the sacrum; three or four bones: The coccyx is the final remnant of whatever tail we may have had in former human iterations. At first it appears to have no real function, except that it supplies the attachment point for a few perineal muscles. For most people, the coccyx is fused directly to the sacrum in a very stable bony connection. For some, however, there is a tiny joint there, and that joint is vulnerable to sprain. This is commonly referred to as a "broken tailbone," though it is actually a sprain in that joint.

The Curves ✪

Each of these spinal regions has its own curva-ture, reversing from one to the next. In utero, we curl into ourselves, creating the primary curve, or *kyphosis* (*kyphotic curve*). Once born out into the world, the sacrum and thoracic spine, because they have a strong bony stability, retain the original prenatal curve. The cervical and lumbar sections adapt with our movements, posture, and the force of gravity to reverse into the secondary curve, or *lordosis* (*lordotic curve*). It's the the counteractive nature of these flow-ing curves that offers us the stability to stand upright for the majority of our life.

While the shape of the vertebrae suggests these curves, gravity is a constant presence, and our center of gravity is shifting constantly. This means that to maintain our curves over time, we have to actively use our muscles to remain upright. A neutral spine is defined as one that inhabits the three curves of cervical (lordotic), thoracic (kyphotic), and lumbar (lor-dotic), supported muscularly from within. It's all too common to see people out of alignment, oftentimes thrusting their pelvis and head for-ward while their rib-spine shifts backward. In these cases, very little muscular work is being done, and instead they are relying on their lig-aments to hold them up. While this may seem efficient from an energy-saving perspective, the joints of the spine take a beating!

Let me be clear about something: we are meant to have a lumbar lordosis. Period. It is THE defining factor in what sets our spine apart from other mammals. We need it to remain stable in our upright posture. If we flatten it out, we lose our shock absorption, we undermine our ability to activate our deep muscular core, we compress our tissues, and we promote long-term damage.

Discs, Joints, and Connective Tissue

In between the vertebral bodies are the *inter-vertebral discs*. These integrate directly with the *periosteum* to create *cartilaginous joints*. These joints aren't free-moving or lubricated like synovial joints; they depend on the pliabil-ity of the cartilage itself. To be able to accom-modate the range of motion we need, the discs have a particular structure. They are not solid like a hockey puck; there is a dense yet flex-ible layer of fibrous cartilage surrounding a soft, gel-like center (think: jelly donut). This center-goo allows for good shock absorption, but it also shifts around within the disc when it flexes and bends in movement. When one side of the disc is compressed as you bend the spine, the goo is pushed over to the expand-ing side, returning to the center when the spine returns to neutral. This movement of gel means the spine has better range than if the disc were solid.

The cartilage layer, as with any connective tissue, is served best by gentle movement and constant hydration. If we stop moving our spine (perhaps by habitually sitting with bad posture at our desk), the tissue becomes chronically dehydrated, and we run the risk of

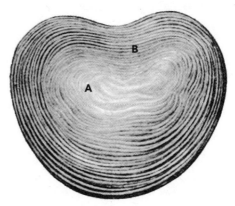

(A) Nucleus pulposus, (B) Annulus fibro-sus (cartilage layers)

Disc Injuries

(A) Herniation, (B) Herniation + bulge, (C) Rupture,
(D) Rupture + fragmentation

losing the pliability of the disc, cracking its outer layer and, eventually, all the goo leaking out. All of this is bad news. We call that initial breakdown and cracking *herniation*. As the fibrous layer thins out, it bulges out from between the vertebrae, oftentimes inflaming the nerve roots exiting the spinal canal. The soft tissue of the area is also affected, creating inflammation and pain loops that are difficult to stop. It can be done! It isn't easy, but with the right care and therapeutic movement, a bulging disc may be reversible.

Without proper attention, however, herniation leads to bulging, which leads to a full rupture, and once again, all the goo leaking out. Just to be absolutely clear, we really don't want that! Once the integrity of the disc is compromised, it will not withstand shock in the same way, will end up far too hypermobile, and will degrade more quickly, and we will end up with no disc at all ... and let me tell you, bone on bone is *no bueno*. Without an integral disc, the space between the vertebral bodies shrinks, soft tissues become inflamed, the nerve roots become irritated or completely impinged, and we perpetuate a pain cycle that is very difficult to reverse. Treat your discs well—you only have one set. The alternative is surgical and it sucks.

While these cartilaginous joints offer us some range of motion, it is at a different set of joints that most of the true movement of the spine occurs. Remember those facets we mentioned earlier? Well, as the vertebrae stack on each other, flat little horns protrude from the bottom of one to land on little horns on the top of the next one down. These *facet joints* are synovial joints that move freely, limited by the ligaments that bind them together, as well as the overall tension/compression of the entire spine/disc/rib system. You'll want to look closely at the skeleton images to examine the difference in the size, shape, plane, and angle of the facets from the cervical to the lumbar regions. ✪

One thing that sets the spinal joints apart from those in the rest of the body is that the ligaments holding them together have *elasticity*. That's right, elasticity. Only the ligaments of the spine can stretch and return to their original size. If you think about it, this is ingenious. Why? Because the spinal column remaining intact is essential to the health of the spinal cord housed inside it. If you're involved in a traumatic accident and your spine is stretched, cranked, or otherwise displaced, it's pretty important for it to be able to return to its original position, or as close to it as possible. If it remains displaced, the risk to the spinal cord is magnified, so the elasticity in the ligaments is a fail-safe. This mechanism has its limits; they can only stretch up to 50 percent of their original length and still be able to rebound. This is great for the long, thick straps of connective tissue that run the length of the front and back of the bones, but it's another story completely for the tiny ligaments that bind the facet joints ... 50 percent of short is, after all, really short. So even with this fail-safe in place, injury is possible at the facets and in the deep short muscles close to the joints if the movement is big enough.

The Rib Cage

The rib cage is a system of separate bones connected to the spine and to each other in such a way that they mostly act as a unit. They connect to the spine in back, while in front a hyaline cartilage framework attaches them to the sternum. It is a closed system integrated with the thoracic spine. This unit creates a great amount of stability to the mid-spine, but it is in fact mobile. Each set of ribs can move independently of one another, which means we may have more range in the rib-spine than we might at first assume. The top two pairs of ribs meet the spine in two places: at the body of their corresponding vertebra and again out at the side pokey bit (the *transverse process*). The remaining pairs of ribs have three joints, first attaching to two vertebral bodies, spanning the disc, and the third joint at the transverse process. This means that there is a lot of connective tissue potentially limiting the movement of the rib, but motion is indeed possible. We just need to be mindful of how we fire our muscles and be thoughtful about where we stabilize and where we focus our movement. It will take diligent work to learn how to fire those intrinsic muscles between the ribs and gain more specific range of motion at each level. Luckily, the work we do in yoga, like pranayama, twists, side bends, and backbends, achieves this particular training.

When you look at the shape of the ribs and the muscles in between them (the *intercostals*), it's pretty obvious that they are meant to move. Our deepest breathing

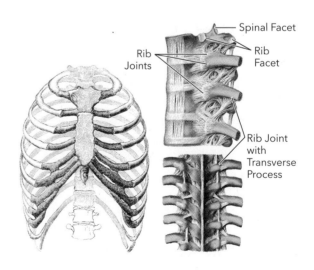

Spinal Facet

Rib Facet

Rib Joints

Rib Joint with Transverse Process

requires the lifting and expansion of the rib system in order to fully increase the volume of the lungs. Our rotation is dependent upon the ribs sliding past each other as the vertebrae rotate on the facet joints. Side bending means that one side of the rib cage compresses together as the other side fans open. Many of us lack dynamic range in the rib joints, but it will be to our advantage to access this movement. If we can soften the tension between the ribs, then our spinal joints will move more freely at each level instead of being rigid in one area and hyper-mobile in another. It is to our long-term advantage to move a little bit at many joints, rather than moving a lot at one or two joints.

Lastly, observe the last two ribs. Notice that they do not make the same connection to the cartilage that unites the others with the sternum. So, the vertebral levels T10–T12 are not stabilized the same way its friends are. These "floating ribs" allow for more movement at those spinal levels, and they require more attentive focus for both stability and movement. If we lack awareness in this region, T10–T11 ends up taking most of our mid-spine movement, leading to faster degeneration and collapse. This is a high-risk area in the very postures you'll use to mobilize the upper ribs.

The Pelvis

The pelvis is a remarkable thing. Though it's not truly part of the axial skeleton, its movements directly impact the spine, so we'll discuss it here. Its shape is strange and can be mind-boggling to consider. The bones sweep forward and back, out and in, up and down at varying angles, so it's easy to get lost when trying to figure it out by looking at a two-dimensional drawing. If at all possible, I highly recommend looking at a three-dimensional model, like Fred, my skeleton. I have videos online that will offer some alternative perspectives and direction as you explore this particular part of the bony anatomy.

The pelvis has two parts, a left and a right side. Each half is a fusion of three bones: the *ilium*, the *pubis*, and the *ischium*. The two halves are joined in front at the pubis by a fibro-cartilage disc. At the back, the ilia offer two upward-facing facets, one on each side, onto which the sacrum fits tightly and is secured by dense layers of ligament. These are the *sacroiliac joints*, or *SI joints*. This engineering, which allows the two sides of our pelvis to move independently, is essential to our ability to move contralaterally as we do, swinging the opposite arm as one leg steps forward. While the SI is essentially stable, it still has a very small amount of movement. Genetic differences, postural stresses, and extreme movements can create hypermobility over time. When the pelvis moves as a unit, the sacrum should move along with it, affecting and moving the lumbar spine in turn. "Where the pelvis goes, the spine follows!" You'll hear me say this repeatedly in yoga classes and workshops. This relationship is a fundamental example of compensation and a primary function of how our spinal core integrates with our lower extremity.

To define a neutrally aligned pelvis, we must first distinguish the differences between the male and female pelvic shapes. The male pelvis (right) has taller, more square ilia, making it appear more box-shaped. The bony prominences known as the *ASIS* in front and the *PSIS* in the back (*anterior/posterior superior iliac spine*—you can see why we abbreviate)

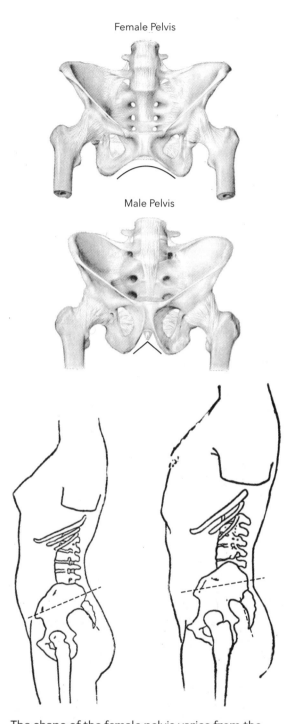

Female Pelvis

Male Pelvis

The shape of the female pelvis varies from the male: the angles of the pubic bones, the alignment of the ilia, and the shape of the ilia and sacrum all contribute to the female pelvis appearing to be tilted forward compared to the male pelvis, even when it is neutral.

are roughly level when the pelvis is neutral. The ischia are tall as well and create a sharply angled pubic arch. The pelvic inlet and outlet are both much narrower in men. In addition, the male sacrum tends to be narrow with a flattish curvature on the posterior aspect, appearing to be very upright with a tucked-in coccyx.

The female ilia (left), in comparison, are shorter, broader, and seem to open up wider in the front, giving the pelvis a more bowl-like appearance. The ASIS is lower than the PSIS when the pelvis is neutral. The ischia are squat and wide and create a round pubic arch. The pelvic inlet and outlet are wider and deeper (front to back) than in males, which is convenient since babies with big ol' heads are meant to pass through there. In addition, the sacrum is much curvier in profile than the male's, and the tail is pointed up and out of the way (again, handy come birthing time). The pitch of the sacrum is also much sharper in females, so that the posterior aspect of the sacrum may be nearly perpendicular to the spine! *All these aspects add up to the female body appearing to have a pelvis that is tilted forward in comparison to the male pelvis, even when it's neutral.* This is a very big deal when it comes to cueing a neutral pelvis.

Since we know that "where the pelvis goes, the spine follows," if we direct our students to lengthen the tail or tuck it down or shift it toward the heel etc., we are also instructing them to flatten out the lumbar lordosis. But the lumbar lordosis is integral to the stability of the spine and the health of its discs and nerve roots. Removing the lumbar curve undermines our deep core strength and stability. It is essential that we start seeing the neutral pelvis as it is engineered and not how we think it should look. We need to remove the instruction of tucking the tail or "lengthening the low back" from our rhetoric in order to reestablish our deep core stability in line with our fundamental engineering and alignment. We'll discuss some of the things to look out for in the next chapter.

NEUTRALIZING THE PELVIS

I'm often asked, "If the lumbar curve is so important, where did this consistent cueing come from?" Well, that is a very good question. While it may be tough to track the exact inception of this information, we can at least identify one of the conceptual origins.

If you can acknowledge that the male and female pelvises look very different in skeletal form and present differently in the average body, then it serves us to ask, "Who first started teaching yoga?" (Men.) "Who were they teaching?" (Also men, or more accurately, boys.) "Who brought yoga to the West?" (Again, men.) But perhaps the most important question is this: "Who came to yoga classes in the West?" (Women!!!)

So, it stands to reason that these men—who had been teaching a practice based on an oral tradition, lessons taught by one teacher and passed on to the next generation of teachers through rigorous and devoted practice—would look at the bodies of the women who came to class and, for the first time, see bodies that varied so much from their well-honed eyes … and see that something was "wrong" with how they were standing. Their bodies weren't strong, weren't aligned, didn't look like the bodies they'd been instructing for eons. It stands to reason that as yoga took hold slowly in the West, the messaging became rhetorical and the culture of a flat back rooted deeply.

In many ways this approach has also been supported by the fact that few of us understand our anatomy, and since we've been told by doctors and parents to "stand up straight," we may get the notion that a curvy spine is abnormal. When even medical professionals aren't well-versed in biomechanics, poor alignment models get reinforced in many areas of our culture.

So if you continue to hear these cues in classes that you attend, remind yourself that it's not really your teacher's fault; they have been given bad information for a very long time, and it has been constantly repeated to them for a long time. That said, it's time WE change that culture. It's time that we take advantage of the current understanding of posture and kinesiology. Now is the time to change the rhetoric and begin a practice of asking WHY we say the things we do, WHY we ask people to move in certain ways, and IF it's not functional, to change it.

Range of Motion

The spine is unique in its ability to move on any plane. Because of the sheer number of joints that make up the system, we can move on more than one plane at the same time. (While the ball and socket joints of the shoulder and hip can theoretically move in circumduction, the combination of all the planes of movement, they are still limited by the long bone/single articulation.) In the spine, the gliding facet joints move in such a way that the total system can take on a serpentine action that cannot be achieved elsewhere. This can cause a problem though, because when great range of motion is accessible, it's much harder to stabilize the area. We need to become adept at both accessing the movement and stabilizing against it. This takes a ton of focus and practice.

The primary actions of the spine are:

- Flexion and extension on the sagittal plane = forward and backward bending
- Lateral flexion on the coronal plane = side bending

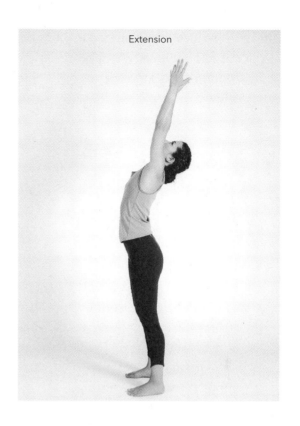

Extension

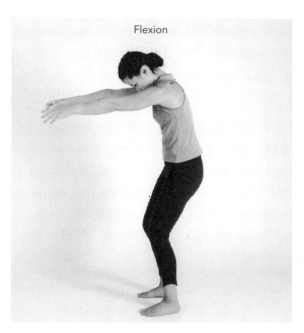

Flexion

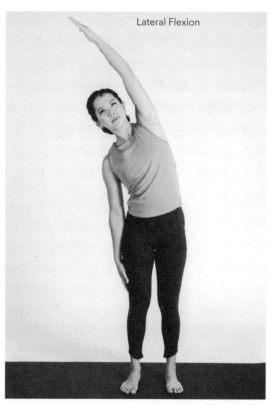

Lateral Flexion

- Rotation on the transverse plane = twisting (defined as one end of the spine being fixed while the other end rotates)

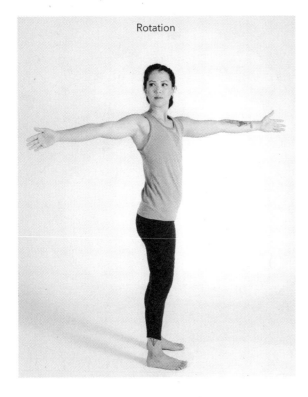

Rotation

As discussed in earlier sections, the vertebrae change shape and orientation from the cervical to the lumbar. As noted, those different shapes have a direct effect on the range of motion at each level. Look again at the models, and since we've already touched on how the processes may impact movement, focus for a moment on the facet joints. Notice that in the cervical and thoracic regions, the left and right facets are on the same plane; you could slide a flat piece of paper in between them. The angle or grade at which these occur may change, but the two sides stay uniform in their orientation to each other. As you move down into the lumbar region, however, the two sides begin to turn to face inward, placing them on two separate planes. This shift is really important, especially when considering the *rotation* range of motion.

When rotating, each vertebra has a finite amount of available movement with respect to the one below it. So, rotation at the spine occurs a bit like a spiral staircase: one bone moves to its max, then the one above continues the movement further, and so on up the chain.

Okay, fair warning! We're gonna talk some numbers here, and it can feel a little technical, but bear with me … this information is deeply insightful and will inform how you practice and teach twisting postures from here forward.

In the cervical and thoracic regions, the facets move with great ease in rotation. The neck-spine is capable of 80–90 degrees total in either direction. That is roughly 10 degrees per vertebral level. The thoracic spine itself is built to achieve something nearly as mobile as the cervical, but it is greatly limited by the ultra-stabilizing force of the rib cage. Therefore, from our twelve thoracic levels, we could achieve about 35 degrees total rotation each way. It breaks down to roughly 2.5 degrees of rotation at each level from T1 to T9, and then a bit more at levels T10–T12. Why the difference at the bottom? Because the last two ribs are "floating"—they don't attach to the cartilage web that connects around to the sternum, so they don't stabilize the way the upper ribs do. All this potential movement is theoretical of course, because many of us don't even try to rotate here, because frankly, to do so is intense work. Our mind prefers that our body finds the path of least resistance, so if we aren't conscientious about specifically activating the thoracic muscles, we will inevitably move in places with more inherent mobility and less resistance. So, where is that? Where will we compensate if we aren't thoughtfully moving from each thoracic level?

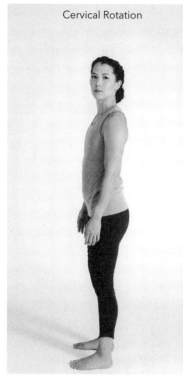

Cervical Rotation

80–90 degrees

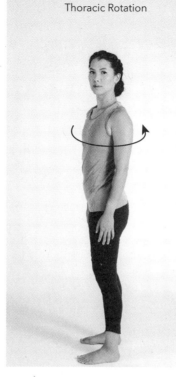

Thoracic Rotation

35 degrees

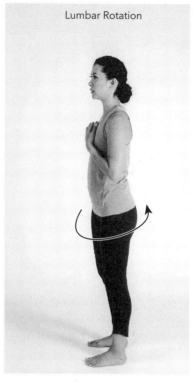

Lumbar Rotation

13 degrees

For many of us, the answer is the lumbar spine. We compensate for the stability of the thoracic spine by seeking out movement from the T10–12 levels and the lumbar spine. If you watch people do twisting postures, especially supine twists where they lie on the floor, you'll notice that there is a significant effort to mobilize the lumbar area. In fact, many times we are instructed specifically to try to keep our shoulders on the ground while rotating the hips. You'll see some particularly hypermobile people get nearly 90 degrees from these seven thoracolumbar levels. Unfortunately, that is a recipe for disaster.

If we take the bony engineering seriously and understand that the form of these joints truly does define their appropriate range of motion, then we must consider it very important that the change in the planes of the lumbar facets means *we should see a profound reduction in rotational range of motion*. From the engineering standpoint, the five levels of lumbar vertebrae should only produce **13 degrees of rotation**! That number may be shocking to see, because as mentioned earlier, we have increased our lumbar rotation a great deal—and become functionally hypermobile. There's a ton of evidence pointing to the fact that this is extremely detrimental over time. After all, hypermobility leads to degeneration, debilitation, and disease.

As a generally hypermobile person myself, I have had to work extra hard to isolate movement out of my lumbar spine and activate the range of motion in my upper thoracic levels. Through diligent practice, I've been able to rehab my low back to the point where I get only about 20 degrees of lumbar rotation. This stability feels amazing!! ☺

	Total Degrees of Rotation (one direction)	Number of Mobile Levels	Degrees of Rotation per Level	Degrees Many Yogis Are Achieving
Cervical	80-90	8	10+	80-90
Thoracic	35	12	2.5 (T1-10) 5 (T11-12)	0-10
Lumbar	13	5	2 (L1-4) 5 (L5/S1)	70-90 (T10-S1) :(So Sad!!

BACK PAIN

Consider this: Only about 10 percent of back pain is due directly to bulging or ruptured discs, yet back pain is one of the primary reasons people seek medical attention. If this is true, what else is causing the pain? Well, it stands to reason that if we are walking around with too much range of motion in our lumbar spine, the soft tissues in the area are being abused on a regular basis. Inflammation in the ligaments and muscles, even the discs and cartilage, will irritate the nerve roots just as a bulging disc might. By learning to tone the intrinsic muscles to stabilize the small joints, and if we habituate the activation of the deep core to decompress the low back as a whole, we can reduce the irritants that cause the majority of our pain. It sounds almost too easy to work, but trust me … my own body and those of many of my students are evidence that this truly does help!

For more a detailed discussion about the rotational range of motion and the studies behind these theories, please read the article by Michael Boyle found at this web address: www.strengthcoach.com/public/1107.cfm?sd=51.

Essentially it says that "rotation training" will contribute to hypermobility, and eliminating it from our regimens can help reverse the trend. If we instead focus on strength and stability in the lumbar spine, we can work to mobilize the thoracic and move more freely overall, with less pain to boot!

One last thing I'd like you to consider with regard to spinal range of motion is this: Because of the angle of the facet joints, the spine has a tendency to side bend when rotating, and to rotate when side bending. In order to keep these movements clean, precise, and non-compensatory, it's important to stabilize against one action while working to achieve the other. Ideally, we'll remain on a clear axis of movement and not blur the edges between the two. If we don't isolate these movements, we are adding greater friction-stress to the discs and increasing our risk of damaging them. Teaching precision in these relatively simple actions will help build awareness and strength in the deep stabilizing muscles of the spine, and perhaps increase our resiliency over time.

Muscles

As mentioned before, the muscular system that moves and supports the spinal column is complex. We'll break it down into smaller sections to make it a bit more digestible.

The core is often referred to as the abs + the low back, and usually we think mostly of the six-pack abs. In reality it is a complex interweaving of the upper and lower bodies. The central object of this confluence is the spine. There are muscular layers from deep to superficial that offer varying degrees of support and movement. The *deep core* is an intrinsic system designed to stabilize the spine before movement of the limbs occurs. The *dynamic core* is the complex of abdominal, paraspinal, and limb muscles that work both directly and indirectly to stabilize certain regions of the spine to allow efficient movement elsewhere.

The Deep Core

Consider this: if you have a long balloon filled with water, and you squeeze it tightly at the center, the ends of the balloon will move away from each other. Keeping this in mind, picture how the muscles of the deep core structures act together to compress the fluid body. This mechanism serves to both decompress the lumbar spine and create an ultra-strong stabilizing force for that area. While the viscera themselves are solid masses, the way they are suspended in our abdomen exhibits a very fluid nature, their relationship to each other has flow and "squish," and the pressure placed on this closed system by the muscles of the deep core acts just as hydraulic systems work in heavy machinery: fluid under pressure is incredibly effective and efficient at moving or controlling mass in gravity.

The fundamental muscles of the deep core are:

- Multifidi
- Transverse Abdominis
- Pelvic Floor
- Diaphragm

The *multifidi* are the smallest and deepest of the paraspinal muscles. They are a series of individual, short muscle bellies that span only one vertebral level at a time. When they contract, their angles actually achieve a sort of decompressive action between the bones. They are designed and enervated to contract in support of the spine before a movement happens at the limbs. This is preemptive, preparatory, reflexive even, but is often undermined by lack of awareness and strength in these muscles. Active, strong multifidi help maintain the lumbar lordosis in its fundamental shape and sacral stability. If multifidi are weak or inaccessible, the lumbar curve can be easily compromised. This is perhaps the most common weakness across our population. Even very strong, capable people can have a hard time accessing the actions of multifidi. In fact, if we have very strong superficial muscles, we will often use those instead, and multifidi just grow weaker over time. Countering this means moving in slow, precise ways until we can relax the larger muscles and re-establish a connection to those tiny intrinsic muscles. Sometimes precise physical therapy is needed to achieve this.

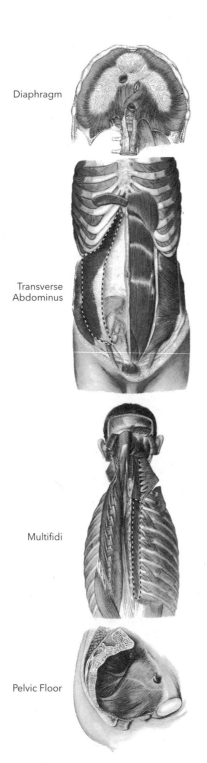

Diaphragm

Transverse
Abdominus

Multifidi

Pelvic Floor

The diaphragm secures the top of the hydraulic system of the deep core, while the pelvic floor supports the bottom. The transverse abdominis and multifidi pressurize from the sides/front/back to the center.

The *transverse abdominis* is the deepest of the abdominal muscles. It attaches in the front at the *linea alba* via a thick layer of tendinous fascia. Its fibers run horizontally around to the back body to attach at the spine via the deepest layers of fascia, called the *thoracolumbar aponeurosis*. Its job on contraction is to pressurize the contents of the abdominal cavity. In other words, it's there to squeeze your guts! Tone in this muscle ensures that the digestive organs are supported and their processes can take place with less interference from gravity. It helps in the acts of elimination and childbirth. It assists in the most efficient breathing techniques. It works in concert with the remaining deep core muscles to decompress and stabilize the lumbar spine.

Recall the image of the water balloon; the same thing is true in the deep core! Pressurize the fluid body of our abdomen using transverse abdominis, and those visceral contents will get squeezed up and down. Why is this important? Because we have the pelvic floor at the bottom and the diaphragm at the top to contain the fluid movement and translate it to spinal decompression and curve support.

The *pelvic floor* muscles are NOT the perineal muscles. They are often confused with each other and get referred to interchangeably, but they are not the same. Please be clear to make the distinction from here on in. The perineal muscles outline the pelvic outlet. If we clench our perineum instead of the gentle contractions of the pelvic floor/transverse abdominis, then we encourage spasm across the base of the pelvis, impacting our sex organs, elimination, and energetic continuity. We can also affect the deep muscular functions of the hips and low back, creating dysfunctions that change how we move and build patterns that are very difficult to reverse.

The true pelvic floor muscles suspend and support your bowel, reproductive organs, and urethra near the pelvic inlet. They are fascially connected to the deep layers of the abdominal wall and the coccyx/sacrum. Our interest with regard to the deep core lies in the true pelvic floor and its ability to counter and contain the internal pressure coming from the transverse abdominis above. To activate these muscles is to protect your pelvic organs, contain your downward energy/prana, and begin to work with Mula Bandha.

To do this, a very gentle pulling straight back of the transverse abdominis will help engage the subtle muscles of the pelvic floor via their fascial connections. There is no need to clench! Clenching will actually trigger deep hip and perineal actions that will undermine our core stability. If doing this correctly, you may experience a sense of the belly and the sacrum pulling toward each other, front to back. These actions prevent the pressurized abdominal organs from squeezing out through the pelvis, and through this resistance, help decompress the lowest levels of the spine. Just as the balloon gets taller, so too does our trunk.

The *diaphragm* is the primary muscle of breathing. It is a thin, dome-shaped muscle that attaches to the front of the spine and the bottom rim of the rib cage at its base, with a thick tendinous patch at the top (the *central tendon*). The dome shape is its relaxed state. When the muscle fibers contract, they pull the central tendon down and flatten out the dome. This action creates a vacuum in the chest cavity, drawing air into the lungs through the mouth and nose. In addition, this action compresses

the abdominal contents downward. If the abdominal muscles are slack, the belly will puff out on inhalation. If, however, the abdominal muscles are contracted, the diaphragm will

Pelvic Floor

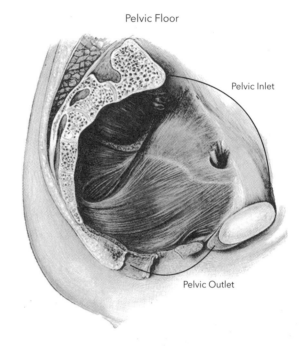

Pelvic Inlet

Pelvic Outlet

Perineum

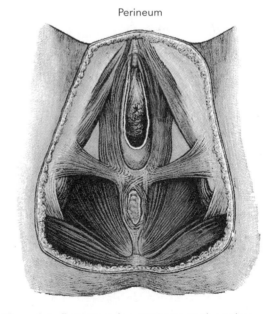

The pelvic floor muscles originate at the pelvic inlet, while the perineum outlines the pelvic outlet.

meet this resistance and two things happen: the increased pressure on the organs helps further decompress and support the low spine, and it forces the ribs to move more in their outward and upward range to further expand the chest cavity for a deeper inhale.

It is this integration and mutual resistance between the diaphragm and transverse abdominis that helps cap the top of the deep core and create the pressure on the fluid body to ensure a decompressive action on the lumbar spine.

RESISTANCE AS EFFICIENCY

Resistance is more efficient than freedom. Say what? This is one statement that needs a physical experience to really grasp. So try this little experiment with me: Either sitting or standing up straight and strong, place your hands near your ribs as if you were doing a Low Plank. Now push AS HARD AS YOU CAN through the air. Do this repeatedly. Push hard! Go fast! I assure you, you will feel ridiculous, but it's fine … everyone around you is worried about themselves, not your display. As you do this, ask yourself, "What am I actually accomplishing?" The answer? Absolutely NOTHING! That's right. You're using a ton of energy and effort to get exactly zero things done. That is the futility of freedom in physics.

Now relax your arms for a moment, shake 'em out. Chill. Then place your palms together in front of your heart in Anjali Mudra. Using the same focus as you did to push hard in the opening exercise, now you will go slow, being subtle. Make sure that your wrists aren't jammed up, allow them to be level with the elbows, this is not a stretch. Begin to press your palms together. Notice just the moment when enough energy has entered the system to feel resistance. Very likely, you'll feel it almost immediately. This is the efficiency of resistance. It takes almost no effort at all to achieve an output from your input.

Keep pressing, very slowly increasing your pressure, your effort. As your work increases, so too does the resistance, equally so in fact, and the more you press, the more the palms will start to shift; they will express a subtle desire to begin to move in a very specific way: upward. If you continue to press, your hands will begin to rise until they reach overhead, without consciously lifting them up there. Once they top out, just for giggles, try to pull them apart. My guess is that there will be a not-so-subtle resistance to that! They may feel magnetically connected, tough to pull apart even. This is the remarkable power of resistance. If you press two parts toward the center, upward energy is the output. Gather into your center to find levity and length. ✪

The Dynamic Core

Besides simply containing our abdominal organs and creating spinal stability, the muscles of the core do actually need to facilitate our movement through space. That's where the dynamic core layers come into play. The abdominal muscles work in concert with the long muscles of the spine, and they even integrate with the hip and shoulder girdle. It's this complex weave of fiber directions and depth of layers that creates the potential for all of the dynamic movements we are able to enjoy in the spine. The muscles we'll discuss constantly ride the line between stabilizing and mobilizing, helping us stay upright and composed while also counteracting the pull of gravity as we continually move off our center of gravity in order to make our way through the world.

Because we are upright a majority of the time, when we are assessing the muscular actions in any particular movement, we have to remember that the muscles on the opposite side of the movement are the ones working. That is to say, the antagonists are using eccentric contractions to control the movements in gravity. Those muscles are contracting, but getting longer. So, if I'm doing a standing side bend, lateral flexion to the right, it's not the right-side muscles that are working to create that movement (see image on p. 18), because gravity is pulling me over to the right ... those muscles are slack! Instead, the muscles on the left side are contracting while slowly getting longer, helping moderate my descent in gravity.

This model changes when we change our relationship to gravity. For example, if I am in Vasisthasana, or Side Plank, with my right hand on the floor and my hips rising up to the sky, I'm still doing a right-side bend, correct? In this case, however, I need to fire those right-side muscles to pull my hip toward my ribs, my shoulder toward my waistline, in order to achieve the lifting action. Keep all of this in mind as we begin to define the actions of each muscle.

The Abdominals

There are three sets of muscles superficial to transverse abdominis that act as both stabilizers and mobilizers of the spine:

- Internal Obliques
- External Obliques
- Rectus Abdominis

The *internal obliques* are the next layer from the inside out. Internal obliques have a fiber direction that runs from their attachments at the pelvis and fascial connection to the thoracolumbar aponeurosis in back, up and inward at a diagonal (or oblique direction, hence the name) to their attachments to the ribs and *linea alba* (the thin white line of connective tissue in front that ties the left and right abdominals together, like a belly zipper!). They function along with transverse abdominis to compress the abdomen, but they also act in rotation of the spine and side bending.

A bit more lateral and another layer more superficial are the *external obliques*. They have fibers that run from their attachments at the pelvis and fascial connections at the linea alba outward and upward to their attachments at the ribs and thoracolumbar aponeurosis. They are responsible for the lateral or side-waistline compression, side bending, and twisting.

Lastly, and most superficially, we find the *rectus abdominis*. These are the multi-bellied muscles that are commonly referred to as the "six-pack" muscles. There are actually four or more bellies on each side of the linea alba, and they run up and down between their

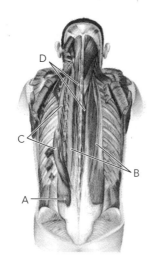

Paraspinal Muscles

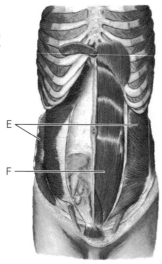

**Abdominal Muscles
Middle Layer**

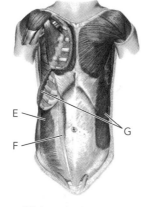

**Abdominal Muscles
Superficial Layer**

(A) Quadratus lumborum, (B) Longissimus,
(C) Iliocostalis, (D) Spinalis, (E) Internal obliques,
(F) Rectus abdominus, (G) External obliques

attachments at the ribs and pelvis. A few important things to note about rectus:

- It doesn't need help to get short from top to bottom if we are standing up (gravity does a fine job of that).

- Its bellies can be fired independently of one another! The upper fibers offer one type of support, while the lower fibers act differently.

- Crunches may be the most functionally useless exercise we can offer it.

Functionally, this muscle must remain toned to assist in the compression of the organs, but in daily life it is most useful for things like climbing trees and rocks—pulling the pelvis up toward the ribs. How many of you do that every day?? If you're not a rock climber, this muscle may show up in workouts as it assists actions like vertical jumping. In fact, I recently tore up some of my lawn in order to plant a flower bed. The repetitive act of jumping up and down on a pitchfork in an effort to tear up the sod left me with the sorest abs I'd had in memory!

From the perspective of your yoga practice, rectus is responsible for lifting the belly deep to the spine in postures like Cat, for keeping us aloft in Plank and arm balances, and for pulling us to standing from a drop-back backbend (flexion from deep extension). Any time you are in a prone or table position, rectus will need to fire to keep the mid-back from collapsing. The upper fibers in particular are integral to keeping the solar plexus area firm and supportive.

This mechanism is also employed when we're upright to help maintain the neutral curves of the spine. If upper-rectus is slack, T10 will usually collapse in extension and we see the front ribs "pop out," allowing posterior compression from T10 to S1. The lower fibers of rectus are responsible for assisting the gentle compression of the low belly and shoring up the deeper transverse abdominis, without actually pulling the pubic bone up toward the navel. So, the low fibers pull back while the upper fibers shorten to tip the front ribs down toward the navel. These two separate actions work together with the deeper abs and spinal muscles to keep our back-spine upright and spacious.

The Paraspinals

The muscles that run along the length of the spine are generically referred to as the *paraspinals*. These muscles are integrated via fascial continuity with the entire back body, along with some upper and lower extremity muscles: from soles to crown, they form what I refer to as the *back channel*. These muscles double as stabilizers and mobilizers, helping keep us upright but also controlling our movement through space. They include:

- **Multifidi and Rotatores**: These are the most intrinsic muscles of the spine. They are the fundamental stabilizers closest to the spinal joints. Multifidi is nearly solely responsible for stabilizing the SI joint.

- **Erector Spinae Group**: Please note that these are actually small bellies that span a few vertebral or rib levels and align to look like one long muscle belly. This design allows us to have fairly finite control of individual spinal levels instead of moving the entire system as one unit. It takes time to learn to control these independently, but it can certainly be done. All of our prone and supine backbends require strong and focused action from these muscles.

- **Quadratus Lumborum (QL)**: This is a very deep muscle that runs from the pelvis to the lumbar spine and twelfth rib. It is a powerful extensor muscle that helps support the lumbar curve in posture and under pressure ... *if* it's strong. It tends to be weak in most people unless they condition it specifically. Boat pose (Navasana) will not be safe if QL isn't strong and activated. Without QL, the pelvis tilts posteriorly and the lumbar spine goes into flexion. This is a very precarious posture with all the leverage of the legs and torso compressing the front of the lumbar spine and stressing the posterior aspects of the lumbar discs.

- **Splenius, Scalenes, Sternocleidomastoid**: These are all neck muscles that help specifically stabilize and mobilize the cervical spine. They are deep (except for sternocleidomastoid) and work in system with and against the shoulder muscles like trapezius and levator scapula.

- **Accessory Muscles**: These include the muscles of the rib cage, like the intercostals and serratus posterior, that may assist in rotation. As we'll discuss in other sections, the muscles that move our extremities also play a role in the spine: psoas in the hip system, latissimus and serratus anterior in the shoulder system.

Bandhas

With regard to the spine, the bandhas play an important role in stabilization. If you consider the curves of the spine, you'll notice a pattern of transitions from one curve to the next. You'll see that from top to bottom, you move from a very mobile section to a more stable section. The cervical is mobile, and the thoracic less so. The thoracic is pretty stable until the floating ribs arrive, allowing far more movement than above them. The lumbar is able to move far more than the fused bones of the sacrum and the limited SI joints.

In terms of stability, we already know that these reversing curves are more stable than if we had a straight column. Recall from chapter 3 that the Law of Compensation says exactly this. However, the *joints where these transitions occur are at substantial risk of absorbing too much movement and becoming hypermobile*. So, it's interesting to me that

the bandhas happen to align nearly perfectly with each of these transition points: **Jalandhara Bandha** at the cervicothoracic junction, **Uddiyana Bandha** just in front of the T10 level (remember that the lowest ribs aren't stabilizers, so the range of motion transition occurs *above* the curve transition), and **Mula Bandha** just in front of the lumbosacral joints. When we activate the bandhas, we use muscles to facilitate energetic awareness, cultivation, and stabilization. Together, the muscular effort and pranic flow help support these fragile junctions.

These bandha locations are even more remarkable if you consider the cultural aspect of the origins of these energy centers. They align perfectly with physiological points of weakness, are necessary to keeping us upright and strong and safe in our body, and were observed in a time and by a people who never cut open a dead body!! They developed an understanding of the bandhas solely from paying close attention to the body as it moved through time and space. From my perspective, this is a perfect example of what we continue to do each day in each class as yoga teachers; we make observations and communicate our real-time knowledge into lessons for individual students.

Experiential Learning

This is the part of class where we get creative: flashcards. Get outside your intellectual brain for a moment and really embrace your artistic side. We've gotta go here because rote memorization sucks. It's not easy for most of us, so any tools we can use to assist the process are important. Flashcards work because they combine our visual acuity with

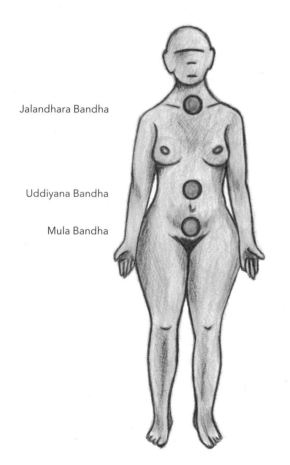

Jalandhara Bandha

Uddiyana Bandha

Mula Bandha

our verbal processors, which reinforces information better than just reading. If you draw your own pictures and write your own words, you get even more information download. Don't worry if you're not a great artist! These could be stick figures—they don't need to be photorealistic renditions in order for you to get the information into your head. In fact, this practice may help you start seeing the stick figure every time you look at your students, which may reinforce the muscle action/alignment principles we talk through in this training.

In the basic Yoga Engineer classes we expressly avoid trying to learn the names of specific structures, but sometimes having more technical language at your disposal can come in handy as you grow more advanced. It's still only a small part of a complex puzzle, but it could be helpful to integrate it into your learning.

Focus on just the names of the **major bones and muscles**. We will learn their specific actions over the long haul by paying attention to the fiber directions between the bones they connect.

- Draw a picture on one side of a notecard and write the name on the other.

- Or write the name on one card and draw the muscle on another in order to make a game of matching the two, like Memory.

- Print out images of the muscles from the internet and paste them onto cards if you don't like to draw.

- Of course, there is always the fallback of using The Anatomy Coloring Book ... an excellent resource, frankly.

I suggest using ALL of these practices over time to reinforce this information.

Limitations

Structurally, the shape of the bones is the first factor in determining the movement of any joint. The bones of the spine have many protuberances and processes, otherwise known as "pokey bits" (that's the technical term, I ASSURE you), that many muscles attach to. These bits create great potential to limit movement through compression, much more so than the ligaments of the spine. (In other words, bone on bone won't move very well.)

There are many thick ligaments that run the length of the spine on all aspects, but *spinal ligaments* are special. They have elasticity that other ligaments don't have. This is a kind of a fail-safe because the stability of the spine is so integral to our survival. The facet joints themselves are limited by the ligaments that bind the joints, but they can essentially still move in any direction. The discs as well have a finite level of flex and compression, which limits the range of each level. As the discs degrade, they are less resilient and supportive, leading to hypermobility. But as discs degenerate, space between the vertebrae is reduced, providing the potential for bony compression that may limit range of motion.

Functionally, we need to consider limitations that maybe, just maybe, we should *encourage* in our practice. This speaks directly to one principle of physiology: "Just because we can go there doesn't mean we should." Because of the propensity to move more in the hypermobile joints, *many of us exploit those places in order to get deeper into backbends or twists*. To prevent injury, we need to become acutely aware of these areas and develop the strength and acuity to support these levels specifically.

As discussed earlier in the bandhas, the levels where we transition from one region to the next are particularly at risk. Besides firing the bandhas effectively when we go deep into backbends and twists, *we need to use even more muscular action to support these levels from "breaking."* We need instead to spread movement across all the joints of the region. The postures are "bends" after all, not "breaks."

Spinal Risk Factors

Each region of the spine presents its own set of potential problems. Bony shape may contribute

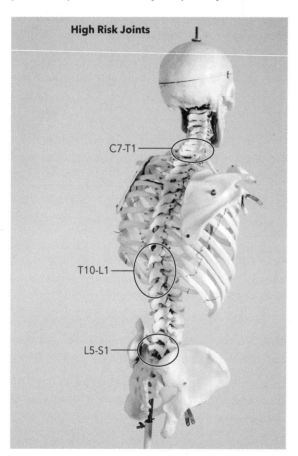

High Risk Joints

C7-T1

T10-L1

L5-S1

These are the levels of the spine where the curves switch directions, as well as where a relatively mobile section meets a more stable section. These relationships set them up for extra wear and tear, according to the Law of Compensation.

to stability or mobility. Some levels have more intrinsic structural stability while others are built specifically to move freely. I think it's important that you look closely at the skeletal images to become familiar with the vertebral shapes so you understand why each risk factor exists. I'll break it down for you so you have a general blueprint and can start amending your current cueing to reduce risk in real time.

Backbends

Backbends are extensions of the spine. Since the lumbar spine in its neutral position is already extended, that means our effort ought to focus in the thoracic region while stabilizing the lumbar lordosis. Our primary risk factors exist at the *break-points*, the joints where intrinsic hypermobility exists:

- **C1**: We need to be very thoughtful as we tip our head back in space. There is no bony support to limit range, so soft tissues are at risk. Muscles can spasm and neurovascular bundles may become impinged or abraded. Maintain adequate contracture of the anterior neck muscles to make sure the space at the back of the skull doesn't collapse.

- **C7**: This is where we transition from the mobility of the neck to the relative stability of the thoracic spine. Even with the stabilizing factor of long spinous processes to limit movement, we need to make sure that Jalandhara Bandha is active to minimize compression between those bones.

To ensure safe extension through the entire neck, begin moving from C7 instead of C1. It's easier to fire the anterior muscles and control the movement. This is particularly true in standing backbends and Camel pose (Ustrasana), but it's also useful in prone backbends, as it prevents the breaking that occurs when you try to look straight ahead. This method keeps the back-neck long and in cohesive curvature with the thoracic spine.

- **T10**: Again, because the ribs at T11 and T12 are floating, there's no extraneous support below T10. This is the transition point from stable to relatively mobile. In most bodies, this level is already compromised by our daily posture; so many of us are walking around with a pelvic thrust and collapsed T10! In backbends,

this is where we will break if we don't have a vital and active solar plexus/ Uddiyana Bandha/upper rectus abdominis.

We need the muscular support of the front body to keep this area long and arching in extension; that will help it curve instead of snapping sharply.

- **L5/S1**: This level is pretty infamous for its fragility. People often complain about the pain they feel in this area. In backbending practice, this level is the last mobile level in the spine; the sacrum is solid, and by design the SI

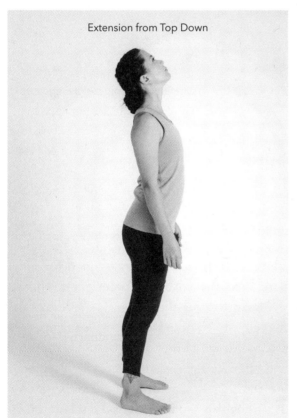
Extension from Top Down

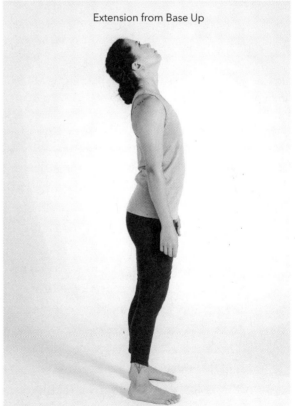
Extension from Base Up

On the left, the head rolls back first, jutting the chin, stressing the throat, and shifting the center of gravity—note the forward compensation in the hips and chest. On the right, extension originates at C7, activating the throat and allowing the center of gravity to remain over the ankles.

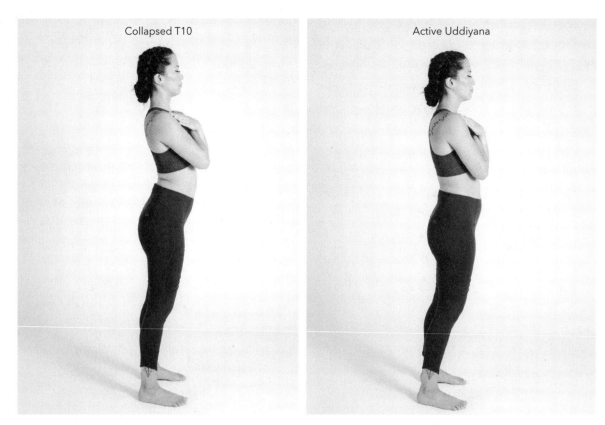

Collapsed T10

Active Uddiyana

On the left, you can see the crease that forms at the base of the ribs as T10 collapses. On the right, the upper abdominal muscles are active, adding lift to the posterior ribs and relieving pressure from the low back.

joints ought not to move very much. If the anterior body is not active in stabilizing this level—or the lumbar spine as a whole—this is the place where the whole system will jam up. Like dominoes falling upon one another, all of the extension energy will back up in T10, then translate to here, crushing the posterior side of the joint and sending inordinate forces into the SI. There is a ton of soft tissue in those spaces, and they are easily irritated by this compression; the nerve roots as well can be directly affected.

To avoid cascading dysfunction, we need to work to stabilize this area with our whole core, while our extension effort is focused above T10.

Twists

Twists require one end of the spine to remain fixed while the other end rotates on the spinal axis. If these rotational forces aren't distributed carefully across a large number of joints, joints that are specifically designed for rotation, then the shearing forces on the discs will build up and their integrity will degrade. It's relevant to note that when discs degenerate, the range of motion in flexion, extension, and lateral flexion are not greatly affected—but rotational range of motion increases as a disc's health is reduced. Consider this carefully because for many students, increasing the fullness of their twists is a direct corollary of their advancement in their practice! We need to have frank discussions about this in class to change the perceptions of success, in order to support their work in the thoracic region.

- **T10**: Since this is where the stability of the rib cage ends, this is where rotational energy will build up if we aren't hyperaware of stabilizing it. In twists especially, we need to treat this area like the less-mobile lumbar spine, helping support its neutrality, limiting the amount of twist that occurs here, or else ALL the rotation will happen here.

Use your thoracic muscles as the engine of the twist, not your arms or your obliques, and you're far less likely to dump your rotation into T10. This is not easy. It's actually rather difficult, which is why so many of us defer to the ease of twisting in our belly. Fight!! Resist the path of least resistance!! Your spine will thank you later.

- **Lumbar**: The low back transitions to the most stable region of the spine, the sacrum being solid and all, and since we get very little movement from the SI joints that the sacrum settles into, L5/S1 takes the brunt of spinal rotations that aren't actively focused up in the thoracic. If you look at the skeleton model, you'll see that the angle at which the vertebra and disc meet the sacrum

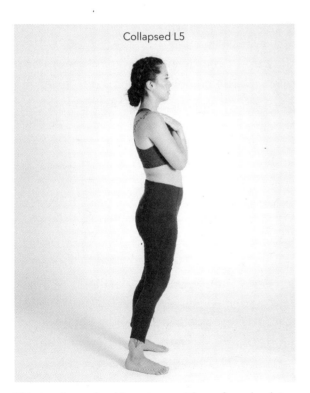

Collapsed L5

This is a "sway back" posture, with profound pelvic thrust. Note that there is a similarity with the previous T10-collapse image: the crease along the low back. In that image, however, the hips were not nearly as far forward. It will take time to learn to see these subtle differences in real time.

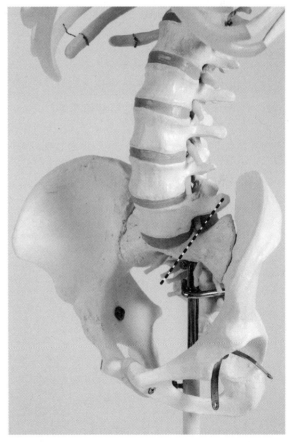

The joint at L5/S1 is not horizontal—it's at quite a sharp angle.

is quite sharp, angled downward toward the front. This angle adds to the risk of instability if it's exposed to long-term, excessive range-of-motion forces. If and when this particular disc degenerates, there is a much higher rate of actual displacement of the bones. (The lumbar spine can literally slide forward off the sacrum, impinging the nerve roots and even the spinal cord.)

Keep your pelvis in a stable position with respect to the lumbar spine, and you ensure that L5/S1 will not absorb so much torque. Activations of the hips will be necessary for this pelvic stability. As you'll discover in later chapters, the lower extremity and the spine are inherently supportive of one another.

Forward Folds

- **Lumbar Discs**: Forward folds are tricky. The posture we hold during most of our day will have a lasting effect on the condition of our discs and their pliability when we come to our mat. The lumbar spine is at particular risk for dysfunctional discs because they bear the majority of our weight, and few of us habitually stand or sit in ways that preserve their health and vitality. That means that when we approach our yoga practice, we must be especially mindful of these levels, or else we risk pushing them past the brink into significant injury. Forward folds are highlighted because in deep flexion, the back side of the disc is exposed to high internal pressure—the soft core of the disc is being pushed toward the expended back side of the disc. If that disc is dry,

altered, cracked, or already herniated, that intense pressure is likely to create or exacerbate bulges, and perhaps encourage a full rupture. The fact that it is the back of the disc is significant because that is where the spinal cord and nerve roots lie. The risk of herniation or rupture is there regardless of the range of motion, but because of those nerves, we need to be hypervigilant in flexion movements.

The key here is acknowledging that flexion in the low back is a high-risk proposition. Any time the lumbar spine is bearing weight in flexion, we must counteract that energy by activating the paraspinal muscles. We need to add spinal extension energy to the pose and direct the flexion energy into the hips. This will help minimize the compression of the front of the discs and the bulging of the back side.

Inversions

- **Neck Spine**: Hopefully it is obvious that the neck is not originally designed for bearing the entire weight of the body. This is in fact the argument that some styles of yoga use when proclaiming that we should never do headstands. While I'll agree that *some* necks ought never to do a headstand, I don't believe that the architecture in general can't do the job. I think massive populations of both yogis and breakdancers would take my side on this. An otherwise healthy neck with a proper curve and adequate muscular support is certainly capable of bearing the weight of the body for short periods of time.

It is IMPERATIVE that we pay very close attention to where we place our head on the floor, that we use our total core to minimize strain in the neck muscles, and that we avoid momentum in getting our hips over our shoulders. The strength in the neck and stability in the curve must be earned slowly, and momentum is the enemy of strength and grace.

- **T10/Lumbar Dumping**: The same risks apply here as they do in backbends. Just turning it upside down doesn't eliminate the crunching compression that can happen if we don't use our core to keep the spinal curves and transitions neutral. T10 and L5 will break and cause damage to the soft tissues if we aren't conscientious about remaining engaged in our central core. In addition, we will hemorrhage energetically if we are dumping here ... because one can't collapse in this area if the bandhas are active and intact.

Keep your deep core engaged the same way you would in backbends. Pressurizing the abdomen will help decompress the lower body up away from the ribs in inversions.

- **SI Joints**: The SI joints are especially at risk in backbending or asymmetrical inversions. Scorpion and leg variations in headstand come to mind. Injury or irritation here is often in conjunction with dumping in the lumbar spine since they are very closely related, just as they are in upright postures. The SI joint is the next mobile point in the system, whether energy is moving from the spine toward the legs (as in upright, weight-bearing poses) or from the legs

toward the spine (as in inversions). If adequate attention isn't paid to stabilizing the base of the spine, or limiting/controlling the extension in the hip, the SI will absorb the excess energy and hypermobility will ensue.

Maintain a deep activation of Mula Bandha and close attention to not letting the hip flexors go totally slack. These actions will help stabilize the SI joints and prevent their total collapse into the lumbar spine.

Common Conditions
Soft Tissue Injury

- **Sprain**: Stretching or tearing of ligaments. Under extreme conditions, like car accidents, the short ligaments go way past their elastic limits and will sprain. In yoga, however, we're usually referring to the ligaments of the SI because they have less elasticity and we tend to move without a ton of momentum. We have to work toward muscular stability around these injuries.

- **Strain**: Overstretching or tearing of the muscle fibers or tendons. These injuries should not be overworked. Gentle contractions and gentle stretching. Yoga practice should only be engaged after about seventy-two hours of RICE treatments (rest, ice, compression, elevation).

- **Spasm**: Hard, deep contraction of muscle fibers that can't relax of their own accord. Spasm can be associated with strain either as a cause or effect. Sometimes contraction of surrounding muscles can help this condition, and stretching should only be done if the area is already warmed up. Bodywork is highly recommended, since spasm can cause really disruptive compensations throughout the body.

- **Whiplash**: Fundamentally a combination of sprain/strain at the facet joints and surrounding muscle tissue. Though often associated with the neck, whiplash can occur at any spinal level. These injuries lead to chronic spasticity in unaffected muscles trying to reduce movement around the injury. We call this *guarding*.

Disc Injury

- **Herniation/Bulge**: If the integrity of the fibrous layer of cartilage is compromised, cracked, or starts to deteriorate in any way, the disc's nucleus will protrude through the herniation and the thinned wall will bulge out past the body of the vertebra. Under the right conditions this can be reversed with physical training/therapy, but you should proceed with caution if you don't have special training or specific instructions from the treating PT or chiropractor.

- **Rupture**: A herniation that goes unchecked, or a severe trauma that results in the complete breach of the fibrous wall of the disc so that the nucleus is no longer contained. This results in zero shock absorption at that level, increased range of rotation, and accelerated degeneration of the the disc overall. The oozing nucleus also causes inflammation of the surrounding soft tissue. Once you reach this stage, it cannot be reversed. Great care must be paid to supporting these levels with muscular stability, and extreme movements around this level should be avoided.

- **Spondylolisthesis**: This is a specific disc-degeneration injury where the fifth lumbar vertebra slides forward off of the sacrum. (It can happen at other levels, but it is most common there.) There is significant risk to the nerve roots and spinal cord itself. Strength in multifidi and transverse abdominis is essential to gaining any stability at this joint, but emphasis on lordosis should only be encouraged when supine. Usually surgical at some point.

8

The Spine and Core: Principles of Teaching and Practice Mechanics

This chapter will highlight how we use our knowledge of the structure and nature of the spine in our teaching and asana practice. All of that data is just sitting there, taking up valuable space in our brain, if we don't have a way to apply it directly to our movements on the mat. In "Principles of Teaching" we'll explore the aspects of teaching that sometimes get overlooked, like observation skills and vocabulary ... what NOT to say will be just as important as what you SHOULD say. In "Practice Mechanics" we'll categorize the movements needed to embody the most common postures encountered in general classes.

Along the way, I'll offer tools and exercises you can use as a teacher to build your skill set in different areas. Breakout sessions to brainstorm vocabulary, practice teaching modules, blueprinting exercises ... all of these will help ingrain the anatomy from the previous chapter, as well as offer insight on how to integrate that information into your own practice and teaching.

Principles of Teaching

With the spine, we need to be extremely mindful of people with hypermobility. They are more prone to injury in yoga than the ones who are stiff. Moderation, integrity, and muscular precision are the names of the game.

To that end, always keep the following points in mind when approaching your cueing of the spine:

- Does the pose at hand require the spine to be stable or mobile? Nearly all postures demand one or the other. If the hips have to move, it's likely that the spine should be stabilized, and vice versa. Isolate in order to integrate!

- If the pose you're teaching requires a neutral spine, cue it specifically. Make no assumptions about your students' inherent posture here. Very few yogis have the updated knowledge about the lumbar curve, so you are responsible for changing those habits.

- More movement in the spine does NOT mean a more advanced pose—it could just signal that certain levels have too much range of motion and there isn't adequate core stability to support proper alignment. Teach integrity, even if it means backing someone out of the pose a bit.

- Blueprint: The spine in its neutrality is the combination of Cow and Cat poses. The curved low back and tilted hips of Cow, the gathered belly and ribs of Cat, the broad open heart of Cow.

When sequencing a typical class, we're often taught to offer counterposes. In the spine, be mindful that most of the spinal discs out there on those mats are already compromised to some extent. Teaching extreme backbends followed by extreme forward folds may not be to the advantage of those tissues. Consider moderating movements, and adding transitions that employ gentle twisting or decompression before making drastic reversals of range of motion.

Observation Skills

When learning to see the body through skilled eyes, you must start at the beginning. If you miss the first step, the following ones won't be as informative. Start at the foundation of the posture. This doesn't always mean the bottom but instead refers to what is integral to the pose. Choose what needs to be stable and what needs to move. Then, teach. Use your blueprints. Teach each part in its stability or movement. Where to place your parts and how to get them there. That is the most fundamental definition of teaching yoga. All the other philosophical, metaphorical, esoteric, and mythological bits will flow naturally into your vernacular once you gain confidence in simply telling people how to move.

Seeing the neutral spine and neutral pelvis comes first. Train your eyes to stop

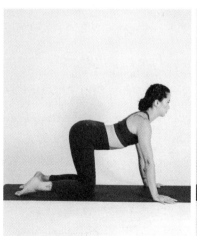 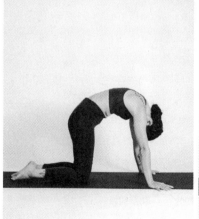 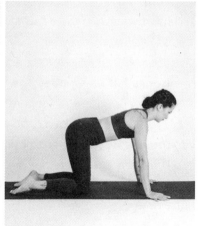

A neutral spine is achieved by simultaneously engaging the pelvis/lumbar actions of Cow with the belly/rib cage effort of Cat. These opposing postures ensure spinal stability through counteraction.

assuming that lumbar curvature is bad and to begin encouraging it in your students—this is of utmost importance. Once your sight becomes accustomed to looking at curves and pelvic points to assess misalignments, you can develop a grab bag of cues to coax your students to reinvigorate their lumbar spine and develop the necessary acuity in their abdominal wall. We'll discuss specific cues and modifications later in this chapter.

Recall from our introductory section that clothing is a fabulous tell for alignment. Wrinkles will show up to alert you to compressions and imbalances. Is your student side bending while in that twist? Are they twisting in that side bend? Do they exhibit a graceful, arching

OPTICAL ILLUSIONS ⚙

When observing our students on the mat, it is imperative that we begin to see the curves of the spine as they actually are, not get distracted by optical illusions. I don't know how many students have come to me saying that they've been told they have a "sway-back," or hyperlordosis, in their lumbar spine. Sometimes another teacher has told them this, sometimes it's a physician. In nearly all of these cases, however, it is not their low back spine that is the issue.

In all my time working directly with bodies, I have only encountered two or three cases of actual significant hyperlordosis. Most everybody else is experiencing one of two things: They are collapsed at T10, allowing their ribs to "pop out" in front and accentuating the look of the spinal extension. Or they have a voluptuous booty with a significantly angled sacrum, extending the visual line of the lumbar curve and making it appear far more extreme than it is in reality.

In either of these cases, telling your student to lengthen their tail or flatten the lumbar curve will result in a release of the deep core muscles and a destabilizing of the lumbar spine. The discs will be compressed at the front and expanded at the back, increasing the risk for posterior bulges. Remember, the lumbar spine is built to be in lordosis—flattening it out doesn't offer it more stability, it undermines it.

Instead, the student with the collapsed T10 needs to activate their solar plexus muscles, shortening the upper abdomen (rectus abdominis) in front and lifting their lowest ribs in back. They need to contract all of the muscles of the deep core to create the compression of the viscera that results in the decompression of the spinal column. In the case of the bootylicious, they ought to check in with their own deep core to ensure that they are decompressing from within and that their solar plexus is active. If both of those are happening, then they should be just fine.

backbend, or are they collapsing at one or more break-points? In forward folds, are they collapsing into their low back instead of working those hips??

All of these are relevant questions when teaching yoga. Note that if you are teaching a vinyasa class, it's gonna be tough to catch all of these nuances if your students are flowing too quickly. Consider teaching one time through your sequence, or at least a fundamental version of it, and go slow, offering the minutiae required to be wholly present. That way, as you begin to link the postures in flow, those actions will already be ingrained to some extent. You'll only need to cue to the most pressing actions, or be able to make individual adjustments on each pass through.

Cueing Principles

In my opinion, the primary awareness we are building, for the majority of students, is that of the three active curves of the neutral spine. This is foreign territory for virtually every person walking (and sitting) around our Western world. Essentially, if we are trying to move the limbs in any posture, we need to keep the spine stable. Its stability is a direct function of those curves being supported by muscle activation. If the spine is in motion, however, we must first make sure that the foundation of the limbs is stable, then activate and move deliberately and intently through the spinal body. So, to achieve either of these, our cueing must include some reference to this principle. When offering postures that move the hip, for instance, you must instruct clearly to maintain a neutral spine while flexing or extending in the hip. Teach support in the spine and action in the hip.

Here are conceptual explanations for the nature of the spine in different posture groups and transitions, as well as sample cueing for a pose in that family.

Along the way, keep in mind the applicable Dirty Dozen points to **eliminate**:

- Feet Together (boooo!)
- Tucked Tail (yikes!)
- Lifted Sternum (no!!)

Mountain/Equal Standing (Tadasana/Samasthiti)

Since Mountain is considered the blueprint for all postures, it makes perfect sense to begin here. Within that blueprint, however, is the spinal blueprint derived from that Cow/Cat combo-pack. So, every time you come to the top of your mat and stand in focused attention, the following alignment principles apply. You definitely need to get used to keeping people here, in standing meditation if you will,

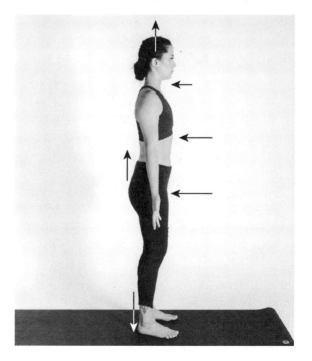

as you learn to look at their body, assess their center of gravity, and help them make adjustments to their foundation in order to support a neutral spine. You'll need to look beyond the optical illusions, focus on the truth that is being told in each individual body, and identify where they actually collapse or blow out.

Cueing Practice

A neutral spine is nearly impossible to attain atop a faulty foundation. So first you must look at the feet, then the position of the hips. I assure you that the majority of your students will have their hips thrust forward and their knees locked or very nearly locked. In order for the center of gravity to remain true, the pelvis must align properly over the ankles. We'll discuss the how and why of this in more detail in later chapters, so for now, please just roll with the instructions for the lower extremity.

> "Stand with your feet hips-width apart. Balance a majority of your weight through the ankles and into the heels. Soften the knees into a micro-bend, or even deeper bend, in order to feel some forward momentum through the shins, and then backward momentum through the upper thigh bones. You want your greater trochanter, the big knob of bone near the top of your thigh bone, to stack directly over your ankle bones. For most of us, that means sitting back quite a bit. Hinge your hips slightly to achieve this, or you'll feel very top heavy and topple over backward."

Trust me on this: the preceding will take a long time to habituate, so you'll need to teach only this portion for a bit, and certainly make hands-on adjustments. Again, we'll detail this later, so for now, please just bear with it.

As you begin to cue the spinal alignment, you'll need to repeat the foundation instructions and then repeat the spine. This can actually serve as a brilliant opening active meditation because it takes a ton of concentration, demands repetition, easily incorporates the breath, and offers time and opportunity for metaphorical/philosophical exposition. That said, start with the basics and repeat. Don't worry about folks getting bored ... they're working harder than it looks from the outside.

> "As you sit back over the ankles, lift the tail toward the back of the heart, activating the low back muscles. You WILL feel this in your low back, it's perfectly natural. Gently gather the low belly back toward the sacrum, firming the organs without lifting the pubic bone. Now breathe into the kidneys at the base and back of the ribs; as you exhale, pull in your solar plexus deeply, compressing the upper belly and supporting the lift of the base-ribs in back. Slight lift in the shoulder blades, broaden the chest without collapsing the back of the heart. Draw your vocal cords back toward the spine, lengthening the back-neck and stacking the head directly above the heart, crown rising."

That's a ton of information!! Thus, the repetition. Eventually it turns into shorthand:

- Feet hips-width apart, soft knees.

- Pull hips back over heels, lift tail.

- Gently gather low belly, deeply gather upper belly, lift back ribs.

- Light shoulders, open chest, don't blow out the ribs.

- Gather throat/vocal cords, crown rises.

Until you detail these though, none of it makes a whole lot of sense. So practice the long-winded version, or one recited in your own voice and words, until all of the principles are embedded in your brain. Then you can riff depending on what you see in front of you and focus on specific cues as you move through practice.

The Bandhas

If you were really paying attention to the cueing above, you may have noticed that we were simultaneously instructing on how to engage the bandha energy while focusing on the muscular actions. Once you teach your students the physical actions, then you can offer them the deeper insight as to the energetic containment they are achieving at each level.

Cueing Practice

The low belly pulling back corresponds with the Mula Bandha. The upper belly/solar plexus aligns with Uddiyana Bandha. The throat/vocal cords support Jalandhara Bandha.

"With eyes closed, gently pull in the lowest belly, compressing your organs toward the sacrum. If you feel into this sensation, you may notice a slight lifting deep in the pelvis. You don't need to clench the perineum, you don't want to harden or actively lift anything. By pulling back gently in the abdomen, you'll automatically engage and lift the deep pelvic floor and contain the downward energy of *apana vayu* (one of the Pranic Winds) with the Mula Bandha."

"Gather your solar plexus deeply toward your spine. Feel the front ribs draw down and the back ribs lift up off the pelvis. Let the breath expand the lungs instead of the belly. The chest can broaden, but don't let the front ribs blow out, don't let the back of the heart collapse. Fill the back body with breath, and on each exhale focus more energy on the containment of the solar plexus. You may feel heat building with each breath as Uddiyana Bandha contains and circulates your prana. Ujjayi Pranayama may be your breath of choice here."

"From a broad chest and anchored belly, draw your vocal cords back toward the neck spine. Lengthen the back-neck, create space at the back and base of the skull, crown rising. The throat will feel open and free, soft palate (roof of mouth) lifted. Breathe gently and evenly, Jalandhara Bandha containing the intake and distribution of prana. No collapsing of the neck, no puking out your energy through a jutting chin and throat."

These are three options on how to approach this, not instructions on how to teach. Some students will be naturally more drawn to the energetic principles of the physical practice, welcoming any esoteric insight you can offer. Others may require a fair amount of hand-holding, ushering them into these concepts slowly, and anchoring it firmly in the land of the physical so they can feel it at the gross level first. Most people build awareness along the way, but offering them the vocabulary to describe new sensations will help highlight those shifts as they occur, making them feel more real and tangible.

Forward Folds

Forward folds are everywhere in asana practice. Every time you flex the hip, you are in a forward fold. Note that: THE FLEXION OF THE HIP DEFINES A FORWARD FOLD. Nothing is said about flexion in the spine. In *most* cases, the effort of a forward fold is to keep the spine neutral and stable to facilitate isolated movement in the hip. As you cue these postures, it's important to emphasize the length and strength of the spine as the hip moves deeper into flexion. It's very easy to lose sight of this when the hamstrings are screaming at you in a mad stretch, but the emphasis cannot be lost!

To this end, we will cue standing and seated forward folds slightly differently. In standing forward folds, we have the work and stability of the legs to support us and gravity to traction the spine, but ONLY IF we engage the legs and properly distribute our weight-bearing. In seated folds, it's easy to assume that we are stable and supported by the earth beneath us, but it is in these postures that the spinal discs are most vulnerable. We want to be hyperaware of the compression that happens to the front of the intervertebral discs in spinal flexion, because the potential for the back side to herniate under these conditions is high, especially if those discs are already compromised.

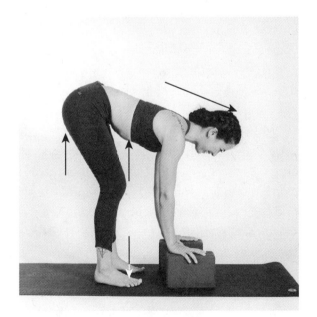

Stability is emphasized in the spine, so that the hip can be the mobile point of the pose.

Cueing Practice

Standing Forward Folds

Mountain transitioning to Standing Forward Bend (Uttanasana) is an example of an active lower extremity, requiring hip joint mobility, while the spine remains essentially neutral/stable. I say "essentially" because at some point in the movement, the spine WILL round out a bit, the lumbar spine finding flexion and the head dropping toward the floor. But this is one of the safer places that the spine finds flexion, IF the legs are working hard and the weight is centered correctly. That is true because of the downward traction on the spine created by gravity. When the legs are working, even if they are bent at the knee, they create a strong framework that the spine can hang from, relieving pressure from the discs instead of compressing them.

> "Reach arms out to the sides and overhead, keep the belly anchored to the spine, lift the tail, gather the upper belly, pull in vocal cords to keep back-neck long … Draw hands down midline as you hinge in the hips, weight forward to keep the back channels of the legs and glutes active … Keep the spine neutral as long as you can, lengthening through the chest and crown, hinge deeply in the hips to touch belly to thighs, bending knees as deeply as needed to achieve this. Finally, let the spine release into gravity, let the head/neck/shoulders go heavy and crown release fully toward the earth. On your next exhale, gather belly more deeply to the spine and the crown will descend more …"

In a flowing sequence, if you effectively communicate these details in the first two rounds, you'll be able to shorthand the instruction for any remaining folds, paying individual attention to students who need continued adjustment or adaptation.

Seated Forward Folds

Again, there is more inherent risk to the spine here than in standing variations. Our goal in these postures should be repeatedly stated: "Bring the crown toward the toes, not to the knees." If downward momentum takes over, spinal flexion is focused into the lumbar spine, and compression threatens the integrity of the posterior aspects of those discs. These poses require focused extension effort in the lumbar and thoracic regions, almost as if seeking a backbend!

We want to keep the chest broad and the sternum long. We want movement in the hip joint, deepening flexion there first, and only when the spine is supported—belly on thighs or on a prop—can we release that extension effort and surrender. Generally speaking, seated folds are active postures that can be turned into more passive restorative postures with the right support in place. Surrender should only be offered to those with inherent hip flexibility or those who use props appropriately. In my opinion, even with props, some very slight lengthening action should remain in the spine, never going absolutely passive.

> "Hips are elevated and legs out in front of you, feet hips-width, knees bent or supported as needed. Lift the tail, gather the low belly in support. Contain your solar plexus and broaden your chest. Use your fingertips behind you slightly to press the floor away and begin to hinge forward in the hips. Keep the spine active and long, don't hunch down. Slide hands forward under the shoulders. Lift the tail to hinge deeper in the hips. This may be a minute movement, it may be imaginary! All of these millimeters count. Use your breath to flood your thighs and hips and spine with prana, filling and clearing, creating space, allowing movement without forcing it. If it feels appropriate, the hands may slide forward, engaging the hands with the earth, gently pulling back to help keep the chest long and wide without cranking. If your belly begins to meet the thighs, you may begin to slowly round the spine, lengthening crown toward your toes, filling the back body with your full and even breaths as the front body compresses.

> "To come out, hands align under shoulders to push the earth away, finding a neutral spine and extension energy before firing the glutes and not the low back to stack the heart over the hips once more."

There are mechanisms in the lumbar spine that will reflexively limit our flexing movements if too much tension is placed on it. The fascia of this area is thick and active; it has its own contractile functions and will actively resist us. If you reach this point and continue adding energy, forcing the movement, you will injure yourself. It may be a disc, it may be muscle or connective tissue. Either way, it's a condition that will set you back, not propel you forward. So ... don't do that.

When rising up to a seat once more, acknowledge that the back muscles are at their longest and, therefore, weakest. Don't ask them to act alone in bringing you upright. Use your arms to find the basic shape of neutrality, then fire the muscles as stabilizers of that shape, THEN fire the hips to do the heavy lifting.

Be gentle. Go slow. Listen to your body, to your tissues, and move as they guide you, flowing with them instead of forcing them to your will.

Side Bending

Because of the shape of the vertebrae, there is a phenomenon in side bending: the spine will try to rotate. It has to do with the angles of the facet joints and how the two surfaces slide against each other. This is important to note, because if we don't pay close attention to the plane on which we move, our compensations will prevent access to the pure and safe form of lateral flexion. If you watch your students do a right-side bend, you'll notice the trailing side (left side) will tend to drop down toward the earth, rotating so the chest collapses slightly. It takes focus and effort to avoid this and stay on one plane of movement.

Why not twist? Well, it won't necessarily set you up for injury directly, but it will mean escaping the work of truly opening up the ribs and stretching the intercostal muscles. By side bending with integrity, you can more efficiently access the full range of the thoracic spine and rib cage, which over time will translate into more effective extension and rotation. It's ironic, I know ... don't rotate here and it will improve your rotation.

ELEVATING THE HIPS

I believe that EVERYONE should elevate their hips to some extent in seated folds. Even those of us with flexy hips should at least prop up our tail on the edge of a blanket. Since the back body is connected by a cohesive track of fascia and connective tissue, tension anywhere in that system can limit movement elsewhere in the system. This is geometry and physics at work, people. Elevating the hips automatically creates a little slack in the hammies and adductors, offering more potential for flexion at the hip.

People with legitimately short hamstrings ought to stack a couple of blankets and sit directly in the center of them. They may also need to bend knees and even roll a blanket under them for added slack and support.

For those with longer, more supple thigh muscles, a folded blanket is still an asset. Single- or double-fold a blanket and place the folded edge to face the front edge of your mat. Sit on that folded edge, right at the edge, so that you can slide forward slightly, so your sitting bones actually slip off the blanket and toward the floor. This will leave your tailbone and the flesh of your glutes propped up on the blanket-fold. This is important!

With your tail wedged up on the blanket, your pelvis tilts to neutral, but the hip flexors themselves can relax slightly. The lumbar muscles will be able to fire without clenching hard, and you will find yourself sitting upright without the strain that notoriously accompanies this posture.

Cueing Practice

"From a stable Mountain, reach arms overhead and bind hands together. Push down evenly with both feet, reach further to the sky with your left hand as you inhale. On exhale, begin to reach the left hand up and over to the right, bending the rib-spine. Keep length in the right side-waist, avoid collapsing, reach ribs upward first, then bend right. Shrug left shoulder slightly. Rotate left arm toward cheekbone, bringing shoulder blade around the armpit. Roll left ribs back, breathing into the fullness of back and side bodies, meet forward resistance of shoulder blade. Imagine stacking left ribs over right ribs while reaching up and past your left ear. On your next inhale, push both feet down and shorten left side-waist, engaging the obliques to raise you back upright."

There is a common cue in side bending that makes me crazy: "Press your hips to the left as you bend to the right." UGH!!! There is an impression that if you do this you are increasing the length of that side channel, but really you are only sending a bunch of energy into the hips while disrupting the rooting force of the legs. This makes it much harder to engage your core fully. It also makes it harder to get full access into those ribs and side bend with integrity.

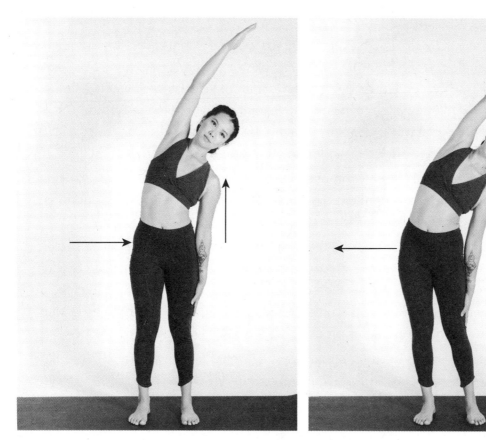

When the hips are stable under the spine, it is better equipped to stay tall while side bending. When the hips are allowed to shift, the bend appears to be deeper, but in reality it is the collapse of the spine downward.

"From a strong Mountain, reach overhead and bind hands. Keep feet hips-width and center the hips between them. Lift the tail slightly, gather the belly. Rise through crown and wrap shoulder blades forward around the ribs. Press down with both feet, inhaling. On exhale, bend to the left, keep the hips centered and tail lifted. Make sure weight is mostly in the heels, don't let pelvis shift forward."

If you try it this way, it's possible, even likely, that you will not bend as far as when you release the hips in opposition. To me, that is a sign that integrity is being fostered and both sides of the waist will remain tall without collapse. Try it this way, then while in the side bend, let the hips move out. Feel the difference. My bet is that you'll immediately feel the release of your core and connection to the ground. You can't be tall and strong without those roots!

Backbends

Backbends are extensions of the spine. There are a few key things to remember when practicing backbends. The first is that the lumbar spine is already in a backbend! That's right, kids, that lumbar lordosis that exists when the spine is neutral IS extension. So, the work in this region ought to be that of simply stabilizing the curve that already exists.

Note that more traditional cueing usually asks you to flatten this curve by tucking the tail. Since that goes against the fundamental biomechanics of a backbend, I strongly suggest that you never do that, and certainly don't ask your students to do it. Instead, you'll cue them to use their deep core to support the curve as it is, perhaps even accentuate it in some bodies, and then instruct them on where else in the spine they can do the work.

Cueing Practice
Lumbar Support

Let's use Bridge pose (Setu Bandha Sarvangasana) as our example, since oftentimes the directions here are overt to lengthen the tail. We're rewriting the book!

"With knees bent and feet hips-width apart, align heels directly under knees so shins are upright. Arms are at your sides, shrug shoulders slightly and pull shoulder blades together toward the spine. Feel how your sacrum meets the floor … begin to pull it toward the back of your heart, allowing the low-back spine to lift away from the floor slightly. You'll feel those muscles engage, this is what we want. On an inhale, gather your belly through your organs, firming them into your spine without flattening out the low back. Maintain these actions for a breath or two, until they feel a bit more familiar and refined. On an exhale, press through the shoulders, arms and feet, lift the hips off the floor without losing that curve in the spine. Do not tuck the tail toward the knees or thrust the pubic bone to the sky. Instead, continue to pull the tail toward the back of the heart. Belly firm, breath smooth,

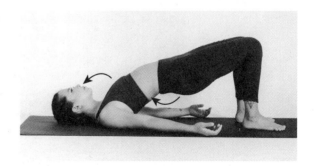

When the tail is pulled toward the ribs, a continuous curve is created, rippling through the thoracic spine and sending the sternum toward the chin.

let the backbend coil behind the heart, lifting the sternum to the chin. Rise up using the actions of the entire spine, buoyant, light; long from the pit of the throat to the knees. Resist the urge to thrust the pelvis—instead, think about lifting the chest and the thighs while letting the pelvis come along for the ride."

In this example, we emphasize the forward tilt of the pelvis and the actions of a supported lumbar lordosis and an actively extended thoracic spine. It's important to get clear that the spine is the action center here, the engine of our movement, while the limbs provide roots through the earth. The lift is achieved by the back spine meeting the stabilizing contractions of the front body, not by gross clenching of the glutes. The scaps and arms provide a strong base that interacts with the floor, but the thoracic spine is doing the heavy lifting of expanding the front-heart and lengthening it toward the chin.

Thoracic Action

There are many ways to approach the direction around the low back curve; the key is that it exists, and that it is supported by muscular contraction. In some way we also need to emphasize that the thoracic spine is where the real work of extension must happen. I said, "coil behind the heart," "lift the sternum to the chin." Once the low back is stable, we need to cue to the action of the upper back. Eventually, this will include instructions specific to the shoulder blades, but we'll talk about that in later chapters. For now, you'll need to develop language that speaks directly to activating the upper erector spinaes, to expanding the chest, to lengthening the sternum (of course, you can't actually do that, but yoga is at least halfway about pretending), to opening the rib cage, to supporting the heart's buoyancy ... see where I'm going with that? We'll offer some exercises for this in the "Vocabulary" section.

Keep in mind that for many people, the thoracic region of the spine is hypomobile ... it is stiff and stuck and maybe even fused! This work will be tough, sometimes moving those bones will actually be impossible, but it is still worth the effort. If we let go and allow the extension energy to go elsewhere, we'll break at our weak points and compress our squishy bits, risking long term damage.

Throat and Neck

Lastly, we need to make sure that we aren't casting our head back in space or deeply arching our

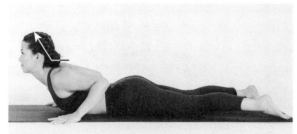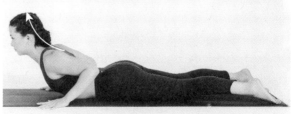

If you look straight ahead in your prone backbends (Cobra family), your neck breaks at a harsh angle. Instead, keep the back-neck long to ensure extension energy flows freely through to the crown.

neck in backbends. You'll often see this in the Cobra family of postures: Cobra (Bhujangasana), Upward Facing Dog (Urdhva Mukha Svanasana), Locust (Salabhasana), even Cow. When this happens, not only do we break at the base of the skull and mid-neck, but our throat is totally exposed and has no muscular support. This results in all our prana puking out through the vocal cords and the soft tissues at the back of the neck getting compressed. Our head feels heavy and our breath is stifled. None of these qualities serves a potent backbend. Instead, we need to activate the anterior neck muscles, keep the airway open and the back-neck long.

"As you find your Cobra pose, lengthening the sternum to the front of the room, gather your vocal cords back toward the neck spine. Create space at the base of the skull. Imagine that you are lifting up from the base of the neck instead of the top of the crown. You want to feel long first; lifting up is the natural reaction to growing long."

I use similar language around the vocal cords for most postures. It creates continuity for an area that few people think much about in daily life. Consider as well that most people have poor neck posture, generally speaking, so gaining strength in those throat muscles will be difficult, but it will have positive ramifications both on and off the mat.

TO GLUTE OR NOT TO GLUTE

There is an almost reflexive desire to clench the glutes in backbends. This phenomenon, I believe, is associated with the constant old-school cueing to drop the tail. For most people, this means clenching gluteus maximus. Obviously, we now know that flattening the lumbar curve is not ideal for the health of the spine, so we could just leave it there … but even if we don't tuck the tail, many students habitually clench their booty. There is a time and place to fire those big bulky bits—strengthening them, conditioning them to propel us through or hold us up in space—but backbends are not that place.

If we think about the entire spine in a backbend, and we consider the energy flowing through that system, we have to acknowledge that we need that energy to flow freely and not get jammed up in any one place. If energy flow gets stuck, we'll suffer from compression in the soft tissues; if compression occurs, energy will get stuck. At the base of the spine, we need there to be an emergency exit of sorts, a place where any excess extension energy can continue flowing. If you are in Cobra pose, for instance, and the booty is hard, but you push into the earth with your hands to gain more height, then the spine will jam up at the base because those glutes prevent movement … movement of bones AND energy. L5 ends up taking up all that energy, and the soft tissues are compressed. You've quite literally set up the rock and the hard place.

If the glutes remain active without clenching, however, the sacrum and tail have just a few millimeters of movement available to them … and that's enough to keep the energy flowing and the bony bits free of the strongest compressive forces.

This principle stands for all the backbend families. Bridge shapes, Camel shapes, Cobra shapes, they all require mellow glutes to prevent jamming up in those breaking points.

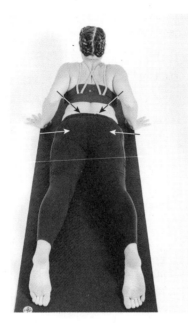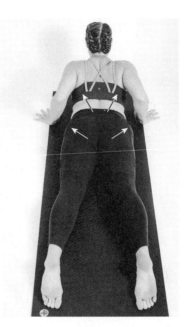

If the glutes clench in prone backbends, the energy of extension jams up at L5/S1. When the glutes are softened while the belly and hip flexors activate, the extension energy flows up through the entire spine.

Twists

Whether you are practicing fiery upright twists or ending class with well-supported restorative postures, twists are dynamic beasts. They don't always look like much on the outside, but each one is a complex interaction of the spine with the extremities. There is ample opportunity to use those limbs in ways that make it appear that we are moving deeper into the rotation, but oftentimes these are illusions. What is really happening in those cases is a series of compensations that will take us out of our integrity and off our spinal axis.

So, rule No. 1 in twists is: Twist actively through the thoracic and keep the lumbar spine stable. That means that rule No. 1a is: No cranking with the arms. If you use your arms to pull you into the rotation, you are much more likely to go slack in your thoracic spine, twist in the lumbar spine instead, and go far beyond its engineered limits. *No bueno!!*

Cueing Practice

Let's use a seated twist, Half Lord of the Fishes (Ardha Matsyendrasana), to examine this. Assume that your body is already in the proper shape, with left leg straight and right knee bent, right ankle crossed over the left thigh, foot flat on the floor.

"Hips are elevated on the edge of a blanket. Make sure both sitting bones bear weight equally. Lift tail toward back of heart, gather low belly to firm the pelvic organs. Rise through crown, deeply gather solar plexus. Right hand slides back behind and just outside the hip, acting as a kickstand to keep us upright and on axis. Left hand makes a fist; place that fist on the front of right shin, and pull straight back toward the heart. This will help you feel more lift as the torso and thigh pull together. Inhale fully and gather belly, exhale long as you rotate right, focusing movement in the rib-spine. Don't let your hand pull your shin across your body; pull straight back toward your spine. Make sure both side-waist lines are equally long and that solar plexus remains anchored."

In this example, the arms are given jobs to do, but neither is allowed to pull your heart further into the twist. The paraspinal muscles are required to do the work, building both strength and mobility over time in an integral way. Nothing is forced through external mechanics; all that movement comes from within.

Rule No. 2 in twists is: Isolate the movement in the spine by stabilizing the hips. If you are allowing shifts in the hips, you are not maintaining integrity in spinal rotation. Remember, one end of the spine must remain stable in order for it to be a twist ... in upright and

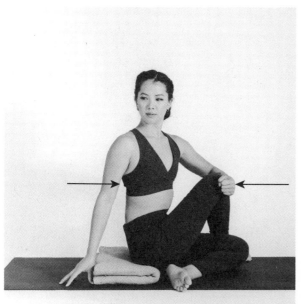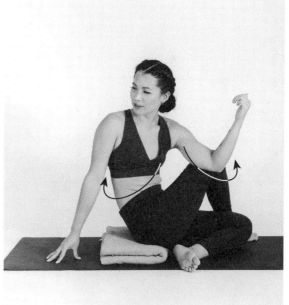

The arm pulling straight back results in the spine pressing toward the thigh. If the arm works as a cranking lever by pressing away from the thigh, the spine is much more likely to spin downward, collapsing into flexion or lateral flexion.

seated postures, this means the hips. Some renowned instructors teach that shifting the hips will save your SI. I do not subscribe to this theory, and I tell you why in the sidebar.

This time we'll talk about a standing twist, Revolved Side Angle (Parivrtta Parsvakonasana). For our purposes, the right back knee is low, the right hand is on a block at shoulder width, and left hand will reach out and up to the sky.

> "From low lunge, right knee on the ground, activate right hip flexors by pulling right knee forward into the friction of the mat. This fires right hip flexors, adding upward momentum to right sitting bone.

We want the pelvis to remain neutral and level ... don't allow the right hip to drop toward the floor. Gather belly deep, left hand on heart, inhale fully. On exhale, begin to rotate heart open, elbow in line with collarbones. Keep belly firm to avoid backbending here; ribs pull back like Cat pose. Buoyancy through right thigh and hip, lift tail, spiral heart."

There's all sorts of actions that the upper extremities can do here to keep us stable, but we'll touch on those in later chapters. For now, please focus on language that encourages the hips to remain neutral, avoiding compensation and keeping the twist isolated and integral.

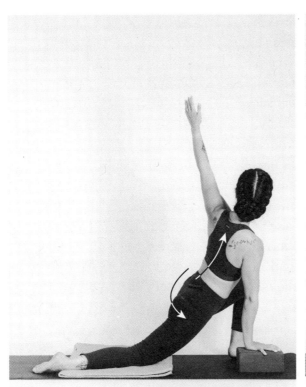 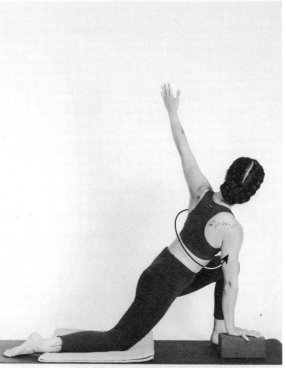

A dropped hip in twists means the spine isn't doing the rotations, and this usually results in a backbend instead. With stable hips, the rotational energy is isolated to the thoracic spine (assuming the belly is active to stabilize the lumbar spine.)

Recall the tendency for twists and side bends to want to hybridize. From a teacher's perspective, this is clear enough when teaching simple side bends or seated twists, but as soon as we get into postures like Twisted Chair (Parivrtta Utkatasana), things get a little more complicated. The deep flexion at the hip in this pose can distort our perception of what we're actually trying to achieve. Twisted Chair is certainly a twist, meaning the hips must stay stable while the ribs rotate, then the arms reach out and exaggerate the visual sense of the chest expansion. On the other hand, if you transition from this shape to an arm balance like Side Crow/Crane, you are neutralizing the rotation in order to get both hands on the ground. All of a sudden you are in a side bend instead of a twist. Many arm balances are taught as twists but are really very deep side

HIPS SHIFTS IN SEATED TWISTS

In seated twists in particular, the SI is put at risk. The more asymmetric the posture, the more torque will be applied to the pelvis. To lessen this risk, some teachers have begun to advise students to allow the hips to shift in these seated twists, relieving pressure while allowing for "deeper twists." I think all this is phooey.

Here's the thing: twists should emphasize rotation in the thoracic spine. If a student has SI issues that are aggravated by these twists, it's likely that the combination of hip external rotation/flexion/abduction is creating tension through the hip-pelvis-low back, and then poor mechanics in their twist is amplifying that tension. If they don't stabilize the lumbar spine, their SI will surely absorb rotational energy, to its peril. Personally, I don't think the answer is to more fully degrade the integrity of the twist by going slack in the hips.

Instead, what if we just go ahead and firm 'em up, distributing that stretchy tension across the entire pelvis so it doesn't dump directly into the SI? What if we also used our deep core to stabilize the lumbar spine and the L5/S1 junction, creating continuity from the spine to the lower extremity? What if we also used our upper body with intelligence and focused our rotational energy into the thoracic spine where it belongs, working from the inside and *not* using the arms to crank us "deeper" into the twist? What if we deemphasize the depth of a twist, and shift the narrative of "mastery" to one of stability, nuance, and refinement?

What if.

I'm only slightly sorry to sound so snarky on this, but come on! Don't teach students to undermine stability. Don't teach students to take the path of least resistance … they're very likely to do that on their own. They came to class to be taught, taught to be better in their practice, taught to find strength and focus and integrity. So do that. Be the better teacher.

bends with only the slightest bit of rotation ... and that perceived rotation is actually more a function of the shoulder coming around the ribs than a true rotation in the spine. Making this distinction is important when it comes to choosing preparatory poses, but is more relevant in terms of choosing the best words that will help students isolate and activate the proper muscles and counteractions to practice the posture with integrity. ✿

Cueing Practice

Watch a student transition back and forth between a Revolved Chair pose to the setup for Revolved Crow. Pay close attention to their spine as they move. Are they remaining in a rotation as they move to the arm balance? How does the movement of the scapula inform your perception of what the spine is doing?

Revolved Chair (Parivrtta Utkatasana)

"From Chair pose, hands together at heart, rotate heart to the right. Hinge in the hips to bring left elbow to meet the legs wherever it lands naturally ... maybe on the inner left knee or inner right knee ... don't try to reach it further across if the spine doesn't twist that far. Keep belly lifted, spiral through ribs while low back is stable and hips are centered."

Revolved Crane/Crow (Bakasana)

"From Revolved Chair (right), reach right ribs toward hip, finding a side bend. Reach left hand out from heart, across right thigh, so upper arm meets outer thigh. Bring both hands to the floor near long edge of mat, slightly wider than shoulders. The thigh may or may not touch the right arm, depending on your

variation. Coming onto tiptoes, bend elbows to lean thigh onto the upper left arm. Lift belly, activate hands and upper back (Cow and Cat!). One foot at a time may leave the earth as your weight shifts forward onto arm(s)."

When observing closely, you can see that the spine unwinds from its rotation and becomes a pretty clear side bend, while the shoulders wrap around and the arms reach for the mat. That wraparound can leave an impression of rotation even though the spine has changed. It's good practice to begin to see the shoulder blades as separate from the rib-spine so these distinctions become more clear in real time. There are a ton of refinements that can be made in all sorts of rotated, side-bent, or reaching postures if these can be instructed separately.

When observing supine twists, recognize that the ribs and shoulders remain more fixed than the hips. As discussed earlier, that can cause problems because the low back shouldn't be the focal point of our twists; there just isn't enough safe range of motion engineered into that system. So, if the hips are the mobile end of the spine, how do you make sure the rotation occurs in the thoracic spine? Well, it may be shocking to hear, but the answer is: flexion in the lumbar spine.

Say what?!?!

I know! I've spent pages and pages telling you that the most stable position for the lumbar spine is in lordosis, and that IS true when we are bearing weight. It is also true that the lumbar spine should remain in well-supported extension when doing backbends ... but when you are in **supine twists**, flexion in the low back will help protect it from over-rotating. Since that's the case, you can ask your students to bring the knees up to the chest, arms out to the side, and drop the legs to one side.

"Lying on your back, arms out to the sides or in 'cactus arms,' pull knees toward your heart. On inhale, gather your navel deeply toward your spine. On exhale, rock onto the right hip, keep knees glued together, don't let them slide past one another; this will keep your obliques firing hard and take the twist up into the ribs. Make sure you keep pulling knees up! Try to get them toward your right elbow … the point is not to land them on the ground, the point is to focus rotation into the thoracic spine and gain both strength and mobility in those levels."

An alternative, and perhaps more restorative, version of this same pose is to begin curled in a Child's Pose (Balasana) on your right side. This version will offer a deep chest opening, offer lots of individual variation on which chest fibers find expansion, and still access a deepening rotation in the thoracic spine.

"Roll onto your left side with knees pulled up to chest. Left arm reaches directly out from the heart, straight on the floor. Head can prop on blanket or block if needed. Right arm reaches toward sky. On inhale, gather navel deeply toward sky. On exhale, right arm reaches back, heart spirals into the twist, belly firm. Gaze may remain neutral or move up to the sky. Keep reaching with fingers, but gently pull right shoulder toward spine and broaden collar bones. Breathe fully and evenly into the ribs and up under collarbones. Breathe into back and side-body. Let your exhales release tension and effort as you soften into gravity a bit."

As you can see, the hips are once again stable, but we still have a flexion in the lumbar spine to help keep its rotation neutral. This allows us to relax a bit into the more restorative form without compromising the support and health of the low back. If we allow the low leg to stretch out long like in the traditional form, then that flexion is lost and we automatically dump into the low back.

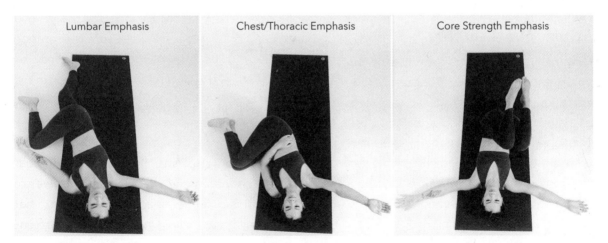

In traditional supine twists, the lumbar spine is emphasized, resulting in a dangerous increase in mobility beyond our 13 degrees. If we alter our twist to support the lumbar spine while opening the thoracic spine, ribs, and chest, we create a much safer rotation. To strengthen in twists, the knees must remain rooted together so the entire pelvis can rotate—not just shifting in the hip joints.

Vocabulary

As we discussed in the introductory chapters, you're trying to be specific without always being technical. How can you use language that tells your students exactly what to move, where to move it, and how to get it there? As practice for building this skill, we'll focus on the terms used to describe the axial skeleton, the spinal muscles, and movements of the spine in the context of practice.

You might consider starting with all the different ways you can emphasize the work of the thoracic spine in backbends. Since this is such a common place for people to avoid, we want to talk about it a lot. How can you do that in class? Follow the next examples to see how I might go about building a repertoire. When you practice on your own, don't hold back! Don't be afraid to push the limits a little and write down things that may not actually be said in class. This is an exercise in creatively expanding the WAY you talk about a part or practice ... so let it be expansive! You can always cross things off the list later.

Experiential Learning

How many ways can you describe the thoracic spine itself? Examples: thoracic spine, rib-spine, heart-spine ...

How many ways can you relate to the heart? Examples: Expand the front of the heart, coil behind the heart, fill the heart with breath, let the front of the heart grow taller, don't collapse the base of the heart, support the heart from below by activating solar plexus ...

How can you bring awareness to the rib cage to increase range of motion and deepen breathing? Examples: Anchor your base ribs, breathe up behind the sternum, breathe back into the kidneys at the base of the ribs, invite your breath behind your lungs, expand the back body/ribs, breathe in between the ribs and shoulder blades, expand the armpits as if you were blowing up little balloons in that space ...

You can make lists, word clouds, flow charts, flashcards ... whatever is in your toolbox to brainstorm words you can use in class to teach with specificity. Find alternative verbiage for some of the technical terminology we've discussed. (This is also a good exercise to be able to interchange technical and lay terms in your own head.) I suggest that you begin by finding word options to use interchangeably for the following parts and concepts, plus adding your own.

Structure

- Spinal column and costals
- Individual vertebrae
- Spinal nerves
- Paraspinal muscles
- Abdominal muscles

Nature

- Neutral spine
- Rib/pelvis agreement
- Range of motion ... this is a biggie!

If you have never done word clouds before, I highly recommend them. Not only are they great for building specific vocabulary, but they have the built-in advantage of associative linguistics. You can see the connections and relationships between words and phrases, helping them to come to life in real time. I love this practice.

In the example given, we've taken a pretty technical term, "Extension," and listed words and phrases that we associate with it. I initially thought, "Backbends!" And then "backbends" triggered all the different backbends that could be done in yoga. I thought about phrases specifically associated with extension activation, so those got grouped together in another area. I considered the deep core, and what that meant or how to use it, but that also led to ideas about the dynamic core, so I used a new arrow to expand the cloud outward. In this way you can build an ever-expanding view of how ideas, words, and phrases fit together and feed off one another. This process is great practice for how it feels to teach a yoga class in real time, instructing basic cues but also observing individual details, and being able to make associations that help you connect the dots from physical to esoteric.

In addition to working with the list I gave, you can brainstorm around a particular posture: imagining all the things a body could do in movement, what parts of the body you'd need to cue, the minutiae of each action and counteraction, the energetics and nervous system impacts. In this way, you continue to build the connections within a posture until it becomes second nature to be able to describe the present moment in florid detail.

Example Word Cloud

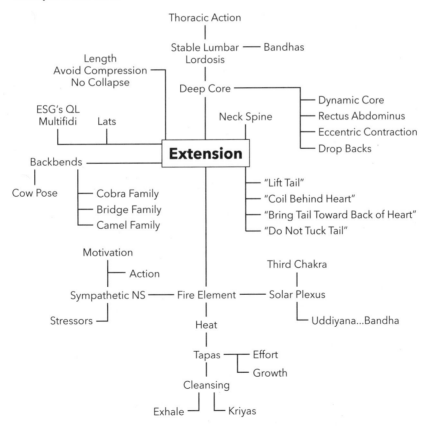

Practice Mechanics

I've created a list of posture categories in which the spine has specific movements or patterns, similar to the "Cueing Principles" categories earlier, in order to outline the fundamental alignment points of each group. Since the spine is an integral part of ALL the postures we practice, the following component points will be applicable to many poses that aren't listed.

As discussed earlier, for most postures, we first need to discern what the fundamental role of the spine is in relation to the extremities: is it mobile or stable? Once you make that distinction, the fundamental alignment and cueing remains the same. Eventually, those cues will become more detailed based on your observations of the folks in class and their individual needs. Your cueing will also get more detailed as you integrate movement or counteraction into the limbs.

Backbends

There are a ton of variations of backbends in yoga. While all of them are extension of the spine, they vary greatly in their relationship to gravity. This is an important quality because it helps define which muscles fire most, on which side of the body, and what those contractions are aimed at accomplishing. Do the paraspinal muscles fire to lift the spine up away from the floor? Do the abdominal muscles fire to control the descent toward the floor? It is precisely this distinction that drives me to separate the backbends into the following families.

Cobra Family

The Cobra family of postures includes all the prone backbends, the ones that begin with the belly on the earth. Cobra, Cow, Up Dog, Locust, Bow, Frog pose (Bhekasana) variations, and Heart and Throat pose are all part of this group. They all require actions in the shoulder girdle and/or arms to be fully embodied, but since we have yet to learn the ins and outs of the upper extremity system, for now we'll focus on the spinal components. All of these postures run the risk of using the arms in a way that jams up the lumbar spine and sacrum, so extra attention must be paid to using the front body to counter the potential collapse in the break-points.

- Hands align under elbows, not shoulders.
- Hands pull back to engage latissimus and traction spine; don't push down.
- Tail pulls toward back of heart; active lumbar lordosis.
- Knees press down to engage hip flexors.
- Glutes remain soft or gently firm, no clenching, no tail-tucking.

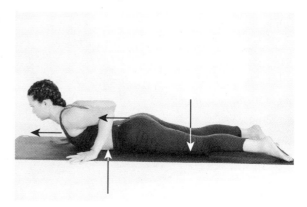

- Belly lifts deeply to prevent collapse at T10 or L5.

- Vocal cords pull in and back-neck lengthens.

- Any lifting of the legs originates from the glute/hamstring junction, not the top of the glutes/sacrum.

Bridge Family

In this group we see the supine backbends, ones that begin with the spine on the floor. Bridge, Upward Facing Bow (Wheel; Urdhva Dhanurasana), King Pigeon (Kapotasana; not the Dead Pigeon hip-opener that's taught as a restorative pose), Upward Facing Staff (Dwi Pada Viparita Dandasana), Wild Thing variations, and Upward Facing Plank (Purvottanasana) all fit into this category. Because the hips and legs are used in many of these to elevate the pelvis, great care is needed to moderate the contraction of the glutes in order to reduce risk of compression at the break-points.

- Neutral lumbar spine; lordosis active; pull tail toward back of heart.

- Belly actively pulls toward spine, preventing T10 or L5 collapse.

- Shoulder blades actively pull toward spine.

- Thoracic spine extends, "coiling behind heart," sternum reaches toward chin.

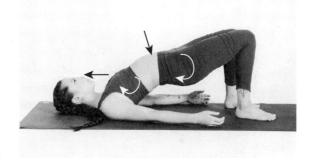

- Glutes and hamstrings activate in unison, no clenching.

- Maintain anterior tilt in pelvis, don't tuck tail or press pubis upward.

Camel Family

This is the family of backbends that begin upright and allow the heart to drop back into gravity, toward the floor. It includes Camel, Standing Backbend (Anuvittasana), drop backs, as well as the lunge-based (asymmetrical) backbending postures like Crescent Lunge (Anjaneyasana) and One-Legged King Pigeon (Eka Pada Rajakapotasana). In the symmetrical postures the most common misalignment is to thrust the pelvis forward, collapsing into the low back. For the deep core to remain intact, the pelvis ought to stay centered under the heart for as long as possible to avoid dumping the entire weight of the ribs into T10 and L5.

- Lift tail; active lumbar lordosis.

- Gather belly deeply to spine, support T10 and L5.

- Shoulder blades hug spine (Camel while reaching back), or wrap forward (when reaching overhead for drop backs).

- Pull thighs backward; don't press them forward.

- Move neck spine from its base, vocal cords gathered; Jalandhara Bandha.

Forward Folds

It's important to remember that forward folds are hip-moving postures! The spine should remain neutral for as long as possible. These spinal cues apply to both standing and seated folds.

- Lift tail; active lumbar lordosis.

- Gather low belly gently, upper belly deeply.

- Collarbones broad without collapsing between shoulder blades.

- Long back-neck, gathered throat/vocal cords.

- Stable, neutral spine; mobile hips.

- Flexion in spine ONLY when spine can traction or be supported with props.

Twists

Twists should always be focused in the thoracic spine, but alignment emphases will vary depending on whether the pose is upright or supine.

- Neutral curves; active lumbar, belly, throat.

- Navel remains centered with pubis, rotation focused in ribs.

- No cranking with the arms.

- Stay on axis; no side bending.

- Hips remain stable, unless in a supine variation focused on oblique strength.

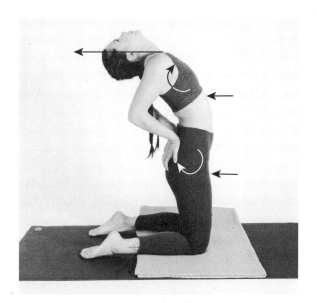
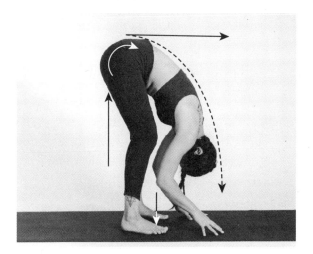
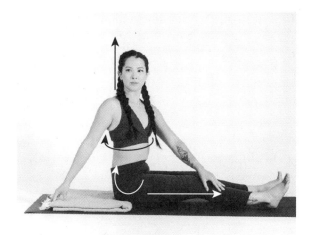

Side Bends

Whether you are seated or standing, keeping the hips stable in these postures will isolate movement into the spine. Be clear about your intent: focus your efforts into the level of the spine that is appropriate to the posture.

- Neutral, active curves; lumbar, belly, throat.
- Weight in heels when standing; no pelvic thrust.
- Keep legs/hips stable; move genuinely through the spine.
- Remain on coronal/frontal plane; avoid rotations of hips or ribs.
- Use obliques on both sides, don't let short-side simply collapse; lift those short-side ribs up off the pelvis.

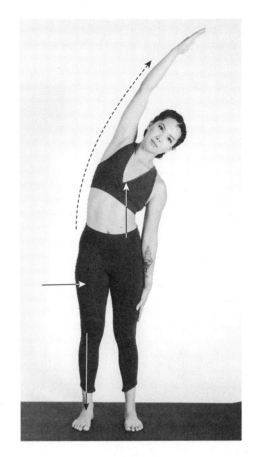

Inversions

Inversions are a special category. The neck is often placed in precarious positions, so great care is needed to ensure that the stressors on these joints are minimized. Strength in the upper extremity can certainly mitigate this risk, but oftentimes props can go a LONG way to reducing pressure and altering the extreme range of motion necessary for some poses.

- Maintain neutral spine, specifically avoid T10 collapse; active Uddiyana Bandha.
- Lots, lots, lots of Cat energy; Uddiyana Bandha.
- Gaze may be toward floor, but do not crank neck; move from the base instead of the skull.
- In backbending versions (Scorpions), maintain active belly and chest; avoid collapse in T10 and L5.
- In asymmetrical versions, don't let hips leave level; use obliques to maintain lumbar axis.

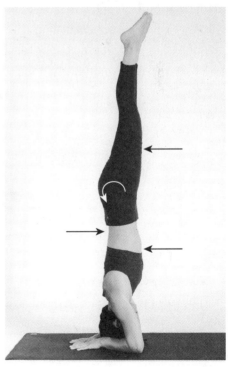

Practice Teaching
Adjustments

Because the spine has so much potential range of motion, and because so few of us pay close attention to our posture in daily life, and because very few of us have developed the appropriate strength to support better posture, I assure you that there will need to be a high level of adjustment for a while. Also consider that many of your students will have been taught to tuck their tail, and it is now your job to fix that. Here is where your rubber meets the road. Your eyes must alert you to specific misalignments, so your voice can offer clear and purposeful adjustments.

In the previous section, you were given the basic alignment points for each family of postures. It's now your job to elaborate, to observe each individual for what needs to be emphasized and altered. At first, you can count on most of your class needing similar adjustments, but once they become familiar with your new, groundbreaking, sacred-cow-slaughtering approach to spinal alignment, you'll have to help them each refine their spinal curves at the personal level.

Neutral Spine

So, what are the primary things you need to be on the lookout for? Remember back to the "Observation Skills" section: *See the neutral curves first.* If you're not seeing this, spend as much time as is needed to tell them what's what. You want to see:

- Hips over heels
- Lifted tail, active lumbar curve
- Gathered low belly, solar plexus; NO blown-out ribs/collapsed T10

- Broad chest, broad upper back
- Ears over shoulders, long back-neck, NO forward head posture
- Easy breathing

The tough one is getting those hips over the heels. For most folks, this will feel totally and utterly unnatural. They won't want to hinge in their hips; they'll keep their knees locked and just lean way back in their heels ... causing them to tip backward because their core can't hold them up. They're just not used to being buoyant in their legs or fluid in their spine. So you'll need to say to them things like:

"Hinge in your hips!"

"Pull your tail back and up!"

"Let the weight settle through the heels, but push your body straight up off the floor!"

"Sit back in space like you're sitting on a barstool!" (That one usually gets giggles the first few times.)

At this stage, I'd like you to try to use your words rather than your hands to make adjustments. It's important to learn these skills because large classes preclude you from adjusting each student individually. You need to be able to see what is happening in multiple bodies and make the tweaks relevant to the most people first, then call out individual cues to those in need.

That said, some people just aren't going to be able to embody these movements immediately, simply because they have NEVER moved that way before. They don't know how it's supposed to feel, and once they feel it, it's so freaking foreign that they immediately go back where they were ... it's like a reflex. That means you may need to eventually offer hands-on adjustments for this most basic of alignments. Once their hips are back, the rest of the instructions will make more sense in their bodies.

Here's how I do it:

I stand directly behind the student and place my open hand on their hips, just above the greater trochanter. I lean to my left a bit as if I'm peeking around their shoulder, using my knee to very lightly nudge the back of their knee in order to unlock it or soften it more. I place my right shoulder on the spine, just between the shoulder blades, keeping it stable (since it tends to already be above or slightly behind the heels). Using my hands, I prompt a slight forward pelvic tilt while also pulling the whole pelvis back in space until those trochanters also line up over the heels.

Almost every time I do this, people are shocked that they have to engage their legs so much. They also feel as though they are sticking their butt out A LOT. Tell them it's okay, acknowledge that it feels vastly different than they're used to, give them props for trying something new! And also, keep repeating your cues as you move around the room making adjustments—otherwise everyone you just touched will certainly let those hips slide back to their reflexive pelvic thrusts. They don't even notice it's happening. Gah, again with all those bad habits!

Okay, so once you get those hips in place, you need to double-check the belly and solar plexus. Make sure that when your students get the low belly pulled in, they don't also lift their pubic bone. This is a great movement to

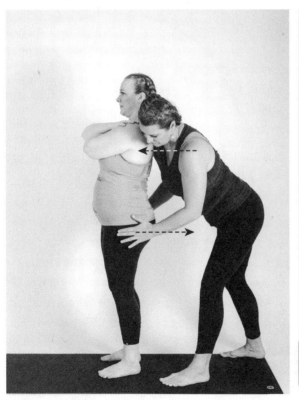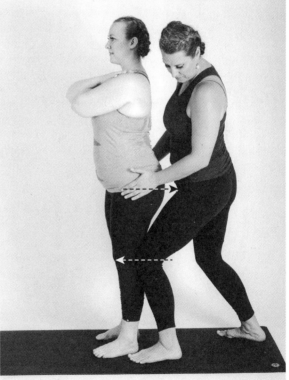

Hands are light, touch is subtle. Make sure you move slowly enough that they can adjust their balance as you go. These new positions will feel very awkward for them at first.

demonstrate in front of the class. Show the difference between gathering the belly and tilting the pelvis. These are also movements where it is helpful to stop class, break down the action, and practice it, so they can feel the difference between the two.

Even more difficult for some to isolate is the solar plexus action. Not many people are accustomed to contracting only one part of rectus abdominis at a time ... for most it's all or nothing. You might want to demo this as well, showing how the rib cage acts like a teeter-totter on the fulcrum of the spine at T10. If the front ribs drop down, the back ribs lift up! That's what we want!! Many people will tirelessly try to keep lifting their "heart" to their chin, assuming that the heart only has one side, expanding the front of the heart at the expense of the collapsing back side of the heart. We need balance so the kidneys and low back have plenty of space. This action is also not familiar, unless they have been practicing really good "crunch" form for a while and can access those upper fibers of rectus. So, yet again, you may need to lay on some hands.

This one can be tricky:

Sometimes I'll place a hand on their solar plexus and back ribs and promote that front down/back up motion.

Sometimes I'll poke one finger into their upper belly and they'll automatically retract and blow up the back ribs. Another way to do this is to pretend you're gonna punch 'em in the gut ... but not everyone takes kindly to that one. It works reeeeally well, though, on those that it works for.

Other times I place my thumb and middle finger of one hand on the front rib-curves and press them down, verbally cueing to drop those toward the hips.

Again, these aren't familiar movements for most yogis. For a very long time they have been told to lengthen their tail downward and to lift their sternum upward. These are very difficult habits to break. Remind them that you are on their side! Learning these new actions will help them stay healthier longer.

I'll also note that these adjustments are similar whether your students are standing

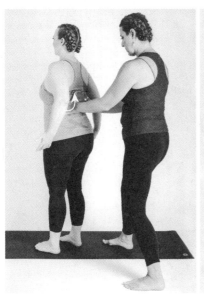
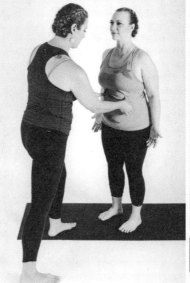
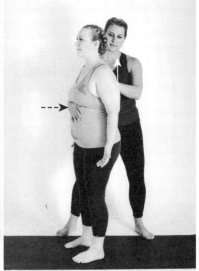

or not. They are also applicable to prone and supine postures. Plank pose is a place where these are usually necessary, so is Bridge.

Lastly, you'll want to eyeball the neck. In standing postures there is a popular tendency for forward head posture. We really want the ears to align roughly over the shoulders. I'll talk about pulling the head back, but sometimes this results in the back of the head retracting and the chin jutting upward, continuing the compression in the back-neck. While a subtle lordosis should be present in the neck, ideally we see the back-neck remaining long and the jaw shifting ever so slightly backward.

If you need to use hands-on adjustments, you could try this:

> I'll stand behind the student and place my hands on the sides of their neck, just about halfway between head and shoulders. My thumbs land lightly on the base of their skull. I use light pressure to pull with my fingers and press with my thumbs, encouraging the middle-neck to move backward and the base of the skull to lengthen away from the neck.

The key to success for all these adjustments, whether verbal or tactile, is this: Ask them if it feels different, confirm for them that it should feel different, acknowledge that it may feel awkward and will take extra work to maintain. Also assure them that through repetition it will all feel more familiar, and eventually it may even come naturally.

Twists/Side Bends

I've put these two families of postures together because they really do relate to one another in practice. Remember that because of the angle of the facet joints, the spine is prone to rotate when side bending and to side bend when rotating. So, you'll need to cue clearly to avoid these compensations—but be on the lookout for a few specific cases.

Seated twists are where I see this phenomenon the most, as students pull the leading ribs toward the hip instead of remaining on their spinal axis. First, ask students to come out of their twists halfway, reaffirm their belly actions, and then twist only from the heart-spine. If you pay attention to each student, it's likely that one of two things will happen: stiff students usually drop their trailing ribs (if twisting right, their left ribs drop and left side-waist collapses), while those with flexy spines will usually drop their leading ribs, giving the illusion that their chest is broad and that they're backbending. Since

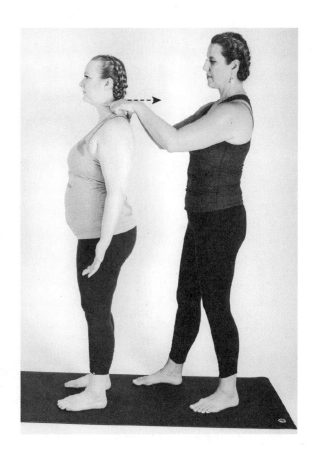

the goal is to get everyone on axis, it can be tricky to cue a correction to the entire class. Situations like this are why it's a great idea to learn everyone's names!! I'll often call out a few people to lift their trailing ribs, and then follow that up with the opposite for the other folks.

Because many students won't already have the acuity to make these fine-tunings the first time you call it out, you will probably need to make some tactile adjustments as well. To do that here:

I like to use pinching motions on the side-waist, indicating a drawing together of the ribs and hip. I'll often say that out loud at the same time: "Pull these ribs closer to the hip to activate those obliques and pull you back on axis."

I'll use the opposite action as well, pressing my fingers away from each other,

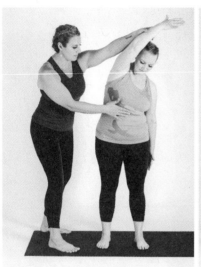
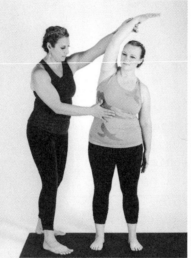
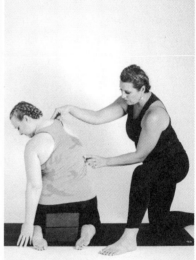

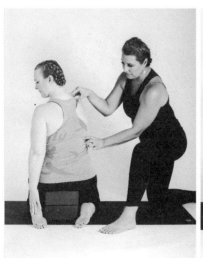
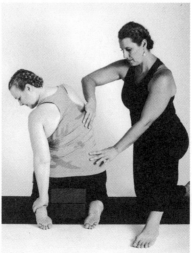
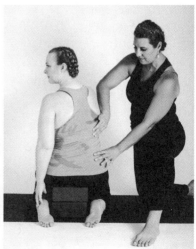

instructing the hip and ribs apart to lengthen the side-waist line.

In some of the extreme cases, you may need to instruct them out of an actual backbend. This is really similar to the movement you made on the neck earlier. Place the fingers on the side-ribs and the thumbs on the back ribs; from here you can steer the entire rib cage in front/back or side-to-side movements to help dial it back onto its axis.

What's fascinating about all these adjustments is that once the spine is on axis and lacks compensations, it will more freely move into the thoracic twist. There is room to spare in those joints when energy isn't being dumped into other movements.

In supine twists, whether the hips are moving or stable, keep your eyes on the spinal axis. There can be a tendency for one hip to rise up toward the ribs, just as the ribs dipped down in seated postures. There's that pesky side bend showing up again! Other than lumbar flexion, the spine should remain on axis, so some cueing to draw one hip away from the ribs may be necessary.

In side bends, I rarely need to lay my hands on a student—verbal adjustments usually work just fine. Keep your eyes peeled in standing side bends for sure, but I find that seated versions are where the heart-spine just totally goes off the rails. Because a hip stretch of some sort is often involved here, and the core has a tough time keeping the lumbar spine stable, there tends to be an exaggerated domino effect from the bottom up. In most students, their heart will collapse toward the floor, turning it into a twisty forward fold of sorts. Instead, we want to use words that encourage the pelvis to stay rooted and the side bend to remain on

one plane, stacking the ribs left over right (or vice versa). I use statements like:

"Pull the bottom ribs through ..."

"Stack the heart perpendicular to the floor ..."

"Spiral the heart as if it could open to the sky ..."

What words could you use to encourage that opening?

Backbends

This is where the habituation of clenching glutes and tucking tails is most prevalent. You'll need to be diligent and repetitious in those areas: "Soften the glutes a bit ... lift the tail toward the back of the heart ... gather the belly to support the lumbar curve without changing its shape." In postures like Bridge, I might say, "Pull your tail to the back of the heart" ten times while holding the pose for five breaths. That's a ton of repetition. It's key, though, because we're talking about changing a deeply rooted belief in how backbends should be done, as well as the physical muscle memory. You have to drill it literally into their heads and their bodies. Turn it into a mantra if you have to, make them say it out loud. Make them use their own hands on their own hips to feel the movements, so they have a tactile trigger as well. Use all the tools.

In addition, it's pretty tough for students to fire their solar plexus and coil in the posterior thoracic at the same time. When making adjustments at the T10 level, it's common to need to repeat the cues and tactile suggestions over and over until they dial in both actions at the same time. I highly recommend the exercise in the sidebar, practicing half of Cow pose with half of Cat pose in order to bring awareness to these combined actions.

HALF COW + HALF CAT

This exercise is integral for introducing the combined efforts of the two poses that best support the curves of a neutral spine. This work will contract and tone the lumbar paraspinals while also firing the upper fibers of rectus abdominis, training us to stay active in both simultaneously.

From a Table posture, begin a series of active Cow and Cat poses, flowing smoothly with the breath. After warming up the entire spine through flexion and extension, find Cow pose and hold it stable for a few breath cycles. Do the same for Cat pose, toning the abdominal muscles without releasing them through at least five breath cycles.

Now find a full Cat pose. Press the ribs up between the shoulder blades, and let the sacrum hang from the low back. This time, maintain the Cat shape of the ribs and upper belly, and on your inhale, pull the tail up toward the sky, activating the lumbar paraspinal muscles and finding Half Cow pose in the low back and hips. Those muscles will be contracting against the resistance of the deep belly, adding tone and strength over time. Your exhale returns you to full Cat, and each inhale moves only the lower body through the Half Cow. Repeat for a total of five rounds.

Cat Pose to Half Cow

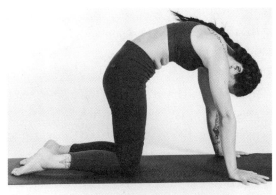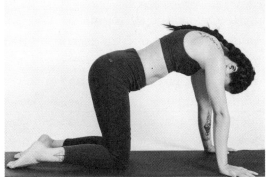

Return on an inhale to Cow pose. Stabilize the hips, maintaining the lumbar lordosis and firm low belly. As you exhale, begin to press through the hands and find Cat pose in just the upper belly, ribs, and neck. Don't change those hips or low back—isolate the movement into the solar plexus and ribs. Your inhale brings you back into a full Cow pose, your exhale will repeat the Half Cat pose. Your movements won't be nearly as large as in a full Cat posture, so don't force it. With each exhale, allow the tension to build between the stability of the low back and the movement of the upper back—this inherent resistance helps increase tone specifically in the upper rectus abdominis.

Cow Pose to Half Cat

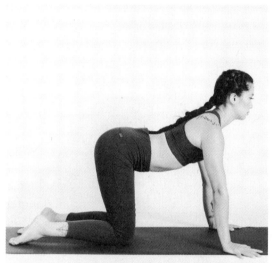 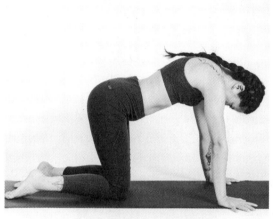

Once you've completed the isolations, return to your typical Cow/Cat flow for another three to five rounds, and assess if anything feels different. It's also interesting to feel what Table pose or even Mountain feels like after this series. For me, I am always more in tune with the compound actions of lifting my tail and gathering my solar plexus.

Once a student knows how to fire these muscles, the key is to make sure that T10 remains supported and doesn't collapse. This requires constant repetition of cues to lengthen through the mid-back and coil in the thoracic. You'll need to reference the shoulder blades here, and while you'll get much more detailed information in later chapters regarding this, you can at least acknowledge that the scaps need to come together at the spine. We can use the shoulder girdle to support the thoracic spine's extension by pulling the shoulder blades toward one another. This is where I get the imagery of the "coil." If the back of the heart-spine is coiling and compressing, then at the same time the front of the heart-spine needs to expand and release. Of course, the sternum isn't actually going to change in length—it's a solid bone, for cryin' in the night—but we can offer this imagery as an impetus to feel the ribs themselves find space. There can be a distinct sense of the base ribs remaining rooted by the solar plexus activation, while the upper ribs spread away from each other. You might offer them the image of the folds of an accordion, some pressing together to facilitate the opening up of others.

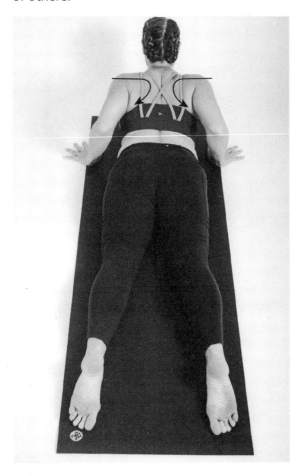

Lastly, we ought to discuss the neck in backbends. It's common practice for yogis to extend really deeply through the neck spine in many of these postures. In particular, Cobra family postures are notorious for this movement, as are postures like Standing Half Forward Fold (Ardha Uttanasana). Pay close attention any time the spine is parallel to the floor, because we have a reflex that drives us to keep our gaze level with the horizon. Remember, if the extension of the neck begins at the top, then the space at the back of the skull gets compressed immediately without any chance for anterior muscular support. Jalandhara Bandha is lost in these cases, and the breath usually gets caught in the compressed throat. In my opinion, these poses don't actually require full extension of the neck, so I often cue students to keep a long back-neck, to keep their vocal cords gathered toward the spine, and to let their gaze fall just a couple feet out in front of them on the floor, instead of trying to look toward the front wall.

If, however, you are teaching a Camel pose, and deep extension is an eventual component of the posture, then you ought to make sure that the movement begins at the base of the neck and not the top. The bony bit will be set up to offer better structural support in the back, and the muscle of the neck will be better equipped to offer functional support in the front ... support all around!!

Forward Folds

Yet again, I'll remind you that forward folds are hip postures. They move in the hip. It is hip flexion. Hips are your prime motivation. So if the hips require mobility, the spine requires stability. Whether standing or seated, the goal is to maintain a long, neutral spine for as long as possible. Eventually, you'll need to release the full actions of the spine, but be very aware of how and when you do this. If standing, you'll need to ensure that the students are truly working in their legs, so the low back muscles can surrender and the spine can traction into gravity. When you're seated, I strongly advise that for anyone who is not remarkably flexible in the hips with supple and long hamstrings, you either retain the spinal extension actions or surrender only to layers of supporting props.

The thing is, the entire back body from feet to crown is connected by deep layers of fascia that create a continuum. This continuum may be soft in some places (usually the lumbar spine, accustomed as it is to collapsing into flexion) and rigid in others (the glutes and hamstrings), but any forces that are applied to one part are translated across the entire track. Those points of rigidity act like resistors in an electrical path, bogging down the flow of energy. In the back channel of the body, those bogged-down points will remain stiff while the more mobile points absorb too much. So forward folds that add stretch-tension to the back channel must be practiced with these forces in mind.

If the hips or thighs are where we want the actual stretch to occur, we must remain active in the spine and direct the stretch into the legs. In a seated fold, for instance, if we simply let our heart grow heavy and drop toward our thighs in gravity, the low back spine is going to absorb much of the flexion energy that could have been focused to the hips. But if the spine remains muscularly active and takes up its slack, then the hips and thighs will absorb the stretch energy instead. In a standing fold, on the other hand, once the belly meets the thighs, we can feel relatively safe letting the spine surrender to gravity. The calves must remain very active to hold us up, directing movement into the hinge of the hip, the hammies get their stretch, and the low back is able to receive gravitational traction instead of a jamming-up of stretch tension.

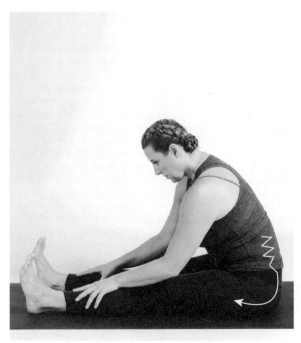
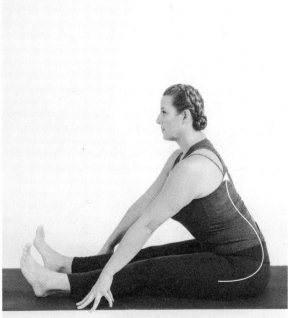

FORWARD FOLDS HAVE FORWARD MOMENTUM

In standing folds in particular but certainly in seated folds too, you want to keep your momentum moving forward instead of backward or down. What do I mean by that? I mean shift the weight of the entire body to the balls of the feet. The knees are soft, sometimes even bent very deeply to add slack to hamstrings, but you need to be holding yourself up with the work of the forefoot. This fires the calves but also encourages the posterior thighs and hips to remain active even as those muscles lengthen. You'll feel the legs engage A LOT, which means that the spine can actually release fully into the pull of gravity: traction, decompression.

Try this: stand in a forward fold as I have just described. Now shift the weight back into the heels and lock out the knees. Feel what just happened in your low back. Did you feel the tension ramp up? Did you feel the belly pull away from the thighs a bit and tension run the length of the spine? Is it tough to let the shoulders and head go completely? My guess is that the answer to all of those questions was yes.

This is physics, my friends. By shifting forward and softening the bend into the knees, you might be adding muscular effort (never a bad thing, I think), but you are also adding slack to the back channel. As soon as you lean back and let the ligaments support the joints instead of muscles, you remove all the slack and leave the tissues vulnerable to strain and sprain. You also pressurize the spinal discs in a way that leaves them at risk … a risk that is significantly mitigated by the traction effect achieved in the forward-leaning version.

The same is true in seated posture: forward folds have forward momentum. In these cases, though, the action is one of avoiding downward pull on the distal spine—the head and the heart. If we give way to gravity, the spine tends to drop into flexion, again removing any slack from the back channel. The low back tissues and spinal discs absorb this energy without the mitigating benefit of contracted muscles. If instead we reach our crown and heart forward toward our toes, and retain a sense of extension action in the low and mid-back, then we can focus the stretch energy into the hips and thighs.

Modifications

In the spine, different people will have different mobility and potential weaknesses. So it's important to note that, nearly universally, action and stability emphases are far safer than mobility-focused work overall. Until you are well-versed in the specific conditions that a student may present with, your best approach is to cue less movement and more stabilization.

As discussed earlier in the forward folds section, reducing slack to the back channel is one way to relieve the system of some potentially harmful tension patterns. Conversely, we can add slack intentionally to allow the individual to better isolate the parts they need to work with, without losing energy to the remaining posterior system. The easiest way to do this in most bodies is to bend the knees. Since the hamstrings tend to be the most dehydrated and least pliable muscles in the continuum, giving them the break is the quickest way to relieve pressure.

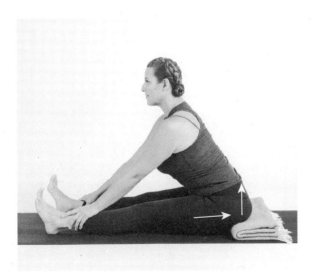

Another way to add slack is by changing the geometry of the pose: add blocks under hands in standing postures, or add elevation under hips in seated variations. With blocks under the hands, we take a small amount of weight energy out of the equation; even if the elbows bend and you begin to fold deeper, the shoulders and arms are removed slightly from the downward energy, so the legs and low back have a lesser burden to bear. By elevating the hips, you change the angle of the leg to the floor and reduce the degree of flexion in the hip, making space to explore movements there that would have already been at their max with hips on the ground.

When practicing Plank variations, it is imperative that students take their knees to the ground if they have *any* trouble maintaining the neutral spine. Typical misalignments include the clenched glutes and tucked tail, hips way too high or way too low, and ribs collapsed toward Earth due to lack of Uddiyana Bandha/solar plexus action. In each of these cases, shortening the lever by eliminating the lower leg reduces the load on the spine significantly. Once the knees are down, the brain has a much easier time learning to recruit the proper pattern of muscles at just the right amplification to hold the whole thing together. Once those activations are established, your students can lift their knees and work to build strength throughout. If they lift their knees and a breakdown occurs somewhere in the system, have them practice with knees down, occasionally lifting them for only an inhale. Over time, this can turn into a flow and build into longer holds.

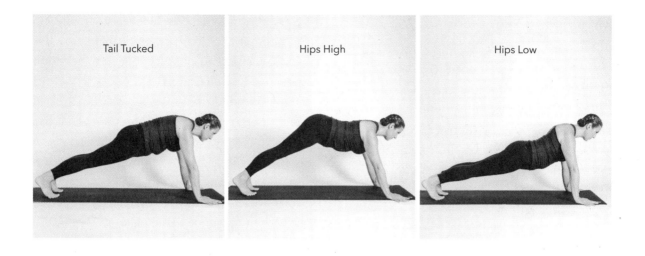

Tail Tucked   Hips High   Hips Low

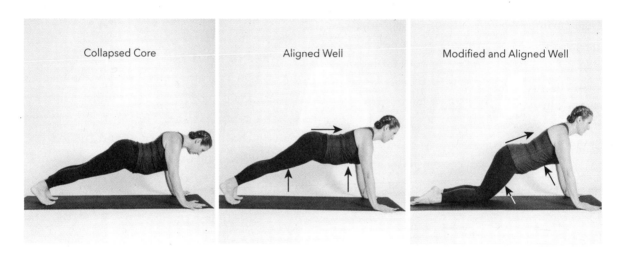

Collapsed Core   Aligned Well   Modified and Aligned Well

If there is not adequate strength in the neck to look up to the sky in backbends, then one should look forward. The act of maintaining upright head posture, pulling chin toward chest, will begin to strengthen the anterior neck. Over time, a student can begin to slowly tip their head back, moving from the base of the neck of course, to alter the range of strength available. This should be done in stages over a long period of time and many practice sessions. One should not rush movements in the neck.

Experiential Learning: Teachers' Work

Practice-teaching is an opportunity to put to use some of the concepts and applications that we've been discussing. It is practice. It is not easy; it will not feel fluid. At first you will look at the bodies before you and see alien objects that you have no idea what to do with. That is the natural state of things, I assure you. Even if you have teaching experience under your belt, we've already begun to question the way you've been taught to do things, we are now rewriting the book ... literally rewiring how your brain sees bodies and instructs them ... so please be gentle with yourselves. Go slow. Start at the beginning, the base, and move just one thing at a time.

In YTT we would now break into groups of three, one teacher to two students. If you are on your own at home, find some friends or colleagues to experiment with. Start by teaching just the neutral spine in Mountain, then work with the details of one of your chosen postures. Offer modifications and adaptations, learn to use new language for this. Make both verbal and hands-on adjustments to get used to the feel of it. This is what practice is for. Take turns in between each pose, allowing practitioners a minute to offer feedback and discuss applications.

While teaching: You need to *teach* the pose in its entirety. Don't worry about fancy transitions or even simple transitions; teach this pose in the most excruciating physical details possible. From Mountain, tell them which part to move, where it needs to go, and how to get it there. Don't worry about how long they are in this pose for this exercise—you want to be able to teach to all the aspects a posture has to offer. You'll adapt this as you go into actual classes, but for this exercise, more is better.

Be sure to pay attention to what is actually happening in front of you. Teach to what you see. There are, after all, two individuals in front of you ... make sure you address any individual alignment issues you see in those bodies. You might consider the following:

- Neutral curves
- Rib to hip agreement; staying on axis—are the ribs shifted left or right, side bends, rotations, etc.?
- If teaching side bends or twists—does spine maintain a solid axis?
- If twisting—hip stability without compensating

When practicing: Honor your own individual shape, but don't make automatic adjustments. If you know you have scoliosis, try to let it express itself so your teacher can learn to see it. It's not necessary to fake misalignments, but for this exercise you must do only what you are told to do, so your teacher has the ultimate feedback for the words they are using. Listen intently and do exactly as you are prompted, nothing more.

When offering feedback, if the teacher has not noticed or mentioned your particular individual needs, bring it up and show them the potential shift in alignment, so they will be more likely to see it next time.

This is an excellent time to gather a group of like-minded teacher-students to explore these concepts and practices. It will help to have a book group of sorts to bounce these ideas off of. Check in on the Facebook page for Yoga Engineer or the Facebook group Yoga Engineer's Manual Book Club.

9

The Lower Extremity: Structure and Nature

The vinyasa. The seat. Each step we take on and off the mat.

Many of us take for granted the ability to stand and walk and climb stairs. We assume that to put one foot in front of the other is a thing we learned how to do as infants, and has been and will remain a constant through life. Unfortunately, we don't pay much attention to our individual patterns of movement; we don't actually know how our foot is designed to strike the earth or understand the mechanics of movement in gravity. What is actually holding us up? What is truly efficient? Obviously, we know how to stand up and stay that way, but are we doing it with any awareness of how we find balance? What are our habits and compensations?

Are you, right now, relying on a chair to hold you up in gravity? If you were to stand up on your two feet, could you become aware of what parts are working to stabilize your joints, what

muscles must fire to strike the chord that is harmonious between stillness and movement? These are important questions.

The lower extremity is built for both stability in its weight bearing and mobility to propel us through space. We depend on it in asana as our base and foundation, but also as the powerhouse to move us fluidly through vinyasa. This makes for a complicated system of both tiny and very large muscles that need to control both finite and gross movement. The continuity of the spinal core and the lower limb cannot be underestimated—they are completely intertwined and have profound impacts on one another in both posture and movement. The joints of the lower extremity are built to perform under all sorts of conditions, sustain many different forces, and absorb shock. There are specific limitations to this system, however, and to engage it inefficiently will certainly lead to degeneration and dysfunction.

An understanding of the interconnected-ness, at the physical and energetic levels, of the toes through the core is necessary for being able to effectively cue your asana sequences. While it may not be integral to know the names of all the myriad muscles that move our bodies, having a fundamental knowledge of the system as a whole and its parts, their interactions and effects on one another, the risks involved and the precautions that can be taken ... these *are* all integral to offering the most cohesive and safe practice to your students.

Use your parts wisely and with deliberation! Don't take them for granted ... a new hip or set of knees will be very expensive. As yoga teachers, we have the opportunity to help each student access a deeper knowledge of their individual differences and how to best align themselves in gravity. The lower extremity is a carnival fun house of distortions and differentiations. No two people have the same shaped bones. Many people don't even match up on their own left and right sides. This means that each person has a particular blueprint for their posture that is likely to differ significantly from their neighbor. It is our job to observe these differences to the best of our ability and offer an individual alignment practice to each one. No two Mountains will look perfectly alike. While fundamental rules apply at the tissue level, we now must begin to consider that each person will need to receive personal insight to their own body and alignment.

There are many different yogic lineages with particular rules about how to place the feet and how to stand. We are hereby wiping the slate clean and proclaiming that regardless of a person's chosen style, their practice is their own, and they deserve to work within the body they actually have. They need not force it into the shape that a long-dead teacher's teacher proclaimed was appropriate, because frankly, very few alignments work for everybody.

Bones

The bones of the lower extremity are some of the most oddly shaped anywhere in the body. They vary from very large (the femur is the longest bone we have) to tiny (the midfoot and toes are made up of small irregular bones). Their shapes are bewildering, offering up tons of surface area that a staggering number of ligaments and muscles attach to. As you read through the descriptions below, look at the images and any 3D models you have available. Eventually, the shapes and attachment points will become so familiar that you'll be able to envision them each time you look at your students' bodies, developing a sort of X-ray vision. Regardless of what the bones are called, being able to identify particular bony prominences in a flesh-and-blood body will help you spot individual misalignments on the mat in real time.

Pelvis. The pelvis is remarkable in its simplicity, yet its shape and contours can be confusing. Its three-dimensional nature is difficult to capture effectively in two-dimensional illustrations, so any access you have to a skeletal model will help here. The pelvis is constructed of two separate halves that join the sacrum (the *sacroiliac joints*, or *SI*) at the back and connect in the front at a cartilaginous joint called the *symphysis pubis*. Each side is a fusion of three different sections: the *ilium, ischium*, and *pubis*. It's important to know these bits because they are the attachment points for most of the muscles of the abdomen and hip. They also provide bony landmarks that will help you observe and assess alignment in your students.

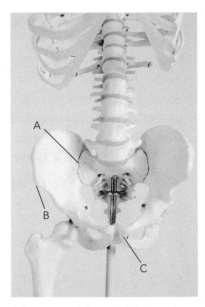 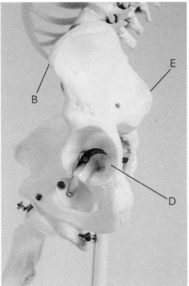 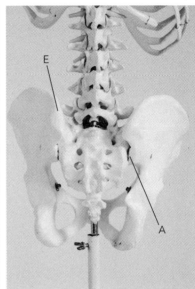

(A) SI joint, (B) ASIS, (C) Symphysis pubis, (D) Acetabulum, (E) PSIS

The *ASIS* (*anterior superior iliac spine* … though you don't *need* to know that) is the bony point often referred to as the "hip point," when in fact it is a pelvic point. Some teachers call these the "headlights," and they become integral to seeing the agreement between the ribs and hips, as well as determining whether a student's pelvic tilt is neutral or not (and by proxy, whether or not the lumbar spine is neutral). We'll go into excruciating detail about that in a bit, and you'll likely be surprised by what you read. Be prepared!

Acetabulum. The socket into which the head of the femur articulates. The front and base of the acetabulum exhibit a cut-away of the bone, leaving a deep divot through which nerves and blood vessels and connective tissue can travel. The depth of the acetabulum may impact the overall range of motion of the hip joint; deeper socket may equal less range. The rim of the socket has a ring of cartilage to act as a gasket of sorts where the head of the femur seats itself into the joint. This cartilage is called the *labrum*.

Femur. The femur is the long bone of the thigh. It is not straight; it bends at the top, delineating the *shaft* and the *neck*, while creating the big bump on the lateral side that we call the *greater trochanter*. The *head* of the femur is the ball that articulates with the pelvis to form the *coxal (hip) joint*. The angle of the neck of the femur is significant, because it can affect the range of motion at the hip joint.

The shape of the femur may differ in many ways for each individual:

- The arc of the shaft can vary both laterally and anteriorly, giving it a bowed shape. Physics tells us that curves are more stable than straight lines, so this makes sense, considering this is the primary weight-bearing bone of the leg.

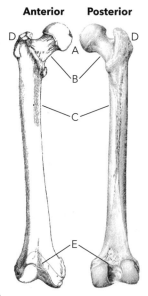

Anterior   Posterior

(A) Head, (B) Neck, (C) Shaft, (D) Greater trochanter, (E) Distal end/Epicondyles

Tibia and Fibula. The *tibia* is a weight-bearing bone of the leg, while the *fibula* butts up against its lateral side to help absorb shock. At the distal end the two bones form the ankle joint by hugging the *talus* bone between them. The top of the tibia has two bony divots called *epicondyles* that the *condyles* of the distal end of the femur sit in and form the knee joint.

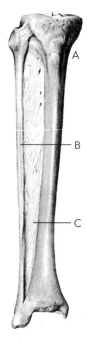

(A) Tibia, (B) Fibula, (C) Interosseous membrane

- The torsion of the shaft of the femur varies greatly. There is a typical torsion of 12 degrees, so that when the head is seated in the acetabulum, the greater trochanter actually aligns behind the midline of the joint. That torsion can be over- or under-exaggerated, so that when the hip is neutral, the knee may not point straight ahead.

- Differences in the angle of the neck of the femur can be present; an angle closer to 90 degrees will limit abduction and maybe external rotation, while an angle closer to 180 degrees may allow for greater abduction and external rotation.

- The shape and size of the head of the femur can vary greatly, impacting its relationship with the acetabulum, and possibly the bony stability of the joint.

Talus. The talus is one of the irregularly shaped bones of the foot and is considered the "ankle bone" due to its articulation with the tibia. It allows for separate movements between the tibia/fibula above it (the *talocrural joint*) and the *calcaneus*, or the heel bone, below it. As significant structural components of the plantar arches, these bones must have alignment for proper posture and gait, though many people lack the muscular acuity to help maintain this alignment.

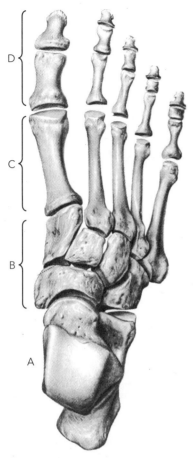

(A) Talus (ankle bone), (B) Tarsals (midfoot),
(C) Metatarsals (forefoot), (D) Phalanges (toes)

Foot: Calcaneus + Tarsals + Metatarsals.
Otherwise known as the heel, midfoot, and fore-foot, these bones fit like oddly shaped 3D puzzle pieces to form both the foot and its arches.

Joints and Connective Tissue

Sacroiliac Joint (SI). This joint is where the sacrum meets the pelvis at each ilium ... hence the name. The surface of each bone has a broad and wavy interface that mirrors the other. You may experience this relationship if you place one of your palms in the other, letting the heel

of one hand seat into the palm of the other. Notice how the knuckles stack above each other and the fingers of one hand slide into the grooves between the fingers of the other hand. If you press together, there is a sort of seal that forms, and very little movement is available between the two surfaces, right? That is a kind of model for the SI joint: broad, textured surfaces held very closely together so that very little range of motion is available.

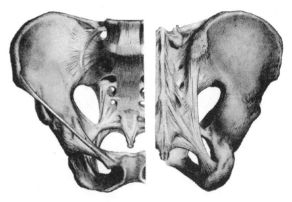

The ligaments of the posterior SI joint are more numerous and substantial.

If you look at a skeleton model, you'll see that the backs of the ilia protrude back from the sacrum by a fair degree, leaving a partic-ularly deep gap, but on a live person that gap has been filled in. ✪ These joints have a dense layering of ligaments that cross back and forth at many angles between the spine and pelvis. It looks like a ton of stabilizing tissue! But when you examine pictures of the front side of the joint, the ligamentous support is far less pro-fuse. Keep this in mind as we discuss range of motion. The SI is built to transfer our weight bearing from the lower extremity to the spine, and to be a transition between mobile joints. It is engineered to remain stable through the typical movements of daily life, but our yoga practice puts a great amount of torsion on these joints, more than they are designed to cope with. This leads almost universally to hypermobility in the SI joints of yoga practitioners.

Coxal Joint. This is the name we use to identify the hip joint. The hip is the ball and socket joint where the head of the femur fits into the acetabulum. It's important to note that the pelvic socket sits on top of the head of the femur—they don't "pop" together securely. When we are upright, gravity is responsible for a fair amount of the joint's ability to function. For that to work most efficiently, our posture must align the pelvis on the femur in a balanced way; otherwise we risk injury to soft tissues. We must use our muscular body to keep this alignment sound, or else the joint will suffer and degenerate over time.

In addition, a neutral hip is integral to how the forces of gravity travel through the knee and ankles. While it's common to assume that our alignment begins at the base of our extremity, I argue that the neutral hip joint ensures the proper stacking of your individual bones as they were engineered. In a neutral hip, the greater trochanter ought to align just behind the midline. Because of the gentle torsion of the femur, this position allows the knees of many people to face directly forward. Individual differences in that torsion, however, may mean the knees will point slightly in or out when the hips are neutral, and so will the feet (outward is much more common than inward, frankly). Many folks out there are walking around (and standing and practicing yoga) with habitually *inwardly* rotated femurs, creating distortive forces down through the knees and ankles.

Encouraging a natural turn-out of the thigh (and thus everything below it too) will bring a better balance to the architecture of all of our standing postures.

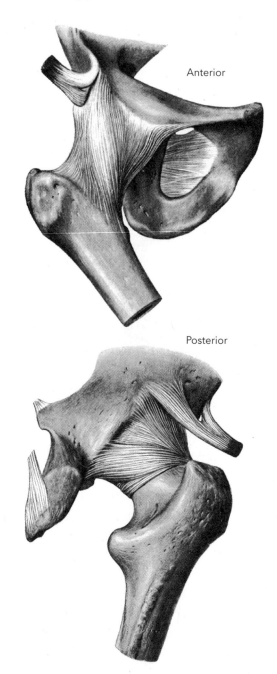

Anterior

Posterior

The ligaments of the anterior hip are more substantial than the posterior, and they are designed specifically to limit extension.

Remember that the acetabulum has a sort of cut-away section near its front aspect. If the pelvis tilts too far back on the femoral head (posterior tilt or tucking the tail), there is less bone to support the weight and balance of the pelvis, resulting in hip instability as well as wear and tear to the articular cartilage and labrum.

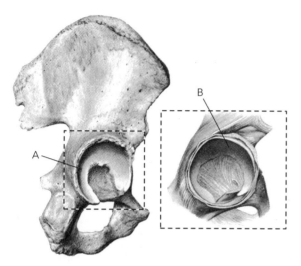

(A) Acetabulum, (B) Labrum

Luckily, the anterior side of the joint is supported by a thick and dense ligament, the *iliofemoral ligament*. This tissue limits extension to help us stay upright ... and, as a bonus, prevents the pelvis from tipping completely off the femur. This is a mechanism to keep us safe when muscle tone is not sufficient, but if we exploit that function, we'll lose muscle tone and the ligament will degrade over time. Stretching this ligament will lead to hypermobility, joint degeneration, and dysfunction. Regardless of whether the stretching occurs during passive misalignment while standing, or if we are seeking strong sensations of stretch during deep lunges, the stability of the hip will be compromised over time.

In contrast, the ligaments of the posterior/inferior aspects are short, small, and don't cover the entirety of the joint. After all, gravity keeps the underside of the joint from bearing much force except in cases where the hip is in deep flexion or abduction. In normal life this is fine, but in yoga we find ourselves bearing weight in these ranges of motion often (like Warrior I and II, Side Angle, Triangle ... plus many others), so we have significant risk of injury here if we aren't mindful of supporting the joint muscularly.

From an engineering perspective, the head of the femur must stay closely connected to the acetabulum to reduce impact stress and maintain the health of the articulating cartilage. If the joint becomes too lax, either because of genetic inheritance or through stretching the ligaments, the impact of moving through gravity will accelerate the degeneration of the joint structures and lead to dysfunction.

Knee Joint. The knee joint is formed by the articulation of the femur and the tibia, the larger bone of the lower leg. It is fundamentally held together and stabilized by four ligaments:

- Anterior Cruciate (ACL) = restricts anterior movement of tibia

- Posterior Cruciate (PCL) = restricts posterior movement of tibia

- Medial Collateral (MCL) = restricts medial opening of joint

- Lateral Collateral (LCL) = restricts lateral opening of the joint

Cruciate is Latin for "cross," and the ACL and PCL do just that. They each connect to the front and back of the joint, crossing in the middle at some interesting angles. As the knee flexes and extends, the cruciate ligaments twist around each other slightly, creating tension that limits movement. This is also true in a flexed knee that is rotating. If these ligaments are overstretched, that tension no longer builds and the knee becomes hypermobile. If you hear someone say "I blew out my knee," they are typically referring to a complete tear of the ACL. In some cases, a patient may opt to not repair an ACL, leaving the knee less stable in bent-knee exercises. It's important to keep this in mind when teaching lunging postures. We'll discuss that in detail in the following chapter.

Collateral refers to the ligaments that attach on the medial and lateral aspects of the joint. Since the knee is not engineered to abduct or adduct, these ligaments do their best to make sure those movements don't happen. Some folks are born with abnormally long ligaments, leaving them vulnerable to lateral laxity. You may see this manifest as "knock knees," where the medial support is lackluster and allows the joint to sag toward midline.

There is a massive amount of other connective tissue surrounding the joint, along with the fibrous joint capsule, but these are the ones to be most familiar with. These ligaments offer the primary stabilization of the knee. While many muscles are available to move the knee, their bulky bellies are above or below it, leaving only tendons to actually cross the joint structure. This means that while we can certainly employ counteractive contractions to keep the joint in a static hold, there is not much muscular stability offered to the joint itself, only ligaments.

The medial and lateral *menisci* (see image in chapter 5, p. 41) are thin fibrous cartilage rims attached to the top of the tibia. Named thusly for their crescent-moon shape, the menisci have curves that seem to wrap gently around the condyles of the femur, actually guiding the thigh bone into a subtle internal rotation at full extension. They create space between the two bones when we're not bearing weight, which helps prevent the fixation that can occur in joints with two relatively flat surfaces, such as the facet joints. They provide some extra shock absorption, though that function is

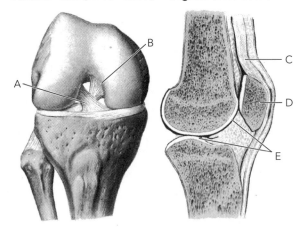

Anterior View (Knee Flexed)   **Sagittal Cross Section**

(A) Anterior cruciate ligament/ACL, (B) Posterior cruciate ligament/PCL, (C) Patellar tendon, (D) Patella/kneecap, (E) Articular cartilage

limited by the soft nature of fibrous cartilage. Since the menisci are not nearly as dense as the articular hyaline cartilage, they can really take a beating if you're living a high-impact life.

The meniscus is also at risk of tearing if the knee is rotated while extended, or from impacts that create shearing forces that the ligaments can't withstand. The medial meniscus in each knee is at higher risk for this, and the injury is often in combination with a torn ACL. By never completely locking your knee, you can reduce these risks to near zero, barring some traumatic impact or external forces.

Foot Joints. There are three plantar arches on each foot, formed by the mid- and forefoot bones:

- Transverse Arch = supports the tarsals of the midfoot + shock absorption, supported by tibialis posterior
- Medial Longitudinal Arch = supports the first metatarsal (big toe) line + shock absorption + balance, supported by tibialis anterior
- Lateral Longitudinal Arch = supports fifth metatarsal (pinky toe) line + shock absorption + transfers weight from heel to forefoot, supported by peroneus longus

As pictured, these arches are also supported by a dense matrix of ligament and intrinsic muscle, so the shape of the foot can be pretty fluid. Wearing shoes that don't allow for proper movement of all of the bones of the foot, or that reduce the muscular recruitment necessary to maintain active support of the foot bones, can result in less functional gait and posture or degenerative diseases of the joints and soft tissues. Oftentimes these failures occur very early in life, and therefore many adults are faced with remediation as they age—or suffer from compensatory posture and degeneration throughout their structural system.

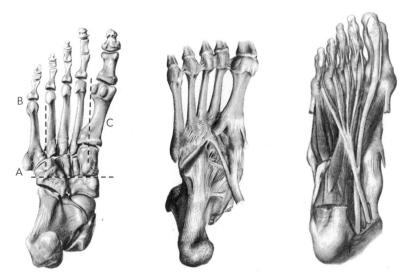

(A) Transverse arch, (B) Lateral longitudinal arch, (C) Medial longitudinal arch, ligaments (*middle*), intrinsic musculature (*right*)

IT BAND: STRUCTURE AND FUNCTIONS

Oh the IT band. So much is said about this structure even though it is not very well understood. The *iliotibial band* (*IT band*; sometimes referred to in other texts as the iliotibial tract, ITT) is the thick band of fascia that begins at the top edge of the lateral pelvis, provides attachment points for the gluteus maximus and tensor fascia latae (TFL), and travels down the lateral thigh to cross the knee. Many folks say that it's there to protect the knee, but only about 10 percent of it actually crosses the lateral knee joint, so how could that be the case? There is evidence that it is separate from the thigh muscle it covers up (vastus lateralis, the largest of the quadriceps), and also evidence that it works fascially with this muscle. So, what's the point of this massive yet mysterious tissue?

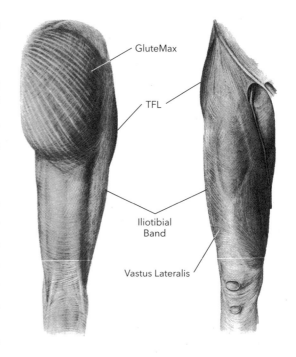

GluteMax

TFL

Iliotibial Band

Vastus Lateralis

Stability.

This very densely packed fascial tract resembles threaded packing tape, like a heavy-duty strap, more like ligament than tendon, connecting the pelvis to the tibia. While it's true to say the muscles that attach to it are abductors of the hip, their position on the body leaves them less as mobilizers in this range and much more in the role of stabilizer to our lateral body. When the TFL and/or the glute max contract even moderately, significant tension is applied to the IT band, creating a strong connection across both the hip and the knee. This is mostly only true when standing upright, however. As soon as the hip or knee are bent moderately, the angles of force on the IT band change dramatically. Remember the earlier discussion about tensegrity? The IT band is a clear example of how tension in one area will affect the entire structural system. The knee is supported not by the thin strands that actually align with that joint but by the entire length of the tract, along with its connections to the ribs above and leg tissues below. Tension is applied to the entirety of that continuum, supporting the cohesion of each and every bone and joint in the system.

But because many of us do not stand with adequate alignment or action in the hips, eliminating the balanced tension that it's designed for, the IT band is typically devoid of its normal functioning. Instead, it bears imbalanced tension (TFL is often locked long or short, while the glutes are either completely flaccid or strictly clenched), doesn't move effectively over the lateral quadricep, and dries up into a sticky mess. Once the tissue is dried out, the intervening layers of mobile fascia between the quad and the IT band also harden and become adhered to one another. Because the lateral line of the facial body interweaves with other functional lines, this adhesion creates plenty of posture-altering changes, as well as functional difficulties. Standing posture, walking gait, even the way you move through your yoga practice—all of these are affected because your whole system is integrated so fully.

Once this adhesion occurs, it's really difficult to relieve, hence the vast market of foam rollers and the like, and the fact that none of them actually achieve long-lasting change. Getting this dense tissue rehydrated is tough, as is separating it from the layers beneath it to keep it mobile, but it can be done. Simply pressing it against those stuck areas and rolling along its length, however, are merely exercises in self-torture. To effectively detach those layers from one another, you'll need to pull them apart, not squash them together. This is where professional bodywork comes in. There is a point in the hardening of fascia where mechanical separation is needed, and the techniques that can be applied across the fibers instead of along them (as with rolling) are far more effective. Cupping can also be utilized, but it's advisable to get some pro treatments for that as well, before trying to apply these tools yourself.

Range of Motion

The lower extremity is a bit of an engineering marvel. From the foot to the SI, bones and joints work to both support our full weight in gravity and propel us through space. To manage this, there is a complex system of heavy bones and tiny ones, large muscles and fine ones. As yoga teachers, we must understand the varying mechanisms within this system. What is the actual function of each joint? How do we optimize our range to be both supportive and mobile? How do we use large muscles to hold us up in gravity, to float, to fly? How do we fine-tune those actions to maintain joint stability, balance, and grace?

First, we need an understanding of the function of each joint or joint complex. Just looking at the body, much less the skeleton, it's easy to notice that the feet are engineered differently than the knee or hip. When you have the opportunity to see the bones in illustrations or in a model skeleton, you'll see that our need for both mobility and stability are met by very different design systems. Through the feet, we have lots of small bones, shaped very strangely (like the heel and ankle bones) in order to provide just the right forces for support as we move in all directions. There are flat articulating surfaces (the tarsals of the midfoot) to provide nearly infinite potential movement combinations to translate forces in many directions. Then we have long bones to direct energy efficiently into those more complex systems (metatarsals of the forefoot). In addition, there are lots of ligaments to hold them tightly together and withstand the ever-present weight-bearing functions of these functional arches. Up through the leg, thigh, and pelvis we have much larger bones, bigger articulations, more free range in the joints. Ligaments still hold it all together, but because the range is more significant, so is the opportunity for inefficient patterns of movement.

We'll discuss the specific muscles that create these movements in the next section. For now, let's focus on the movements themselves at each joint or complex. Keep in mind that all of these movements are defined from a neutral anatomical position, or Mountain.

Coxal Joint. The nature of a ball and socket joint is that it can move in any direction, on all of the planes of movement:

- **Flexion** = pulling the thigh bone forward toward the chest. We see this movement more than just about any other in our yoga practice. Consider how many forward folds happen in one single Sun Salutation (Surya Namaskara A)! Often flexion is limited mostly by musculofascial restrictions because the back of the joint has very little ligamentous support.

- **Extension** = pulling the thigh backward. This movement is employed in backbends and standing postures. Because

of the thick ligaments on the front side of the hip joint, this movement is significantly limited. Those ligaments can be offered a tiny bit of slack with external rotation, so if you combine the two movements, you will reduce the risk of stretching the ligament while slightly increasing potential for extension.

- **Abduction** = pulling the thigh out to the side. We use this to get to postures like wide leg forward folds. Notice, though, that we rarely employ this range in isolation. That's because bony shape as well as some musculofascial restrictions can prevent much lateral movement. (See "Horizontal Abduction" in this list for more details.) Muscularly, we often employ abduction as a stabilizing action as opposed to a gross movement.

- **Adduction** = pulling the thigh in toward midline. Since the neutral hip leaves our thighs pretty close to the midline, this action is also limited. Often we're talking about adducting *from an abducted position to neutral*. Exceptions are deep crossed-legged poses like Eagle (Garudasana) or Cow Face (Gomukhasana). (Consider that some amount of flexion is required to achieve that cross-legged position.)

- **Internal Rotation** = rotating the thigh so the quads (on the front) point in toward the midline. This is usually used as a stabilizing action more than a gross movement. The exception is in the Hero pose variations where the knee is bent and the heels go wider than the knees. These postures tend to be more passive in nature, allowing gravity to move us into internal rotation as opposed to asking muscles to create that action directly.

- **External Rotation** = rotating the thigh so the quads point outward, away from the midline. The Warrior II family of standing poses is sometimes referred to as the "externally rotated" postures because of the way the thighs are taken off neutral compared to the Warrior I family. It's not totally accurate, though, as you'll see next in "Horizontal Abduction." External rotation is actually only used in smaller, supportive roles to help stabilize the hip in those postures. The exception is in the seated family of "hip openers," where deliberate rotation is needed in combination with flexion and abduction to get the thigh to the earth or the foot up onto the opposite thigh as in the Lotus variations.

- **Horizontal Abduction** = combining flexion with abduction; bringing thigh to hip height, then drawing thigh out to the side. This is the actual range we employ in Tree pose, all of our Warrior II standing postures, wide leg forward folds, and seated hip openers. Often it's confused with external rotation but is in fact a particular movement all its own. As you'll soon see, this confusion is reinforced by the fact that the "external rotators" are the muscles that contract to create the abduction portion of the movement.

- **Circumduction** = taking the hip through its full range of motion, combining all three planes, moving in a sweeping circle. Some folks call this a "frog kick." It's not really used in specific yoga postures, but we use it sometimes in warm-up exercises or cool-down unwinding.

Knee Joint. The knee moves on two planes only. The knee should NOT move laterally or medially, though genetics and long-term forces can result in "knock knees," a medial deviation of the knee. Note that the range of motion at the knee is defined in reverse from the other flexion/extension joints in the body.

- **Flexion**: A bent knee is a flexed knee.

- **Extension**: A straight knee is an extended knee. Be clear that there is a natural neutrality for the bones that may not be sufficiently supported by the ligaments, and therefore, a *hyperextended* knee may occur, wherein the knee bends backward. (hyper = too much)

- **Rotation**: A locked knee should not rotate, but if flexed, the hamstrings can rotate the tibia internally or externally (medially or laterally) because of the way they wrap around from the posterior thigh to their attachments on the front of the tibia.

Ankle Joint. The ankle is where the tibia and fibula hug the talus to form a hinge joint. The ligaments that hold the talus and tibia together exist up above the actual joint. These are what get injured in a "high-ankle sprain." The more typical "ankle sprain" occurs at any of the lateral ligaments between the fibula, talus, and foot bones. The true ankle joint (*talocrural* joint for those who geek out on this stuff) has only two movements on the sagittal plane:

- **Plantarflexion** is "pointing the toes." The sole of the foot is where you would "plant" your foot on the earth. Get it? Plantar surface. So when you activate the plantar surface, we call it *plantarflexion*.

- **Dorsiflexion** is what we typically call "flexing the foot": pulling the toes toward the knee. It is thus described since the foot in the standing position has a top and a bottom, instead of a front and back like the leg and body above it. That top side is called the *dorsal* side, just like the dorsal side of a fish or whale (hence, *dorsal fin*). So when the top side of the foot is activated toward the leg, we refer to it as *dorsiflexion*.

Foot Joints. The midfoot and forefoot are responsible for the remainder of the movements we make with our foot. We define the *midfoot* as all joints between the talus and metatarsals, while the *forefoot* includes the long bones and toes.

- **Inversion** is when the sole of the foot turns in toward midline. The back foot in a Warrior II pose is inverted. Some people are limited in this action by soft tissues, but if you've sprained your ankles repeatedly, there tends to be hypermobility here.

- **Eversion** is turning the sole to point outward, away from the midline. There are thick ligaments on the medial ankle (the *deltoid* ligaments, so called because of their shape) that restrict this movement for most folks.

- *Pronation* and *supination* are terms you may hear from your students,

especially if they are runners. Pronation is the combination of inversion and plantarflexion. Supination is the combination of eversion and dorsiflexion. I don't think it's important for you to understand these fully because, frankly, the terms aren't used properly in most instances, and they only serve to confuse both you and your student. That information is best left to the act of buying running shoes, not practicing yoga (even if the running store folks also have a wonky perception of the technicalities of these terms).

Because of the number of joints that form the foot, many intrinsic muscles are involved. As you'll see in a moment, there are many muscles in the calf as well. These are the primary mobilizers of the foot and ankle, the ones that move us through space. These take a ton of effort to learn to work intelligently and strategically, but it can be done. Some massage or manual therapy is necessary for many folks to ensure these muscles have optimal blood flow and neurosensitivity. This can be done with the aid of golf or tennis balls, massage tools, manual massage, and passive range of motion of the toes and midfoot. With this extra attention, you can regain thorough dexterity in your feet, improve your balance, and refine your gait. All of these shifts can have positive compensatory effects upstream through the legs and spine.

Keep in mind that while these muscles do create movement, they also act as stabilizers for our arches. They also work in concert with the channels of muscle up the thigh and into the spine to keep us upright. The calf muscles in particular are referred to as *postural muscles* and will remain active, even go into spasm if needed, just to keep us from collapsing. They're kind of a big deal, but we tend to lack awareness of them. Just about all of us would be surprised to find how sore and tender our calves are in a massage ... it's because they're working overtime for us in gravity! Give them a break, stretch them out, and offer them a warm soak on a regular basis—they'll thank you with more fluid movement, strength, and agility.

HOW THE FOOT RELATES TO GAIT ⊙

It is a true pity that while most of us have been walking around for decades, we really have never thought much about how we walk, much less how we are meant to walk. In a walking gait there are so many things that go wrong that we'll leave it to your imagination. The fact is that it is rare to see someone in good posture, with their weight balanced and their limbs doing as they ought. You'll notice that the three arches were described in terms of their two primary functions: absorbing shock and transferring weight and force to other parts of the foot. We have been given some pretty sophisticated tools but no instruction manual on how best to use them.

Well, here ya go!

Humans are intended to propel ourselves through space with an active softness in most of our joints. That is to say, we are meant to rely on our muscles contracting to move our bones. The effect is one of a slight bounciness or even a subtle glide across the floor. But many of us instead rely on the ligaments to meet their max tension while our muscles go mostly slack, locking out at the joints and dumping into our connective tissue. This is inefficiency at its worst.

Each step should be a fluid sequence of subtle actions and placements. Remember this: Heel, Pinky, Big Toe.

1. **Heel** = heel strike. The forward foot should land at the centerline of the heel, foot actively dorsiflexed until connection with the floor is made.

2. **Pinky** = lateral transfer. The weight of the step now moves up the lateral foot, not on its outer edge but along the lateral longitudinal arch under the fifth metatarsal, to the root of the pinky toe.

3. **Big Toe** = toe-off. Weight is then transferred across the ball of the foot, almost a rolling motion, to the root of the big toe, which presses actively into the floor to propel the whole body forward.

This entire series provides the base of action, each movement creating angles of tension and force up through the remaining extremity in fairly precise ways. If you keep your knees soft and your heart/ribs aligned over your pelvis, these steps will help you engage your calves, quads, hamstrings, and glutes in a fluid manner that avoids the typical slap-foot, locked-knee, flinging quality of most strides out there in the world. Through these actions you're more likely to feel a bit like you're ice skating; at first you may even experience a subtle side-to-side sensation, until your hips and lateral stabilizers reawaken to their purpose. The glide reveals itself as your joints become accustomed to more and more subtle softness.

How does this apply to yoga? If you can become more aware of the recruitment of the feet and ankles in your daily activities like standing and walking, you are more likely to have dexterity of engagement while taking on your standing and balancing postures—not to mention the added strength of the intrinsic muscle that will help support your transitions.

PS: Running is a whole different gait, so don't go trying to skate your way through the 10K.

Muscles

The nature of our everyday posture is such that many students (and probably ourselves too!) have lost much of the awareness and tone in our stabilizing muscles. This leaves the big guys, those heavy hitters who are really built for weight bearing and propulsion, to try to also hold our joints together and maintain balance. That lack of awareness and misappropriation of effort often result in gross compensatory misalignments. My hope is that if you understand which muscles need to activate for each function, you'll be better equipped to teach your students the refined movements necessary to find and hold postures with both grace and dexterity.

When studying the movement of the hip, you could memorize the muscles and what action they do, or you could look at the illustrations and pay attention to the directions the muscle fibers run in. Those lines drawn in aren't just for show ... those lines are reflective of our actual muscle striations and represent the fiber direction in each belly. As discussed in our introduction chapters, every muscle works to bring its attachment ends toward one another along the fiber direction. So these pictures offer helpful information!

An example: One essential rule for the entire body is that muscles that have an oblique fiber direction will create rotation. If you look at the drawing for glute max, you'll notice the lines are diagonal, so you should automatically assume they'll create some sort of *rotation*. If you then figure that this muscle pulls the lateral femur toward the sacrum, you can define that rotation more clearly as *external*.

Remember those questions that help you define the work of any muscle:

1. Which joint does it cross?
2. Where does it attach?
3. If the two ends are brought closer together, which bone will move, and in which direction?

Fair warning: Many muscles of the lower extremity will create more than one action. You'll need to pay close attention to the details of HOW they cross a joint. They may even cross more than one joint, and in so doing will move them all. When this happens, consider separately their action at each joint. It will hopefully feel a little less confusing that way.

Muscles that cross the anterior hip create **flexion**:

- Psoas + Iliacus (prime mover): Both muscles are hip flexors, but because of a subtle oblique path around the femur, they also act as external rotators. These two muscles are often lumped together as "iliopsoas." I think that's a crock of hooey. While they do share a common tendon and insertion point on the femur, they have different origins on completely separate parts of the body and very different belly structures. Psoas originates on the spine as multi-fingered strands and is long and relatively thin, while iliacus originates

on the pelvis in a broad swath with multiple fiber directions and lies much closer to the joint. By shape and length alone, it seems they would have different jobs to do, one acting more as a stabilizer and the other a mobilizer. Also, while the pelvis and spine are deeply integrated in many ways, they are very much separate, and therefore the muscles' contractions will have subtle but distinguished effects on the core's movements.

Of the two, psoas is generally the more well-known. Here again, I'm gonna get a little bit snarky, since psoas's notoriety is often associated with an insistence that it is very short, and therefore our yoga practice should aim to stretch it at every turn. Well, I'll admit that this muscle is often dysfunctional, but rarely is it actually short in the average human walking around out there. (See the next sidebar.) In my

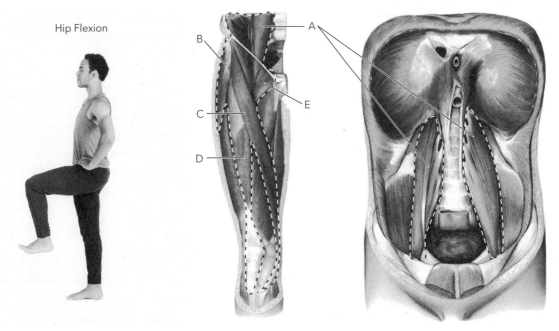

Hip Flexion

(A) Psoas (iliacus, adjacent), (B) Tensor fascia latae/TFL, (C) Sartorius, (D) Rectus femoris, (E) Pectineus

opinion, the greatest function of this hip flexor is to actually flex the hip, you know, like when you walk or march or lift your leg out in front of you for any number of yoga postures that ask you to balance. A widely misunderstood function, however, is its ability to pull forward subtly on the lumbar spine, an action that won't cause the gross movement it has been accused of, but instead will play a vital role in counteraction in the mid-spine and deep core. When you activate Uddiyana Bandha through the anterior abdominal wall or simply fire the rectus abdominis, psoas can counter any potential over-flexion by pulling the lumbar spine into subtle extension, helping create even more abdominal pressure and spinal decompression. Few people engage it as such, and even fewer people take it to the extreme that is often cited as cause for too much lumbar curve. (Please also refer to the sidebar for a debunking of this one.)

Both of these functions require the muscle to be both strong and supple, allowing a wide range of both subtle and powerful contractions to accomplish whatever you need at the time. Regrettably, this is one common problem: weakness. Many people can't get their knee up to hip height without significant compensations helping them along. If you ask them to flex a straight leg out there ... well, good luck to any but the most active and devoted yoga practitioners. It's hard. Like, really hard.

So, instead of stretching, we need to activate it. We need to get blood flowing to it so the fascia can soften up and spasms can let go. Many of us also need direct manual therapy on it to help deactivate any trigger points that may be present and inducing that chronic spasticity. So work it, teachers! Work it, don't stretch it. We'll discuss ways to do this in both overt and stabilizing ways in the following chapter.

As for iliacus, due to its origination on the inside bowl of the ilium, its primary action is on the pelvis, not directly on the spine. Of course we could reference my adage that "where the pelvis goes, the spine follows," in which case it seems reasonable that iliacus and psoas be lumped together. If that were the case though, why is it that psoas is more well-known? Iliacus should move the pelvis, right? Shouldn't it be the one running the show?? Shouldn't it be the one we're all trying to access to fix the system? Hmmm ...

If you consider for a moment the reality of any yogi who has been practicing for a long while—or for that matter, consider that many of the students who walk through your door have likely been in a fall or car accident at some point or taken gymnastics or dance as kids—then you can assume that nearly everyone in your class has some level of SI instability. That instability means that when iliacus contracts, it will move the pelvis without moving the spine, at least not at first. The SI will eventually reach its mobile limit, but not before more movement has occurred there than it was designed for. Since there is already a tendency for the paraspinal muscles to be weak and insufficient to stabilize a hypermobile SI, a dysfunctional iliacus can cause some particular issues all its own.

Both of these muscles are prone to weakness, spasm, and activated trigger points. Both can have impacts on the low back in both posture and sensation. Both are significant to pay attention to, but for different reasons and in different ways.

- Rectus Femoris (synergist): This muscle is one of the four quadricep muscles of the thigh. It is the only one of those four bellies that crosses the hip joint, leaving the others to move the knee exclusively. It is long and rather thin, offering some leverage for big movements of the hip in flexion, but not particularly strong ones. It's prone to both weakness and stickiness, leaving it ripe for spasm if overworked too fast.

- Sartorius (synergist): A very thin, very long muscle that wraps around the anterior thigh, crossing both the hip and knee. Its oblique angle means it is also an external rotator. Also prone to stickiness, it can contribute to pain patterns after too much work or stretching.

- Tensor Fascia Latae (TFL) (synergist): While its literal name is tensor fascia latae, I tend to refer to it as "Bane of Our Existence." This short, dense muscle is situated on the anterior lateral hip, and only by virtue of its angle of insertion into the IT band does it contribute to flexion of the hip. Mostly it's there as a stabilizer and to apply tension to the IT band itself in support of the lateral quadricep. As it does so, however, it tends to develop righteous trigger points that can refer to the hip, low back, belly, groin, and knee. It's a bugger.

PSOAS AND SITTING

You'll often hear that psoas is short because of how much Americans sit these days. It is this argument that is used to promote deep stretches to the hip flexors, like lunges and deep Warrior postures. You'll notice lots of students letting the weight of their hips drop in gravity in low lunges and high lunges, Lizards (Utthan Pristhasana), and Monkeys (Hanumanasana) … but the truth is, psoas's dysfunction is rarely in its length.

If you look at the actual sitting posture of the average person, do you see a 90 degree angle at the hip? Is that person sitting upright on a neutral pelvis and stacking their vertebrae in the neutral curves? Are their feet flat on the floor with their knees stacked directly over their ankles? If you look at the average person sitting at their desk or in their car or in front of their TV, do you see anything approximating "good" postural alignment for any more than mere minutes? I mean honestly, even as I sit here writing this paragraph, I just had to rearrange my pillows behind me because I feel like a jerk, writing about proper posture while sprawled out on my couch like a beach-goer getting sun!

The fact is that even those of us who are deeply aware of what ideal alignment is are not prone to maintain it under any but the most stringently observed circumstances. Nearly all of us will do one of two things in turn:

- We will let our hips slide forward, tucking our sacrum under us, stretching our legs out long, probably crossing our ankles (unless we are driving, but I won't put that past everybody). We'll let our upper back rest against the chair-back and jut our head forward over our chest. Our arms will reach out long for a keyboard or steering wheel.

- Our hips will sit near the center of our chair, and our tail will tuck under. Our chest will collapse down toward our pelvis, bowing our entire spine back in space just like a baby in the womb, letting our face press forward toward our screen. The base of our skull will crush the top of the neck, and our arms will hang right in front of us, hinged at the elbow like we're imitating a T. rex.

If either of these sounds familiar, or even as you're reading this you realize that you are engaged in some hybrid of the two, it turns out you too are human. It's just what we do! Most of us are so habituated at such a deep neurological level to let ourselves go in gravity that it is the most reflexive thing to do.

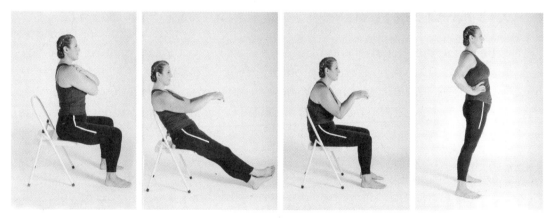

Psoas is only truly shortened when sitting in perfect posture, which for most folks is infrequent.

That said, looking at either of those models shown in pictures here, I ask you this question: Is the hip in any appreciable level of flexion? If the answer to that is NO, well then … I suppose psoas's length isn't greatly impacted by the reality of *the average person's common sitting posture*.

Adding to this strange anatomical drama is the particular mythology about psoas pulling so hard on the lumbar spine when we stand (because of its shortness, of course) that it is responsible for the sway-back epidemic sweeping the nation. I don't believe that is true at all—in fact, most people with anything approximating hyperlordosis experience it because their pelvis is shifted forward when they stand, resulting in a collapse of the lumbar spine as the ribs drop in gravity with nothing under them for support. In this posture, the pelvis actually lands in posterior tilt and the hip in extension. That leaves both psoas and iliacus to stretch over the bony pubic arch to reach their insertion on the femur. Translation: neither muscle is short in standing—both are lengthened.

So you see, there is little in the common postural reality that shortens psoas and demands that we employ gravity and deep lunging postures to stretch it back out. In fact, what it needs most is work.

Okay, so now I must humble myself and add one particular caveat; the crossed-leg sitting posture. If you are not habituated to sitting in chairs, don't work at a desk or stand for a living, or happen to be a yoga teacher who finds themselves in all sorts of floor-sitting situations on the daily … it's likely that you'll end up seated in a variation of Easy (Sukhasana), Accomplished (Siddhasana), or Lotus (Padmasana), or even curled up in a ball. In these cases, well, I'll admit that your psoas is in fact shortened by deep flexion and external rotation. In these bodies, gentle stretching of psoas and iliacus is certainly appropriate, but it still isn't necessary to go into extremely deep, unmitigated gravitational stretches. These muscles will still need work and tone and blood flow, considering that their shortness is not an active contraction but a passive positioning.

Muscles that cross the posterior hip vertically create **extension**:

- Gluteus Maximus (prime mover): This is the big one. Attaching along the lateral edge of the sacrum, coccyx, and sitting bone, glute max has the most potential mass of any muscle in the body. For its size though, it only has a few neural units, and therefore we lack much finite control over how many fibers will fire at one time. That means folks are likely, especially as they are just getting into practice, to mostly fire it as "all or nothing" for a while. Nuance is achievable, but it takes tons of practice and requires learning how to recruit all the extensors as a complete system. We need to avoid outright clenching to keep the SI safe from disruptive forces and to leave some space for our L5 to micro-adjust if needed.

- Gluteus Medius (synergist): The posterior fibers of this muscle assist in extension, but because of the way they originate on the lateral ilia, they function much more as stabilizers than mobilizers. If you look closely, you'll see there are actually three separate fiber directions, two of which are oblique and oppose one another. This is indicative of a muscle that, when fully contracted, actually counteracts itself, reinforcing its function as a stabilizer in rotation, extension, and flexion.

- Hamstrings (prime mover): There are four separate bellies that form the hamstring group. Only three of them cross the hip, attaching to the lateral aspect of the ischia at the ischial tuberosity. Notice just how lateral that origin

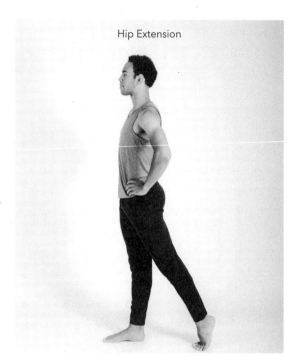

Hip Extension

is ... it's unlikely that you'll actually sit on it, even though it is on the "sitting bone." Notice too that I've labeled both the glute max and hammies as prime movers. That means that either muscle group *could* move the hip into extension on its own, and oftentimes that is exactly what people do: recruit one group or the other. Unfortunately, that isn't a very efficient way of moving the thigh, especially as we do in yoga, reaching our legs out long behind us in backbends and balancing poses. Those actions are leverage-heavy, so to execute them with strength and grace, we require the cohesive use of both muscle groups in concert.

- Adductor Magnus (prime synergist): This is the largest and potentially strongest of the adductor muscles. Because of its relatively broad origin along the bottom of the ischium, it is more posterior than any of its counterparts, and this provides the leverage necessary to make it a powerful

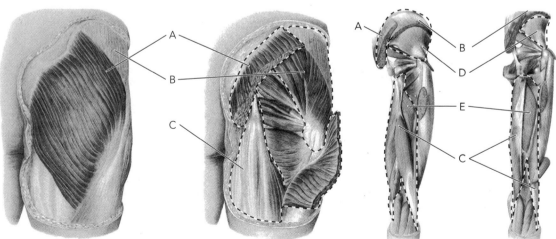

(A) Glute max, (B) Glute medius, (C) Hamstrings, (D) Glute minimus, (E) Adductor magnus extensor. In some bodies, it will work way harder than hamstrings in extension. Femoral shape and alignment will affect how these muscles get recruited. In fact, there is a common strain suffered by numerous yogis and teachers: "the hamstring attachment." It's tough to heal and tends to reoccur. Nearly 100 percent of the time, upon examination, I can say with complete certainty that they have in fact not injured their hamstring in any way, but they have pulled the adductor magnus at the sitting bone. (Visuals and sidebar describe these in the "Risks" section.)

Muscles that cross the lateral hip create **abduction**:

- Gluteus Medius: As described earlier, glute med has three fiber directions on the lateral hip. The middle fibers contracting will create abduction. All the fibers firing together will increase the power of that abduction, but they will also stabilize in flexion/extension and internal/external rotation. The key thing to remember here is that while gluteus medius can move the hip in abduction, it is engineered as a stabilizer more than a mobilizer. As humans, we don't employ nearly as much lateral action as we do forward motion ... unless you play field sports like soccer or football. So, most of the time, it's much more functional to use this muscle for small adjustments and balance, or else you risk activating trigger points and sending it into chronic spasm.

- Gluteus Minimus: Much like its slightly larger cousin, minimus has multiple fiber directions that originate on the

Hip Abduction

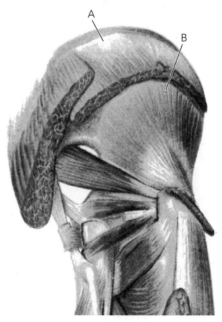

(A) Gluteus medius, cut (B) Gluteus minimus

lateral plate of the ilium. It is smaller and more anterior in alignment than medius, and so it will contribute more in flexion synergy and abduction. Again, it's really designed for balance and stability more than mobility.

- Tensor Fascia Latae ... we meet again. Because of its alignment on the lateral hip, TFL will contribute to the abduction synergy of medius and minimus. It is easily irritated by too much gross abduction and will make sure you know it's pissed off. Emphasize stability without clenching in all of these muscles.

Muscles that cross the medial hip (groin) create **adduction**:

- Adductor Magnus, Adductor Longus, Adductor Brevis, Pectineus, Gracilis: All of the adductor muscles start at that pelvis and insert along the *linea aspera*, a bony ridge that runs the length of the posterior femur. Pectineus is the shortest and most anterior, making it a synergist in flexion. Magnus is the largest and most posterior, making it a powerful extensor. The others are varying lengths but mostly act as adductors. The thing to observe about this group is that the bellies tend to be

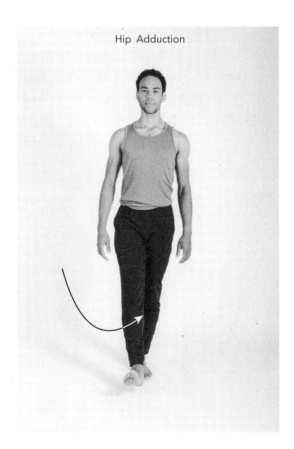

Hip Adduction

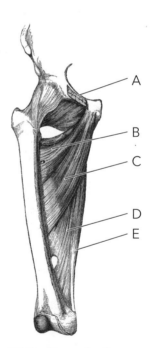

(A) Pectineus (cut),
(B) Adductor brevis,
(C) Adductor longus,
(D) Adductor magnus,
(E) Gracilis

broad (except gracilis, which is long and stringy), and they lie upon one another from front to back, reminding me of sails on a sailboat. This relationship sets them all up for potential adhesion to one another along those flat surfaces, which means that stretching them can become quite impeded by varying points of stickiness.

Muscles all over the hip joint can create **internal rotation**:

- TFL: Its oblique fiber direction pulls the greater trochanter forward, rotating internally.

- Adductors: This is admittedly a very confusing one. If you just look at the pictures, or even a model skeleton, it looks like we'd be pulling the back of the femur forward, but that's not the case in reality. I'm gonna ask you to believe me on this. Because of the angle of the neck and the various arching angles of the shaft of the femur, the forces combine to create internal rotation. This is the rationale (even if it ends up misguided) for some teachers squeezing a block between the thighs to send it back behind you in forward folds.

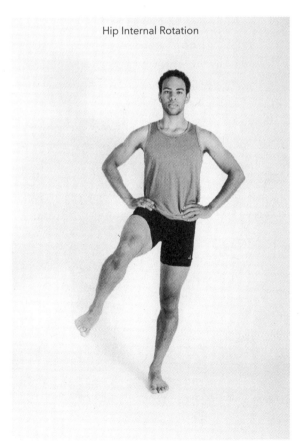

Hip Internal Rotation

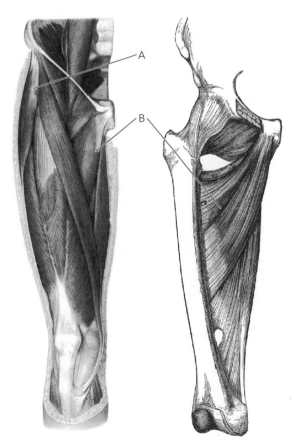

(A) TFL, (B) Adductors (glute med/min's anterior fibers assist; hamstrings may assist rotation in certain alignments, not pictured)

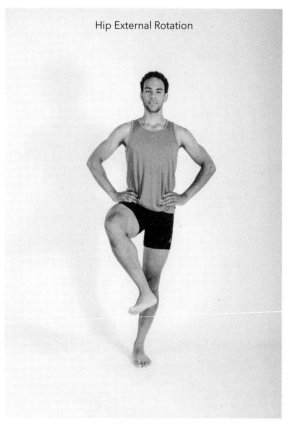

Hip External Rotation

- Glute Med: The anterior fibers of medius line up with TFL, and they work together to assist internal rotation. The problem is that many people are standing around with their hips internally rotated all the time—most aren't in neutral. So, both medius and TFL are in a shortened position, leaving them prone to spasm and trigger points.

Muscles that cross the posterior hip horizontally or obliquely create **external rotation**:

- Glute Max + Med: As described previously, these muscles have dual actions. Remember, though, that glute med acts more as a stabilizer in this range, while glute max can be a pretty powerful prime synergist to the external rotation-contractions of psoas and iliacus on the anterior side. These also act as the prime synergists that create the

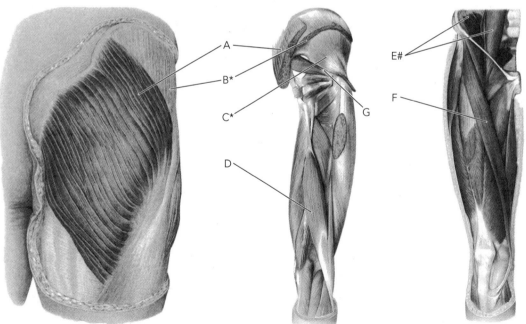

(A) Glute max, (B) Glute med (*posterior fibers), (C) Glute min (*posterior fibers), (D) Lateral hamstrings, (E) Iliacus and psoas (# separate muscles with shared insertion tendon and shared actions), (F) Sartorius, (G) Piriformis

horizontal abduction action described in the range of motion section.

- "Deep Six" muscles, including piriformis: The deep six are a system of small interweaving muscles that run essentially from the sacrum and pelvis to the greater trochanter. Their horizontal alignment sets them up for some very direct synergistic work in both external rotation and horizontal abduction, but their relative size and proximity to the joint capsule make them fine-tuners and stabilizers by nature instead of prime movers. Many people have lost awareness in them completely and require rehab-level exercises to regain healthy recruitment.

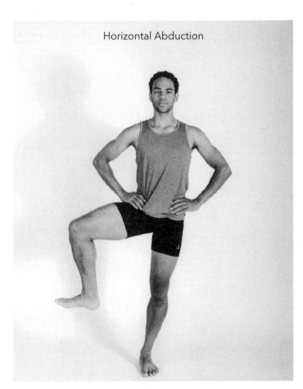

Horizontal Abduction

This movement is the combination of flexion and abduction. Once the hip is flexed, the muscles of the posterior hip all engage to create the horizontal abduction.

Many of you may have heard about one of the deep six muscles in particular: piriformis. This muscle is indeed special, because of its relationship with the *sciatic nerve*. The sciatic nerve is the largest nerve bundle in the body and just so happens to run from the sacral plexus, behind the hip joint, and down the thigh and leg. At the point it runs through the posterior hip, it will travel one of four paths:

1. Under piriformis, where it can get compressed against the other deep six muscles.

2. Over piriformis, where it can get compressed against glute max.

3. Split in two and wrap around piriformis, where it can get compressed by either the deep six or glute max, or even both at the same time.

4. Punch a pathway through piriformis, where, well, it's gonna get irritated by pretty much any contraction of the muscle at all. Oy.

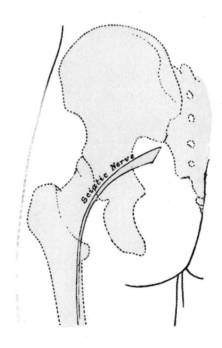

So, the health and functionality of this muscle can have direct impacts on the nerve that serves the entire lower extremity in some way. Here again, though, some assumptions have been made in many exercise fields, yoga among them, that piriformis requires stretching to keep it healthy and give the sciatic nerve some room. I'm not so sure that's the case in all those bodies out there.

- (and iliacus/psoas + sartorius, which have an oblique direction on the anterior hip)

Muscles that cross the posterior knee create **flexion**:

- Hamstrings (prime mover): The hammies flex the knee, but they also rotate it. The insertion tendons wrap from the back thigh around to the lateral and medial tibia. Since the hamstrings are made up of separate bellies, they can fire independently and thereby rotate the flexed knee. Remember, the knee ought not to rotate if it is extended.

- Sartorius (synergist): This long thin muscle crosses from the front of the pelvis to the medial knee at the tibia. Because of its length, it is not a strong extensor but will also contribute to the rotation of the knee when it is flexed.

- Gastrocnemius: This is the calf muscle that crosses the knee joint from below. It is the heart-shaped muscle you see near the top of the calf, especially defined on cyclists. Its proximal end splits in two, and each side wraps up around the medial and lateral femur. Because of this split, those fibers take on an oblique alignment. Since they are a single belly however, they fire concurrently, so they act as a stabilizer to knee rotation instead of a mobilizer.

Muscles that cross the anterior knee create **extension**:

- Quadriceps (prime mover): This group is made up of four bellies (quadri-ceps, get it?). All four meet at a common tendon, in which is embedded the *patella*, or kneecap. The largest of the

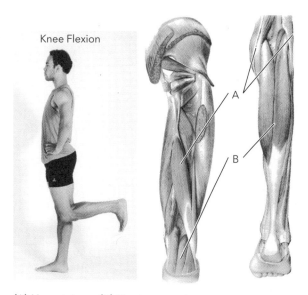

Knee Flexion

(A) Hamstrings, (B) Gastrocnemius

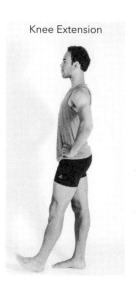
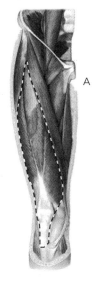

Knee Extension

(A) Quadriceps (rectus femoris, vastus lateralis, vastus medialis, vastus intermedius)

four is *vastus lateralis,* and it is so far lateral on the anterior thigh that it actually wraps around the femur to butt up against the hamstrings. The IT band lies over and integrates with the fascia of vastus lateralis in a vain effort to add stability to the muscle track. If you pay attention to the thighs of your students, you'll see that very few of us have uniform development of all of the muscles of the quads. This can be genetic in origin but can also be influenced by our posture and gait. If we aren't neutral in our hips, our entire extremity will compensate in various ways to try to more efficiently carry our weight through space. These compensations may result in uneven tone in the quads and almost certainly affect the tracking of the patella in its groove on the femur.

Muscles crossing the posterior knee at oblique angles create **internal and external rotation** of the *bent knee*:

- Hamstrings: The tendons of hamstrings wrap around the side of the leg in such a manner that they will rotate the tibia when the knee is bent.

- Gastrocnemius: Because of the way the top of this muscle splits and wraps around the sides of the femur, when it is activated (both of the heads simultaneously), it can stabilize rotation at the knee.

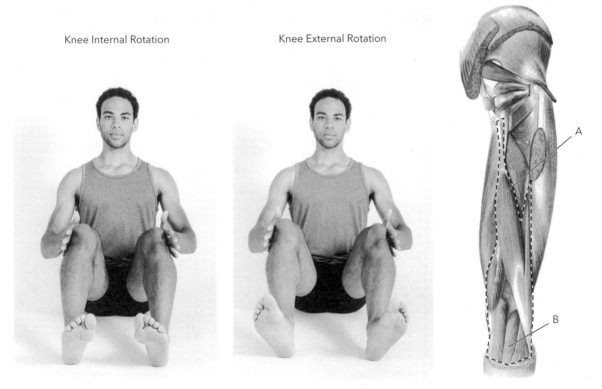

Knee Internal Rotation

Knee External Rotation

(A) Hamstrings, (B) Gastrocnemius (stabilizer only)

Muscles that cross the posterior ankle create **plantarflexion**:

- Gastroc: Upper portion of the calf muscle.

- Soleus: The principal muscle of plantarflexion. It is overlaid at the proximal end by gastroc, and they merge fascially to a common tendon, the *Achilles*. It is via this tendon that the two muscles can powerfully plantarflex, an essential action in walking, running, climbing, and standing upright. These muscles are postural muscles, meaning they are so necessary for our upright posture that if they fatigue, their response is to go into spasm

instead of relaxing. Most of us exist with a chronic state of low-level spasticity in our calves for this reason.

- Tibialis Posterior: An unsung hero of the calf muscles. It is a synergist in many functions of the ankle and foot and gets little love from us. Its position very deep against the posterior tibia makes it difficult to stretch and to massage, but there are a few secret access points we'll cover in the next chapter.

Muscles that cross the anterior ankle create **dorsiflexion**:

- Tibialis Anterior: This is the prime mover in dorsiflexion, though some

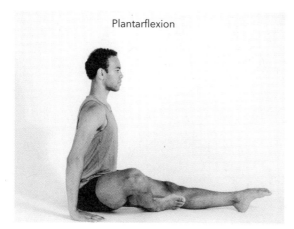

Plantarflexion

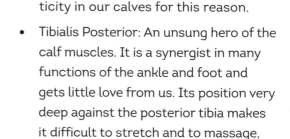

(A) Gastroc, (B) Soleus, (C) Tibialis posterior

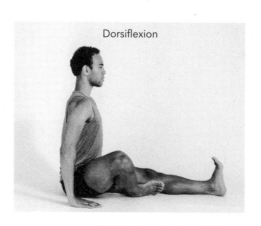

Dorsiflexion

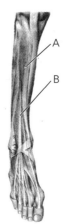

(A) Tibialis anterior, (B) Extensor digitorum

of the toe extensors may contribute. You'll see tib anterior bunch up on the front of the shin in contraction. Though it attaches along the lateral length of the tibia, near the ankle it crosses over to the medial arch to insert at the base of the first metatarsal. It is part of a fascial continuum that acts as a stirrup for the arches of the foot.

- Extensor Digitorum: This is a synergist to the actions of tib anterior. Deeper extensor muscles can also contribute.

Muscles that cross the lateral ankle create **eversion**:

- Peroneus Longus + Peroneus Brevis: These are the lateral muscles of the leg, running along the length of the fibula to the foot. Longus's tendon actually crosses the sole of the foot to connect near the tib anterior insertion, completing the "anatomical stirrup" mentioned earlier. It adds support to the arches of the foot, as well as trying to stabilize the ankle and moving it in eversion.

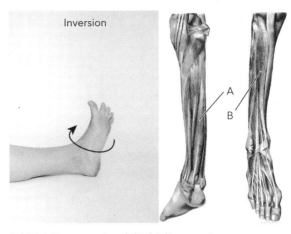

(A) Tibialis posterior, (B) Tibialis anterior

Muscles that cross the medial ankle create **inversion**:

- Tibialis Anterior: Remember, this muscle crosses over to the medial foot, so when contracted it will pull the sole of the foot up the midline.

- Tibialis Posterior: Tib posterior's track takes it along the medial ankle to the bottoms of the tarsal bones. In contraction it will pull the sole of the foot up to face the midline, but it also helps support the transverse arch of the foot when standing.

Bandhas

The interaction of the midfoot and the heel/ankle is what forms the physical structure of *Pada Bandha*, or Foot Container. Though the bandhas are energetic centers, they are profoundly linked to and aligned with the musculofascial body. This means that both physically and energetically you can make connections from the soles of the feet up through the legs, across the pelvis, and into the *Mula Bandha* (Root Container) as discussed in our spine section.

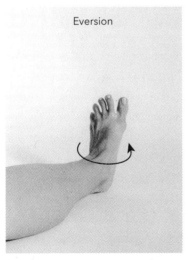
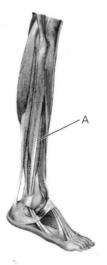

(A) Peroneus Longus and Brevis

So, Pada Bandha really provides the roots of the Root Container. Without the actions of the extremity, Mula Bandha has a really rough time engaging properly, and not only while bearing weight. Seated postures are served by Pada Bandha just as much as standing postures.

A side note: A collapsed foot has trouble finding balance, but so does a locked-up arch. You must be able to find the balance between mobility and stability to create the optimal energetic and structural lift. This balance can only be achieved by working with both the long muscles of the calf and the intrinsic muscles of the foot.

Experiential Learning

When I was in massage school, I found that using different methods and learning tools helped me ingrain more information for the long haul. Reading is only one way. Looking at the visuals offered here is another. I found that making flashcards myself and going through them repeatedly at different times in different places helped me immensely, and I am anything but an artist with a pencil. Remember, you don't have to draw these things; you can find images online and print them out, then affix them to your flashcards.

There are other methods for tactile or experiential learning too! If you learn best by doing, consider finding a friend to be your model, then use washable, nontoxic markers to draw the muscles directly on their body. You can also use tape (I like the multicolored electrical type) to outline the various muscles on their hips and legs. In school, we also used clay to shape out the various muscle bellies and groups.

Whatever works for you, do that. Get playful, get creative. There is no wrong way to do this. ✪

I'm sure you have noticed that there is a ton of material to learn in this section. The lower extremity is super complex! So, I suggest breaking it down into smaller bits. Start with the bones. There aren't that many of those. Make sure you can interchange the technical name for the lay terms on those. Like, femur = thigh, and so on. Once you have that down, you can move on to the joints, describing them in terms of the bones that articulate to form them, and perhaps noting important ligaments that hold them together. Maybe then you can include any specific limitations those ligaments provide. Finally, you can work with the muscles. There's little need to recall the exact name of every minor muscle in this vast and complex matrix. I think it's most important to know what joint the major players cross and their primary action there. If you wanna make a nickname for them because the Latin is too technical … be my guest. Just be consistent if you can. Develop a system that makes sense for you, and then as you integrate this information into your teaching you will have a stronger framework to draw from.

If you really want to take it to the next level and dive into deeper understanding for yourself and your students, there are a few "buzzword" muscles that get a ton of hype in the yoga world. You should be aware of them and what they do, and maybe even why the hype should be believed or not. Psoas and piriformis are two that I called out specifically in the sidebars earlier in this chapter. Perhaps you can go back through the chapter and pick out some specific tidbits about the following muscles that maybe don't get the attention they should. What is important about these? Is there specific work or attention they need in practice? Maybe at this point you don't even answer those questions directly, but you could ask them as you move in your body in practice. If you bring your attention to them in real time, what do they tell you they need?

- Iliacus
- TFL
- Adductor Magnus
- Tibialis Posterior

Limitations
Common Bony Limitations

Angle of the Femoral Neck. The angle of the neck of the femur to the shaft can be measured precisely, but that's not what we do here. For our purposes, we will make a layperson's observation: When the angle is closer to 90 degrees, abduction will be reduced as compression between the greater trochanter and the ilium happens quickly ... there's just not much space. If the angle of the neck is closer to 180 degrees, there is much more space between the trochanter and ilium, allowing for much more abduction before you reach compression.

For people with bony compression in the hip, it does them no good to continue to strive for more movement. This effort will not result in longer muscles, it will only serve to compress the cartilage and likely shred it to bits. Practicing "hip openers" is a tricky business that requires the practitioner to build a deep awareness of the difference in the sensations of stretch and compression.

Misaligned/Misshaped Acetabulum. All of the preceding is moot if there is a profoundly deep acetabulum or if its angle in the pelvis is abnormal. If it's really deep, the neck of the femur will compress against the edge of the socket in external rotation, abduction, or internal rotation regardless of the angle of the neck. Flexion can be compromised if the femur is adducted too much in this case as well. As expected, all of these conditions are reversed if the acetabulum is very shallow, increasing instability at the bony-support level.

If the angle is wonky, then forces may be placed on the head of the femur in imbalanced ways, leading to compression points within the socket itself or between the femur and the labrum.

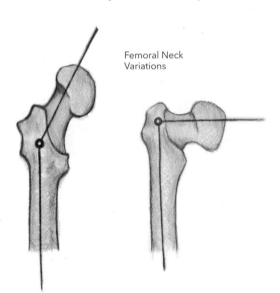

Femoral Neck Variations

Closer to 180 degrees, more range of motion may be available at the hip joint. Closer to 90 degrees, there is likely to be reduced range.

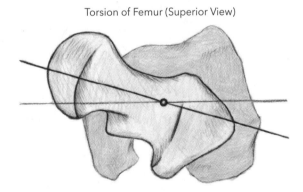

Torsion of Femur (Superior View)

The torsion of the femur will determine which direction the knees will point when the hip joint is neutral.

Torsions of Femur and Tibia. Torsions of the thigh and leg bones will affect the alignment of the trochanter to the knee and/or the knee to the foot. We commonly think that the toes pointing straight ahead is neutral, but that is rarely the case when accounting for individual differences. In truth, for many people this alignment may be significantly internally rotated at the hip and place profound stress on the hip/knee/ankle over time. Notice in your students if their knees point straight ahead, roll in toward midline, or point outward.

The neutral hip aligns the greater trochanter slightly behind the midline of the socket. Once the hip is neutral, then you can see if the knees point straight ahead or if the feet do. For many people, neutral hips leave the feet in a "duck-foot" stance, and that is perfectly okay. They will benefit significantly long-term if they practice with that slight turn-out.

Distortions of the Talus. There is usually a deep notch in the front of the talus that the tibia fits nicely into when you dorsiflex your foot. The depth of that notch varies from person to person, and some people lack this space completely. For them, the talus is solid bone. Without that space to settle into, the tibia and talus reach their compression point with very little movement; more bone equals less range of motion. This hard end-feel may result in the ankle being unable to move past a 90 degree bend.

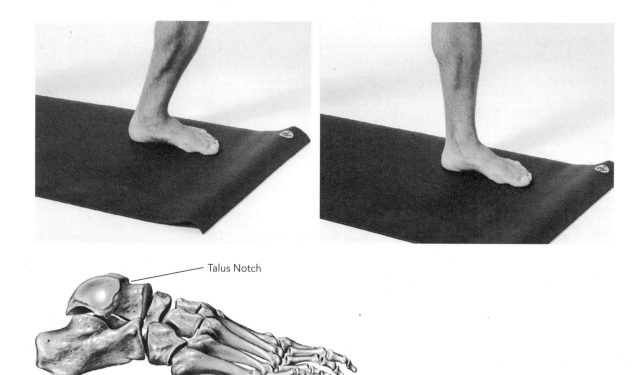
Talus Notch

Without a notch at the front of the talus, the tibia will not be able to move past 90 degrees.

WHAT POSTURES WILL A DISTORTED TALUS IMPACT?

This is a very important question, because it proves that even a tiny deviation from average will have a significant effect on an asana practice. Consider the fact that any time you are weight bearing and need to bend your knees, a forward momentum naturally occurs through the shins—the zigzag pattern of the legs as your center of gravity adjusts. In order for the shin to press forward, the ankle needs to dorsiflex. If the talus is overgrown or lacks that notch, the ankle *can't* dorsiflex much, and balance will be compromised, usually eliciting compensatory patterns elsewhere in the system.

Consider postures like Downward Facing Dog, Standing Forward Fold, Squat, Chair, etc. How will these postures be affected by this limited range of motion? Try this in your body. Go into Down Dog, and once aligned in your own natural shape, bring both ankles to a pure 90 degree angle. Notice how your alignment changed. What if this was your only option, with regard to your feet and ankles?

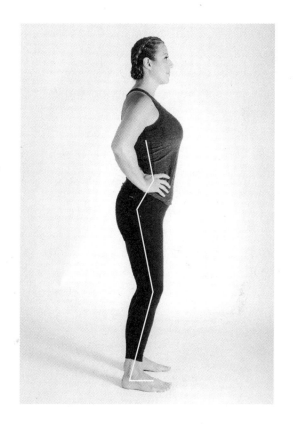

You may also see students who can't plantarflex fully (point their toes), so that their ankles can't come flush to the earth when sitting in postures like Prayer, Rock (Vajrasana), or Hero (Virasana). If the arches are particularly high, the bones may be too rigid and misaligned to allow the talus and calcaneus to move in full range here. Other bony distortions of the ankle or soft tissue may also be a culprit.

Common Soft Tissue Limitations

Hip Extension. Muscle is usually the first barrier in this action, but if your hip flexor muscles are supple, then you will eventually reach the ligament level. You don't want to stretch the ligaments. There is no functional reason to hyperextend your hip, and plenty of reasons not to. External rotation will offer the ligament a small bit of slack in cases where you really need to access more extension, like Hanumanasana (Monkey/full splits), but I honestly recommend using a little flexion/forward tilt in the pelvis to avoid stretching that ligament or cranking the SI joint. It's perfectly fine to have a little backbend in those deep asymmetrical postures if they're well supported by the functional core.

Hip Flexion. The most common limitation here is compression of tendons or bursae between the femur and the pelvis. There are many tendons that travel across the front of the pubic arch, and many muscles that attach directly to it or to the anterior iliac spine, providing ample opportunity for squishy bits to get squished. Add in the fact that bursae are present anywhere squishy bits travel over hard

bits, and you increase the amount of connective tissue that can get irritated and cranky. There is also a ligament that spans the gap between the pubic tubercle and the ASIS, creating a flat channel that much of this tissue travels through, so any irritation or inflammation will result in less space in that channel ... a perfect storm of potential compression!! If that ligament gets hard or tough or sticky, if any of the tendons or bursae get cranky, or if your individual bony shape creates compression in this area, hip flexion will become annoyingly painful. The problem is, we flex the hips A TON in yoga (and everyday life, for that matter), so being mindful of reducing the incidence of irritation here is key to maintaining a healthy and pleasant movement experience.

Hip Internal Rotation. If you are profoundly stiff in the iliofemoral ligament, your internal rotation could be limited. It is more likely that muscles like glutes, sartorius, and psoas are rigid, spastic, or stuck to surrounding structures. They don't even really have to be short if they are tough and lack pliability. The structure of the hip is necessarily complex in its layering of muscle and connective tissue, leaving ample opportunity for compression and lack of movement to wreak havoc on their functionality. Internal rotation is already not a place we have profound range, so it doesn't take much soft tissue dysfunction to impact that movement.

Hip External Rotation. If your individual bony shape is built for external rotation, then this action may be limited instead by the adductor muscles. Since the adductors are the primary internal rotators, they are the muscles most likely to inhibit external rotation when they are stiff or short. The manner in which the adductors lie against each other makes

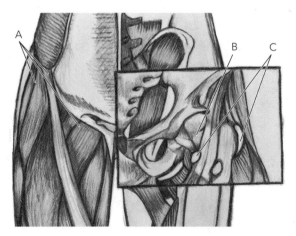

(A) Hip flexor tendons, (B) Hip ligaments, (C) Bursae

them incredibly prone to adhesion, which creates limitations in their fluidity. The shortest adductor, *pectineus*, lies very close to the groin, acting more as a stabilizer than a mobilizer, but since it overlaps mobility muscles like psoas, iliacus, and sartorius (all external rotators), any stickiness or dysfunction can significantly impact external rotation.

Knees. The ligaments of the knee limit lateral and medial movement, rotation and extension, though many people have the ability to hyperextend due to congenital factors and/or poor posture.

The cruciate ligaments in particular are at high risk for stretching if pushing the limits of our range of motion, so we really need to be aware here. With healthy ligaments, you should have a broad ability to flex the knee, but when weight bearing, you need to self-limit this movement. See the "Risks" section later in this chapter for more detail.

Patellar tracking is also an issue if our conditioned hip position is not actually neutral. Since many of us tend toward internal rotation in our everyday posture (feet more parallel than they ought to be), the angles that the quadriceps pull on our kneecap are askew. This poor alignment leads to extra and uneven wear and tear on the cartilage of both the patella and the femur.

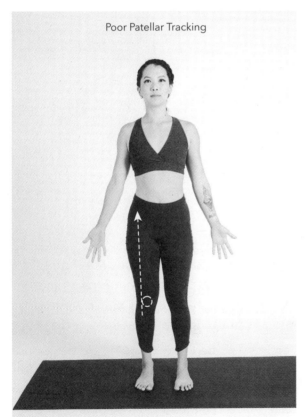
Poor Patellar Tracking

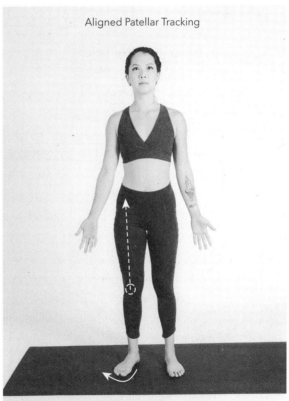
Aligned Patellar Tracking

If feet are forced parallel, the quads no longer pull the kneecap directly up the groove in the femur. Instead, there is lateral deviation, leading to wear and tear on both surfaces.

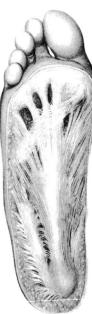
Plantar Fascia

Ankles and Feet. We usually think of the Achilles tendon as the primary limiter of ankle dorsiflexion, but the deeper muscles of the posterior compartment, tibialis posterior in particular, also have profound impact on this movement. The deep fascial track from the posterior muscles across the heel can get thick, stiff, or stuck. All of these can limit dorsiflexion because of tension or adhesions that elicit pain as they are stretched.

The plantar fascia, or connective tissue interwoven from various points on the sole of the foot, can be very restrictive in some bodies. Many issues can arise here, sometimes inflammatory, sometimes spastic, that cause mild to severe pain and limit the ability to bear weight after rest periods, or affect the way the foot dorsiflexes. Its disability is often associated with dysfunction in the muscles and connective tissues of the calf and shin.

Ligaments or anterior muscles are often the cause of limitations in plantarflexion, but bones may be a factor as well. The back of the heel can feel uncomfortably compressed in deep plantarflexion if the posterior musculature is sticky or inefficient at shortening. Stiffness or chronic misalignment of

KNEE SURGERY

Ligaments that have already been surgically replaced may significantly limit the flexion of the knee, as they are typically made deliberately tight in order to "stretch to fit." A PT should urge patients to work on this, and in my opinion, barring any other factors to the contrary, flexion exercises should be used over time to stretch them into a broader range of motion. You may see students in class avoiding this movement due to this restriction, but unfortunately it is outside our scope of practice to challenge this too much. Instead, we can refer them to their doctor for more information or suggest more PT input to get them back on track.

Postsurgical scar tissue can also contribute to significant reductions in range of motion. It may be contributing to stretch tension or compression patterns. I have also had clients who developed postsurgical bone spurs that created pain in certain movements. Remain aware that many factors are potentially at play here and the picture can be pretty vague.

It isn't your job to make sure they are pain-free in all movements, but offering modifications is key. Extra props may help these folks a ton. Offer elevation in seated poses, extra padding under knees, blankets at the back of the knee joint when kneeling, or a folded yoga strap in deeply flexed-knee postures like Lotus and its cousins.

the ankle and midfoot resulting from long or short ligaments, or ones with sufficient scar tissue, could have impacts on one's ability to access Pada Bandha, keep the pinky-edge of the back foot rooted in standing postures, or leave heels on the ground in deep squatting postures.

Common Conditions

Typically, injury in the lower extremity is of the sprain/strain variety. But many congenital issues can lead to other forms of joint degeneration, which will be accelerated by poor posture, gait, and alignment. This means that we must build hyperawareness in the tissues near our joints to ensure that we are moving in our best range of motion and stretching in our muscles and not in our ligaments. We also need to understand that weak muscles are at the most risk for injury in our practice. Building a balance between strength and length in our muscle tissue is integral to preventing strain injuries. In this section we'll focus on descriptions of conditions that may walk through the studio door, so you can get familiar with them and their relationship to yoga. We'll wait until the "Practice Mechanics" section of chapter 10 to dissect what to say, how to teach around these, and cover any modifications or adjustments.

I think it's very important for you to be aware of the following list of conditions, and their potential ramifications, in order for you to competently offer modifications or exclusions to your students' practice. But I'd also like to highlight the fact that yoga teachers are not diagnosticians. Unless you are a physician specializing in musculoskeletal conditions, you do not have the credentials to tell a student what their injury is. In my opinion, you can let them know that you may think a particular pain is related to this or that, but you MUST refer them to the right physician for proper diagnosis. This list is certainly not exhaustive, and it's likely you'll hear of other conditions from your students, but at least you'll have a general idea of the most common presentations.

Ligaments and Connective Tissue

Hips. In the hip, preventing injury means being okay with the limitations of extension imposed by the *iliofemoral ligament*. To push past this is inviting the stretching and long-term degeneration of the ligament, its support of the hip, and potentially harmful hypermobility. The *labrum* is also at risk in this scenario, as hypermobility adds extra stress to this fragile cartilage. Bony compression between the *acetabulum* and the neck of the femur can significantly limit range of motion and can lead to injury to and deterioration of the labrum. Once chronic, this condition is called *femoroacetabular impingement* (FAI). The alignment and shape of the acetabulum in conjunction with the angle of the neck of the femur will determine an individual's risk of this impingement in normal ranges of motion.

In either a sprained ligament or a torn labrum, pain can be local or diffuse, can radiate from the damaged point, or can show up in an entirely different area (called *referral*). Common referral patterns include the groin, lateral hip, SI, low back, and pelvis. Neither ligament nor labrum regenerate once they are injured, so establishing a strong resistance to hyperextension can save you and your students years of pain, potential surgery, and rehabilitative therapy.

HIP REPLACEMENTS

As a recent recipient of a total hip arthroplasty (that's the fancy word for the new titanium/polyethylene implant system that has replaced my bum hip joint), I can tell you one thing: pain sucks, and a lack of pain is way better.

My own injuries and pain began when I was very young … so that's a long story you don't need to hear right now. Suffice it to say that many people were very shocked to hear that I was getting a total hip replacement at the age of forty, arguably younger than the average. I am so glad that I did though! I had a seamless recovery of less than six weeks—seven days with a cane, back to doing massage in three weeks, and teaching yoga in six—which was most definitely served by a ton of strengthening pre-hab, energy medicine, dietary supplements, and a ton of emotional support along the way. You can read more about this in my two-part article at YogaEngineer.com. ✪

I bring this to your attention for a couple of reasons: hip replacements are happening much more frequently and at younger ages, and your yoga practice can be both an injury-inducing culprit and/or a tool for avoiding hip injury. As practitioners and teachers, we can get into a mindset that "deeper is more advanced," or "further is better," or "more sensation means better work." None of that is true. All of those ideas are at the root of many yoga-practice fallacies. If we can shift our perception of practice to one that emphasizes action, integrity, and stability, we can begin to move our physical practice out of the danger zone.

The structure of the hip is built for stability first; adding mobility to it must be done thoughtfully and within the context of our personal skeletal structure. We can build asana sequences that utilize our inherent tensions for *decompression* in our joints, instead of continually grinding our connective tissues between our bones. Our yoga practice should focus on growth, not just depth.

If you have students in class who have had hip replacements, be sure to note their age, how long ago they had surgery, and how much asana or other activity they've been doing since. The techniques for this surgery have changed drastically in the last few years, so those having gotten an "anterior approach" will typically have near normal range of motion, barring any scarring that impedes movement. Those with a "posterior approach" have more limitations but are likely to be well versed in these. In either of these cases, increasing range of motion is not really the best thing for their yoga asana practice to attempt. That needs to be addressed in physical therapy. Our job can be about building awareness in the surrounding tissues, finding the full support of the stabilizing muscles, and emphasizing integrity in every posture.

Knees. In yoga asana, injury to the knee is usually caused by one or more of the following:

- Repetitive or traumatic hyperextension (cruciate ligaments)

- Chronically taking the knee beyond the ankle in lunges (cruciate ligaments + patellar tendon)

- Rotating the tibia too far or while at poor angles to the femur, as in deep seated postures like Lotus (meniscus + collateral ligaments)

In high-lunging postures like Crescent Lunge and the Warrior families, all of the body weight is translated through the femur and into the cruciate ligaments of the knee. With proper alignment the weight translates efficiently to the tibia and foot, but if the knee moves past the ankle, the weight-force bypasses the "turn" down the leg and shoots out through the front of the knee tissues. Because the quads and patellar tendon are not in their midrange in this position, the forces jam up in the cruciate ligaments and can create micro-traumas by overstretching them or creating too much friction between them.

Once the back knee is taken down to the floor in a low lunge, the hip bears the burden of our weight and shifts the center of gravity. Now it is safe to bend the knee past the ankle, because in this position the hips absorb the gravity instead of the knee.

These ligaments are also at risk in hyperextension of the knee. Any time you are in a straight-legged standing pose, make an effort to keep the knees unlocked to avoid hyperextension, which stretches the cruciate ligaments and creates instability in all ranges of motion. Many teachers will cue to "lift the kneecap" during these postures in an effort to support the knee, but think about that for a second … lifting the kneecap is contraction of the quadriceps. The quadriceps are knee extensors, so firing them will extend the knee … not exactly the action necessary to prevent hyperextension, eh? (Don't worry! We'll discuss better ways to handle this in the following chapter.)

The articular cartilage on the top of the tibia and the menisci are at high risk for degeneration, since they're absorbing all the shock of every step we take. If our alignment is off by even a little, this tissue gets abused. The cartilage on the back of the kneecap is also at risk of degeneration. Sometimes it is abused by direct impacts, like falling on our knees (like every single one of us has done at least once, right?). Most trouble that arises here is from the wear and tear of everyday use. Referred to as *chondromalacia*, this degeneration can be amplified and accelerated by poor patellar tracking on the femur. If the quads are imbalanced or more sticky on one side than the other, or the femur isn't seated in its socket in a neutral position, the kneecap gets pulled at odd angles to its natural groove. This will wear down the articular cartilage on the kneecap in uneven patterns, eventually rubbing right on through it to leave you with bone-on-bone action. As I'm sure you would assume … that is painful. Folks with this condition will need to pad their knees with extra cushioning each time they come to the floor. You should also consider offering them hip-neutralizing instruction to see if changing the pull from the quads might reduce stresses on that system.

Tendinitis is common in the front of the knee, along the patellar tendon. Because our yoga practice often brings us down into kneeling positions, this tendon has the triple threat of physical compression (between the bones and the ground), overstretching (the knee gets deeply flexed, maxing out the length), and overwork (the quads are the primary mover from flexion to extension as you come out of the pose). These can combine into a perfect storm of irritation and inflammation. I advise *always* using a blanket to cushion the knees, alleviating some compression and friction. In addition, maintain good lunge alignment to reduce the piling-on of overwork/overstretch that can accompany poor form in high lunges. Lastly, if your student does end up with tendinitis, rest is best! Practicing with this inflammation will only exacerbate the condition. Rest, hydrotherapy, bodywork (once the acute phase has passed)—these are a better approach to healing.

"Shin splints" are common to any practitioner who also does high-impact exercise. This condition is often caused by inflammation of the connective tissue sheet that runs between the tibia and fibula. With each impact, the fibula bows slightly to help absorb some of that force. If that interosseous tissue is hard and dry when that impact occurs, or if the bone bows more than normal, the fascia will get irritated or torn, creating an inflammation response. It is also possible that severely adhered musculature in either the anterior or posterior compartments can cause inflammation to that tissue and cause pain. It's tough to modify for this in yoga, but self-massage or rolling out, along with stretching techniques, can help mitigate the effects.

COMPARTMENT SYNDROME

While common shin splints are a painful nuisance, it's important to recognize that there is a severe form of this injury that needs to be addressed immediately. Since we live in a world where our students may be involved in all sorts of other sports and athletic pursuits outside of their yoga practice, I think you should be aware of a condition called *compartment syndrome*.

Often caused by a direct blow to the shin, but sometimes through repeated shock absorption (such as in dance or gymnastics), it is an intense inflammation of the interosseous membrane between the two bones of the leg. Because some very integral blood vessels and nerves travel through this area, severe inflammation can cause real damage. Acute compartment syndrome is considered a MEDICAL EMERGENCY and should be treated as such. If a student comes in complaining of pain in the shin or leg, reports a history of being recently struck in the leg by any object, and exhibits hot, red, swollen tissue in the anterior shin, send them to the ER immediately. You are not a diagnostician, but this is not something to mess around with. Send them to a doctor and let them do the rest. You must refer them to someone with proper credentials; you can't make them go, but you need to impress upon them the likelihood that real risk is involved. Hopefully it's not so bad, but better to have someone else make that call.

Ankles and Feet. The plantar fascia can get irritated by too much tension and stickiness from the surrounding musculature (including the calf), or too much force being applied to a collapsing arch. This is called *plantar fasciitis*. Clients may complain of sharp, shooting pain when they bear weight, especially first thing in the morning or after sitting down for a while. For some people the pain is on the sole of the foot, while others may experience symptoms beginning on the back of the heel just where the Achilles tendon attaches.

There are varying approaches to this condition, some assuming it is inflammatory, others treating it like a chronic fascial restriction. I personally tend to apply a heat/massage/mobility model, paying close attention to the calf/shin muscles as well as the intrinsic plantar tissues. You might consider offering the whole class some time to massage their own feet, roll out the calves and shins, and mobilize the ankles. I'll offer more specific ways to do this in the next chapter.

Muscles

Psoas. As we discussed in the sidebar regarding psoas and sitting postures (see p. 145), those who habitually sit in chairs are not really likely to suffer from short psoas muscles. Those who sit in cross-legged postures most certainly will. Since the cross-legged camp is shortening the muscle in a passive way, it remains a question whether it is short but strong or short and weak. Likely, the latter is true.

So for now let's assume that most of us do not engage it the way we should in our daily life; therefore it's typically very weak. It might also be tough and taut and even spastic. This does certainly require some form of release, but stretching just may not be the appropriate treatment. Psoas needs blood flow, it needs tone. It needs to learn to fire at the appropriate times. For this, we need to *contract* it, not stretch it. We need to engage it in stable postures first, then ask it to work for us in more dynamic ways as it gains functional strength to actively flex the hip.

Avoiding deep gravitational extension is paramount to building a healthy psoas system. Understanding the role that it can play in our spinal neutrality and core stability can also help us engage it more usefully and keep it toned and responsive.

Abductors. These are fundamentally *stabilizing* muscles. We can tell this by how they have opposing muscle-fiber directions within the same belly; are short, squat muscles close to the joint; and are situated in a place that doesn't allow for dynamic range of motion. In this case, to strengthen them, we should be using them as they were designed and stabilize! Practice balancing poses, perhaps with some movement incorporated to access all their fibers over time (Tree to Warrior III to Half Moon, as an example).

Don't do work that takes them to their shortest length repeatedly, like "fire hydrant" leg lifts or "clam shells" or "lateral leg extensions" or any such nonsense. Because adduction is limited in range, we need to be cautious about shortening a muscle that we can't effectively lengthen through its counteraction. There is no good way to stretch these; we can only "roll them out" or offer them massage.

Adductors. The adductors get overlooked much of the time in favor of the groups they assist in flexion and extension. These muscles don't get used much in the average activities of daily living because we rarely move from side to side. That means that most people working the nine-to-fives have weak, possibly tight adductors that need to be contracted to get strong and healthy.

Then there are the dancers, athletes, yogis, and weekend warriors who use these muscles by expanding their range of motion to include lateral movement, but not necessarily in a healthy way. There is an injury that occurs in yoga especially that is often self-diagnosed as a hamstring strain: in the tendon, near the insertion to the ischial tuberosity. Yogis describe a recurrent, painful point that aches constantly, is aggravated by stretching, and felt when they sit down on their sitting bones. Here's the thing ... it's not their hamstring; it's their *adductor magnus*. This muscle attaches as far back on the ischia as you can get, and it doubles as an extensor along with the hamstrings. Because of its position and action, it is often confused for its neighboring muscles, and it is just as prone to strain because of all of the forward folding we do.

Some complex geometry exists at the hip joint when you go into a deep forward fold. If the femurs internally rotate too much (this is

pretty easy to do, since sometimes we're actually instructed to press our inner thighs to the back wall), the angles created make a little slack in hamstrings and emphasize the adductor magnus instead. Few of us are aware that the adductor attachments lack the muscular action to control the movement, and we don't add the counteraction needed from glute max. Adductor magnus ends up overworked and strained, and we continually reinjure it because we try to protect our hamstrings instead. A subtle balance between active internal and external rotation at the hip will help protect this muscle in forward folds.

Risks to the Lower Extremity

SI Hypermobility. You may or may not have noticed that we skipped right over this joint in the range of motion section, but we did, intentionally. Functionally, the SI is not meant to move much. But because of the asymmetrical nature of many of our standing and seated postures, most yoga practitioners will inevitably overstretch the ligaments of the pelvis, which results in hypermobility. If it's minor, you may not even feel it. If it is severe, there may be inflammation and pain, stiffness and sensitivity in certain movements. There may even be nerve irritation and trigger points that create seemingly unrelated pain patterns. To minimize the development of SI hypermobility, or to slow down further degeneration, you'll need to remain diligently aware of the stability of your pelvis as a whole, using counteractions so hip extension is supported and compensations are absorbed through the entire system: thigh, hip, SI, low back, deep core, etc.

Torn Labrum. There are many ways the coxal labrum can get torn, but in yoga it's

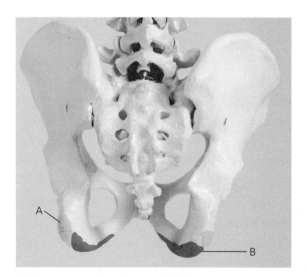

(A) Hamstring attachments, (B) Adductor magnus attachments

often due to compression—deep hip flexions and rotations at angles that aren't in tune with your own bony structure. Mostly, folks come to class having already torn this tissue and only exacerbate the condition in their practice. Pain may be felt locally at the hip, groin, or anterior pelvis, but many people also experience referral pain to the SI, low belly, low back, lateral hip, and inner thigh. Once the coxal labrum is torn, there is no really good fix. Minor tears can be maintained for years if you are thoughtful about limiting your range of motion and avoiding movements that elicit a sharp or pinching pain. Surgery is the only "cure" for severe tears.

Dysplasia. *Dysplasia* is the head of the femur not fitting securely into the socket. Oftentimes this is due to genetic factors, but it may happen over time as a result of hypermobility in the hip. It can lead to increased degeneration of the labrum and articulating cartilages of the hip, as well as alignment issues downstream that will affect the knee and ankle. Students may say things like, "It feels like my hip will pop out of the socket." It's extremely important to teach these students to hold back from their deepest range of motion and to exercise more precise counteractions to build off the deep stabilizers of the hip.

Knee Hyperextension. Hyperextension in the knee is both a sign of and a risk for ligament sprain or permanent destabilization of the knee. Offer plenty of cueing to keep knees micro-bent, counteracted, and supportive. Offer props in postures like Pyramid and Triangle for those folks with extreme hyperextension.

Tendinitis. Inflammation of the tendons is most common in the adductor or hamstring attachments at the hip (forward folds), patellar tendon of the knee (poor alignment in lunges), and the Achilles (overstretching, squats, lunges). This condition really does require rest and self-care. When coming back to practice, students need to be more precise in their alignment, keep the affected tendon's muscles active while stretching, and maintain their ice/heat/anti-inflammatory treatments through their first few weeks back in action.

Turf Toe. This is an inflammatory condition of the ligaments and tendons of the big toe flexors (sole of the foot). Often it is precipitated in practice by active lunges that challenge the strength and stamina of the sole of the foot. Off the mat, it can be caused by dance, sprinting, or agility exercises. Since this a sprain-strain injury, the RICE protocol is called for: rest, ice, compression, elevation. Sometimes a boot is prescribed by a physician to ensure immobility and limited weight bearing.

Relationship to the Spine

Because of the structure of the sacroiliac joint, the lower extremity and the spine cannot be separated functionally—adhering to the Law of Compensation, "where the pelvis goes, the spine follows." The femur begins to act as a lever on the pelvis, so the forces you apply to the thigh will translate almost directly to the spine. This is where I reiterate the need to consciously stabilize the spine while moving the hip, and vice versa. In order to build the awareness to keep all the structures safe, it's best to isolate the different parts, learn to control them well, then reintegrate them once you are proficient.

Since extension in the hip is so limited, there is an increased level of compensation at the spine in this range. To control for the spine compensating, the abdominal core must engage precisely to maintain the lumbar lordosis without cranking into a compressive hyperlordosis. This is a sweet dance of finding the muscular limits of our hip without going into the ligaments, while also finding the length of a decompressed and fully supported lumbar spine. Remember, you can decompress the lumbar spine significantly by engaging the upper abdominals and supporting Uddiyana Bandha. We rarely decompress by tucking the tail or flexing the lumbar spine itself.

This relationship works universally in backbends as well. When you do your Cobra family postures, prone backbends that lift up out of gravity, it's necessary to keep the gluteal contraction moderated. If you clench the glutes, you essentially create a brick wall that jams up around the tailbone and sacrum. This means that all the energy of your pose can get concentrated into the L5 area, and compression becomes inevitable. But if you fire the hip flexors slightly, the gluteal action is moderated, and the tail has an escape route. Now the legs and energetic roots are very active, but you can access a lengthening of the spine from the center out through the ends (using the Uddiyana model and a precise action in the upper extremity), instead of a compressive force from the ends in. This principle holds for all the backbends really, but I think it's easiest to feel it out in the Cobra family.

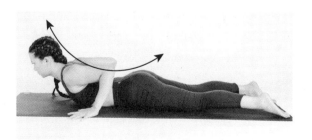

In the Bridge family, supine backbends that lift up out of gravity, it's really tempting to use the glutes to thrust the pelvis to the sky, but this can cause that same jamming into L5. If you moderate this action and use a combo of the hamstrings and glutes to lift the thighs, but keep the neutral curve in the lumbar spine, you have the opportunity to shift the energy of the pose up into the thoracic spine and sternum while also relieving the compression at the sacrum. The spine becomes a more balanced curve from tail to neck, and the legs become the engine that drives the chest closer to the chin.

In spinal rotation, the pelvis tends to follow along in rotation as well. This is another example of movement we want to isolate into the spine while stabilizing the pelvis, instead of allowing the pelvis to rotate just to look and feel like we're going deeper. To ensure we are not going into our most lax places and avoiding the real work of spinal twisting, we need to keep our lumbar spine and pelvis united and active. Using the edge of a blanket to elevate the hips in seated twists not only offers some relief from the hamstrings pulling on the pelvis, but it also gives you a tactile cue to whether your pelvis has remained stable. The pelvis should remain parallel to the blanket as you move through the thoracic spine. This requires the firing of both the adductors and abductors to find lateral stability, and deep core action, to isolate rotation into the ribs.

Because many of our standing postures involve asymmetrical legs, we have to consider what is optimal pelvic alignment, so that both the hip and the spine are safe and our work is effective. Lunges are a great way to figure out what subtle shifts in weight bearing and core actions can offer in terms of alignment. It can look like a complicated mess at first, but when

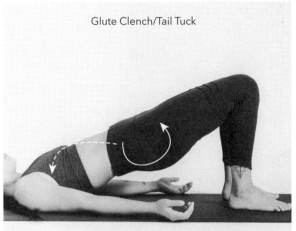

Glute Clench/Tail Tuck

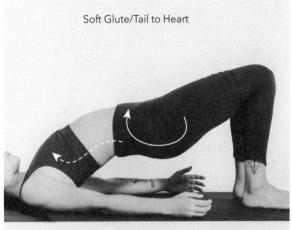

Soft Glute/Tail to Heart

broken down one action at a time, it comes to make sense. Let's do a practice session here and observe these actions.

Experiential Learning

When we are in lunges, the flexion in one leg and extension in the other present us with a potential torsion of the pelvis (front leg supporting a neutral pelvis, back leg pulling toward anterior tilt), as well as rotation (often the back-leg side is pulled back, creating an "open" feel toward Warrior II alignment). These are all fine forces—if we manage our hip and core activation effectively. Otherwise, they can wreak havoc on the SI and lumbosacral joints.

To bring action into our stance means employing counteraction at both the hips and the spine. So, from a high lunge with right leg forward, play with these various opposing actions and shifts in weight bearing to see how the alignment of the pelvis and low back are affected, as well as deep core engagement:

- Weight in right heel, upright spine → Notice how much effort is required by the entire front leg and what

tendencies there are in your spine. Is it naturally in neutral, flexion, or extension?

- Shift your entire weight forward and back → Feel how the work in the legs changes as the thighs rebalance your weight.

- Pada Bandha active in back foot vs. pulling heel back → Notice how much upward energy can be generated by pressing through the ball of the foot instead of the heel. There is often a profound lift, stacking heel over toes, active arches, light shin bone and thigh, all translating to a lifted pelvis overall.

- Pull left thigh forward underneath you, pull right thigh back underneath you → The action of scissoring the legs (they won't move much, but the deep muscles will certainly activate) counters the sense of the feet pressing away from the core, and it adds to the levity of the entire upper body. Note: there is now a connection made from Pada Bandha to Mula Bandha.

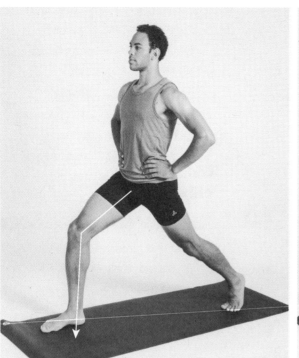
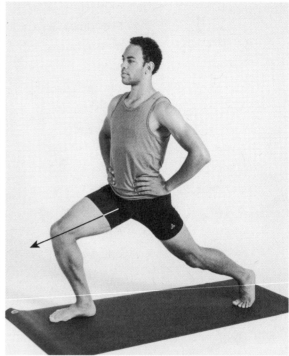

When the knee is centered over the heel, energy grounds efficiently through the knee to the ankle. If the knee aligns past the heel, all of the body weight-energy moves straight out through the knee ligaments, increasing risk of degeneration and injury over time.

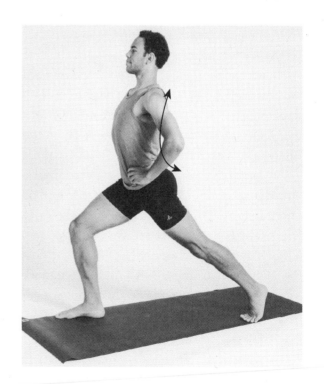

- Use your back leg like a very strong kickstand Instead of relying mostly on the front leg to bear your weight, try allowing the left thigh to press forward as if it could tuck under the pelvis, then lean the entire core body onto it a bit. Notice how light the front leg can be when the back leg takes more of the workload. (Subtle! No need to overdo this and overstretch hip flexors.)

- Practice lifting the tail energetically, or perhaps physically for some of us, to engage the low paraspinal muscles Does this make it easier to gather your low belly toward your spine? Tilt the tail down, move back and forth between the two, and examine the differences.

- Drop knee to a low lunge using different hip actions → At first drop left knee down with whatever momentum comes naturally. Did the right knee shift forward? What happens in the low back? Now try coming down without letting the right knee come forward of the ankle. Is there a difference in how you have to engage the thighs and hips and low belly? Repeat the slow dropping and lifting, tapping the knee lightly to the mat and back up again.

- From a low lunge, hands on blocks, shift weight back and forth between the right leg and left leg → Is there a shift in how your side body responds to these altered forces? Is one side-waist shorter than the other, or do you maintain your spinal axis? What core actions need to come into play to do that?

- Wag your tail; do this while stabilizing the ribs, and then allow the ribs to move with the pelvis as one unit → What is the difference in weight bearing? Does the core respond the same way when the ribs are stable?

- From a high lunge with hands on blocks, take left foot flat to the mat for a Warrior foot → Notice if that movement can be done solely in the hip joint, or if the whole pelvis comes along for the ride, twisting the low spine.

These exercises will help build your insights on how the lower extremity affects the spine and core in various ways as we move through our practice. Keeping our compensations at the forefront of our mind will ensure that we bring attention to them in class, noticing our own reactions as well as clearly observing these common maladjustments in our students. The following chapter goes into sweet detail about the cues we can develop to help our classes grow through these internal observations and actions.

10

The Lower Extremity: Principles of Teaching and Practice Mechanics

This chapter will focus on the teaching aspect of the lower extremity in our yoga practice. Now that you have some knowledge of the individual differences you can encounter and the potential ramifications of those differences, we'll discuss how to apply that knowledge directly to the mat. Just as we did in the spine chapters, we'll examine and discuss common misalignments, modifications, and adjustments. We'll also pinpoint specific ways to talk about the lower extremity. Since there are so many joints that impact one another, we'll need to find ways to address postures from the ground up, both physically and energetically.

Principles of Teaching

Just as in the spine, we need to be particularly mindful of people with hypermobility in the joints of the lower extremity. In the spine there are a couple of commonly weak points, so too in the hip, knee, ankle, and foot. Folks with weakness in the stabilizing muscles of the major joints will be at more risk of injuries than those who have finite control of those contractions. Our language will need to reflect the sense of counteraction and muscular support that can prevent hypermobility injuries.

We need to learn to see a person's bony blueprint even if they aren't already standing in it. We need to get comfortable asking people to adjust themselves on the mat for more centered support of their core. We need to notice when students are aware only of their legs or only of their spine. Most folks aren't going to naturally make the connection between their feet, legs, and core—we need to learn to see those disconnections and then speak to them directly. We need to instruct the principles of isolating our effort in order to integrate the whole system.

Here are some things to consider with regard to the lower extremity and its role in the greater practice (some of these will seem familiar, I'm sure):

- Does the pose demand action or stability in the hips? How does that relate to the spine? Remember, usually a pose is mobile in one while active in the other, especially in the act of transitional movements or vinyasa flowing sequences.

- More movement in the hip—like hyperextension—isn't indicative of a deeper or more advanced practice ... it's just a sign that your student isn't supporting themselves effectively in gravity.

- Compensation in the hips is the enemy of integrity in the spine. Make sure there is agreement between the two regions.

- Maintain the energetic cohesion between the foundation and the core. Whether you are teaching a standing pose or not, make sure that the feet, legs, pelvis, and spine all communicate with each other. It's usually a conversation that flows back and forth, not a one-way monologue.

Observation Skills

Now that we are adept at seeing the spinal alignment, we need to become familiar with the integration of the lower extremity. Initially, it's not so tough to look at the spine and see what's

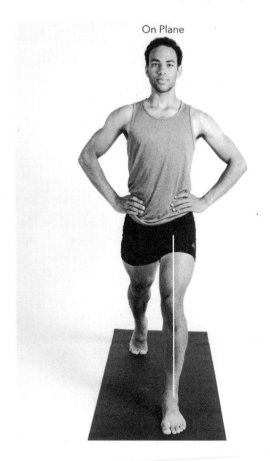

On Plane

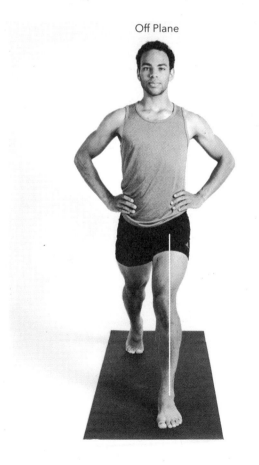

Off Plane

off. Nor is it too tough to see where the legs need to shift. What may seem more daunting is predicting how shifts in one area will affect the other. Can you see the entire system to determine if problems in the spinal alignment actually originate in the lower extremity?

Get in the habit of going through a little checklist to ensure you have seen the alignment of the spine in relation to the hips. Look for the following, whether in standing, lunging, or supine postures.

Heel-Knee-Hip Plane. In the standing poses, whether they are Chairs or Lunges or Warriors, you want to be able to see the heel, knee, and hip on one continuous plane. A common deviation from this is a bent knee drifting in toward midline. If you press that knee laterally, back in line with the hip and ankle, oftentimes the pelvis will come into agreement with the ribs.

If the back leg looks janky in lunges, like the knee is knocked in toward midline, you'll need to check a couple of things: Is the back foot wide enough, and is the hip internally rotated? I find that usually both of these things are happening simultaneously.

Pada Bandha. If the arches collapse and Pada Bandha is not engaged, the lines all the way up to the spine will suffer. If significant deviation exists in the heel-knee-hip plane, then the Pada Bandha may be the culprit. Make sure you observe the actions of their feet in addition to making adjustments from the hip. There should be no overt signs of gripping the toes or forced gathering of the inner arch, but instead a general lightness through the entire center of the foot.

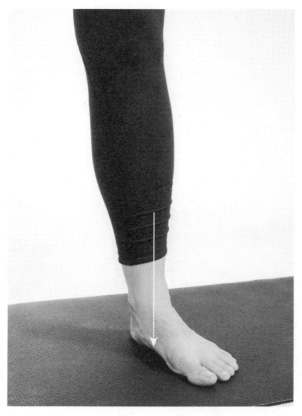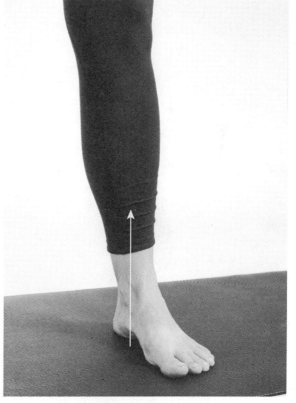

Rooting through the big-toe root and the outer heel provides rebound to the arches.

For some folks, depending on the shape of their bones, they'll have a nearly impossible time activating Pada Bandha unless they allow a slight turn-out of the feet, sometimes one foot more than the other. Usually, this turn-out neutralizes the hip joints and automatically fixes any issues with the heel-knee-hip plane. You'll very likely need to encourage this, since they're unlikely to recognize that they need it.

Heel to Knee to Hip Alignment. This has a few subcategories:

- **Feet Hip-Width.** You are most likely to find aligned hips if the feet take most postures from hip width. Watch where students place their feet when lunging or setting up standing postures, but also help them find a true hip-width stance for symmetrical postures like

forward folds and Chair. These poses lose a ton of energy if the feet are too narrow, because the adductors and quads take over and the glutes go slack.

- **Knees Hip-Width.** If your feet are as wide as your hip joints, your knees should also align with your hip joints. If the knees knock in in any posture, you're not as stable as you could be. Use subtle external rotation from the hips to ensure that the line from foot to knee to hip is straight, and that left and right thighs are roughly parallel to each other. This is true in both straight- and bent-knee postures.

- **Toes Turned Out.** Notice that we are discussing the HEEL-knee-hip alignment. Parallel edges or even arches aren't

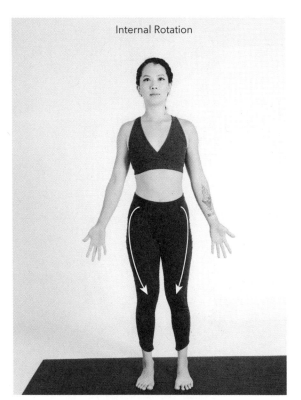
Internal Rotation

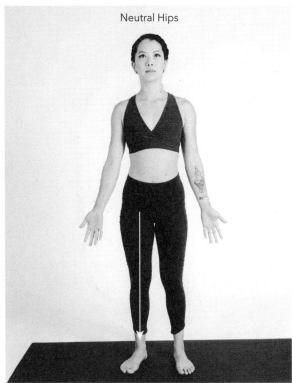
Neutral Hips

Feet parallel is actually internal rotation for many hip joints.

necessarily the most grounded or best aligned feet for the individual. If there are significant structural torsions in either the femur or the tibia, the direction the feet point and the direction the knees point may not agree. If the hip is neutral in rotation but a femoral or tibial torsion exists, the knee may point straight ahead while the feet turn out. Or vice versa, or some other combination. In many cases, the feet may need to point outward to keep the knees in safe alignment throughout a flow.

Pelvis/Rib Agreement (Find the Axis). Make sure that the ribs and pelvis line up. Are the ribs forward of the pelvis? Are the ribs off to one side? Are you in a side bend? Offer cues that help dial in the axis of the spine to ensure that compensations are minimized. Some students will find it difficult to isolate movement of the ribs from the pelvis, so hands-on adjustments may be necessary.

Tail Bone Trajectory. In asymmetrical poses especially, it's common for the pelvis to hike up on the forward-leg side. Here is a principle that nearly always stands in these cases: we want to make a powerful connection between the coccyx and the back heel. That is not to say we pull the tail down toward the heel, but we make rotational adjustments instead. In order to stay on axis, we need the tail to hug toward the back leg, not just shift over to one side, as if the whole sacrum is turning like a dial until the "arrow" of the tail meets the midline. This is a pretty fine-tuned kind of adjustment and may require some hands-on help at first.

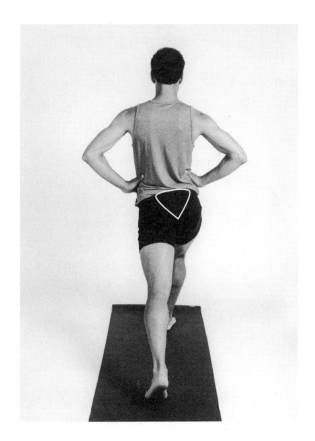
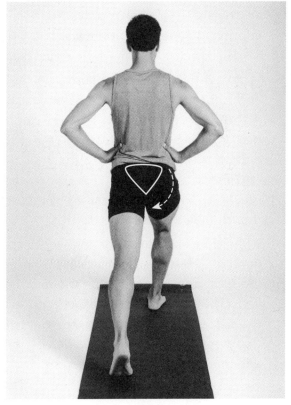

Experiential Learning

To build your observation skills, you'll want to enlist a friend or two from your Yoga Engineer community as models in order to train your eyes to look for the visual cues we just noted. Do not limit your observations to these points, however. Start there, but remain open to seeing the body that is actually in front of you, the bones it actually has, and the real-time imbalances that may arise. Use their clothing and bony landmarks as indicators of these imbalances.

In groups of three if possible, one student takes a low lunge, knee on the ground. Two observers watch and take note of the effects of the leg/spine relationship as the student makes precise shifts: Weight forward, weight back, shift into the left leg, and then into the right leg.

BONES DEFINE HIP-WIDTH

Remember those optical illusions we discussed in the spine chapter? Well, something similar can exist here in the lower extremity. Ideally, as you observe the lineups of heels and knees and hips, as you question whether the tailbone is aligned, as you determine whether knees need to press out or in toward midline, you are "seeing" the bony body with your X-ray vision. Perhaps you are able to see the energetic flow as well, tracing the prana from the earth to the core and back again. What you *don't* want to work with is the contours of a person's flesh. That can be misleading information and throw both you and your student off track.

Hip-width is not thigh-width. Thighs have curves and contours. Some curve more on the inside and some on the outside. Even though thigh bones curve and bend, the hip joint remains just wide of the pubic arch, a bony framework that doesn't change with age or weight or hormones. Your two fists (actual fists) placed side by side in front of your pubic bone approximates your own personal hip-joint-width. If you drop those fists down to hang between your ankle bones (ankles, not arches or big toes), those ankles will align under the neck of the femur, idealizing the weight bearing of the upper body on the legs. Use the bones, my friends (see images on p.49)!!

For most postures, that hip-width stance will be more ideal than feet near midline. Keep an eye on this in asymmetrical postures, anything with one foot back. We have a tendency to ride the midline when we step back or forward, so be vigilant. There are some cases where the front foot may need to step even wider, if the shape of the femur requires that to achieve a more stable hip joint. Be mindful that the bones, not the variables of soft tissue, are your keystone to fundamental alignment.

Wag your tail; do this while stabilizing the ribs, and then allow the ribs to move with the pelvis as one unit. Engage the feet in different ways; press more through the ball of the foot, and then through the heel. In low lunge, press through the back shin. Note how these changes reverberate through the entire system: legs, pelvis, core, ribs, even shoulders and neck. Are these physical changes or pranic ones? All of these observations will help us make more practical adjustments down the line.

Vocabulary

In class we don't want to overwhelm our students with an inordinate amount of technospeak. Since I know you are just soaking up all of this information like a sponge, you can't wait to get into the studio and show everyone all the things you're learning! Unfortunately, we all have probably experienced some form of that class, whether it's anatomy or philosophy or Sanskrit or metaphors that get so lofty and lengthy that we honestly can't follow what they're saying. In order to avoid that, let's take some time to work through, in both creative and systematic ways, some methods for describing movements, actions, intentions, energetic flow, and placement of the lower extremity in our asana practice.

In the spine chapter, we did this with word clouds, and like I said, they're one of my favorite ways to study and build on an idea, perfect for creating connections between subjects that superficially may not seem related. This time, let's use a flowchart. I think this format helps make more specific connections, ways to present the same information differently.

An example (see Flowchart on the next page): Let's say we're going to step back from a forward fold to a lunge. We need to know what part is moving, where it's moving to, and how it's gonna get there, right? What are all the options we can use to describe this particular movement, from technical to specific to esoteric? It's a very simplistic example, but it will offer an idea of how this tool works. Can you use this template to change the language you might use in a similar sequence?

Using this method, outline descriptors for other actions, posture refinements, or transitions. Some possibilities:

- From Mountain, reaching arms overhead
- From Prayer, transitioning to Cow/Cat
- From Downward Facing Dog to stepping forward to lunge

There are endless options for this exercise. If it works for you, you can build a deep reservoir of cues for any movement in your asana practice.

If you are working with a group in YTT or have gathered some like-minded Yoga Engineering students, there are other ways to approach this. Using the various tools we've offered so far (flowcharts, lists, word clouds, etc.), brainstorm words that can be used in class to convey the information we've learned about the bones, muscles, and range of motion of the lower extremity. Include descriptors for the knee and the foot.

Each group will begin with a commonly taught posture—lunge, Warrior I, Warrior II, Triangle, etc.—and expand the descriptors and instructions available for each focal point: feet, knees, hips, and spine. There are a ton of approaches to this, so get creative, go with your gut, avoid the most common cues, and be specific.

Example Flowchart

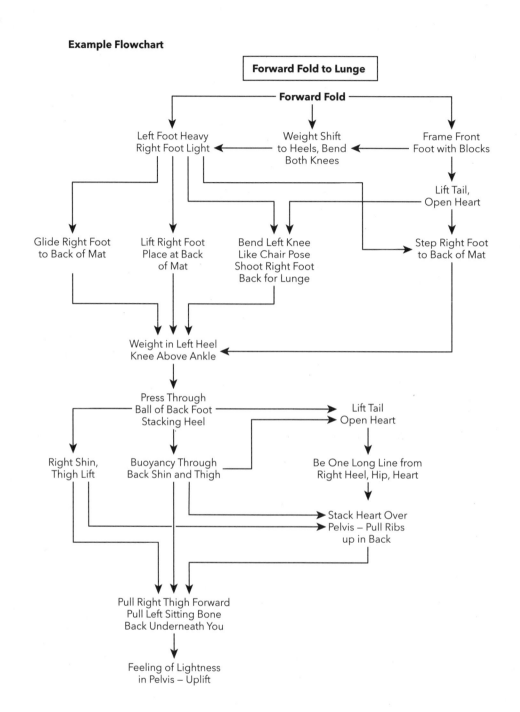

Forward Fold to Lunge

Forward Fold

Left Foot Heavy
Right Foot Light

Weight Shift
to Heels, Bend
Both Knees

Frame Front
Foot with Blocks

Lift Tail,
Open Heart

Glide Right Foot
to Back of Mat

Lift Right Foot
Place at Back
of Mat

Bend Left Knee
Like Chair Pose
Shoot Right Foot
Back for Lunge

Step Right Foot
to Back of Mat

Weight in Left Heel
Knee Above Ankle

Press Through
Ball of Back Foot
Stacking Heel

Lift Tail
Open Heart

Right Shin,
Thigh Lift

Buoyancy Through
Back Shin and Thigh

Be One Long Line from
Right Heel, Hip, Heart

Stack Heart Over
Pelvis – Pull Ribs
up in Back

Pull Right Thigh Forward
Pull Left Sitting Bone
Back Underneath You

Feeling of Lightness
in Pelvis – Uplift

Cueing Principles

In any given posture, there are 100+ items that you could focus on and deliberate on. Okay, that may be an exaggeration, but when you're up there in front of a class, seeing all you can see, noticing all the little things that each person does differently and all the tweaks that are possible, it certainly feels like there are that many things to cover. You can simplify this, though. If you have a theme for your class or a peak pose that you need to get to, cue the details that are most relevant to that pose or theme. This will create continuity between postures that may otherwise seem unrelated.

Remember that in cueing the lower extremity, you must *consider the compensations for the movements on the spine and core*. In standing postures it is common to cue from the bottom up, but this isn't always the most efficient use of your time and breath. If you have already taught the base one time through, it may be more effective to really pay attention to students' spinal stability. But if you are teaching a twist, you may need to emphasize the stability of the base in order to move more efficiently in the spine. Always consider your intention. What needs to stabilize? What needs to move? Which must come first?

In the lower extremity it's also important to think about **momentum**. Momentum is the enemy of strength! If your students are launching forward from lunge to forward fold or Warrior III, then they are working against their ability to build strength deep in the hips and core. They are missing out on the opportunity to increase their balance, grace, and fluid movement. At first, breaking these transitions down into small increments will feel robotic, but in building this stamina over time their movements will actually become more fluid, and the thrusting, leaping actions will diminish. Isolate to integrate!

As introduced in chapter 6, a number of ubiquitous cues have filtered down through the oral history of the modern yoga practice. Please be mindful of rhetorical cueing. Regurgitating the words we have heard over and over is a natural practice, especially as a new teacher, but the longer you are in front of a class, the more thoughtful you can become about the cues you use. Hopefully you will begin to observe the specific movements of the bodies in front of you, and you will not speak only out of habit but will respond to the misalignments you actually witness.

For many teachers, this begins with a deeper awareness of what you feel in your own body as you practice on your own or demonstrate postures in class, recognizing your own habits for weakness or clenching, the places you tend to misalign or forget about completely. After all, if you feel those in your own body, it's very likely that someone else out in the room is also experiencing it. We can't rely on this forever though, because if we're mostly tuned in to our own body, we can't be readily observant of our students. There comes a time when you have to walk away from your mat at the front of the class and trust your words. Trust your previous experience, trust your eyes, trust your deeper understanding of what the body needs from these movements and actions.

In the next section I describe in greater detail a few of those oft-used phrases, and I either support or discredit them. Be especially aware of these, but it would be good practice to consider others that you hear in class regularly and analyze them on your own. Are they truly accurate? Are they really useful? Do they have a functional purpose, or are they designed mostly to make it sound like a teacher knows something technical?

I'm also adding to this list some principles I think are really important from either a physiological or an energetic perspective. They are pretty much the same thing, so we'll address them as such. These are ideas that could help specifically support the principles of counteraction and prevent compensation. These are cues that I have seen actually improve my students' awareness of buoyancy, lift, and integrity. All of those qualities combine to build strength, fluidity, and grace.

Tucking the Tail (or variations on this)

Write down some variations of this instruction, all the ways you hear this cue in class ... then burn them! A ceremonial flushing of this totally ridiculous instruction will be good for the soul, and really good for future yoga practice.

Just in case you missed this in the spine section: If I ever hear of you using this phrase (I will certainly know it through my mystical yoga teacher-of-teachers ways), I will smack you with cosmic lightning whips, just as Sri Iyengar did with his stick. Whether referring to the perceived spinal decompression, or emphasizing the extension of the hip for more stretch in the hip flexors, this instruction is inappropriate nearly 100 percent of the time. No good can come from this cue. The spine follows the pelvis ... tucking the tail is essentially a posterior tilt of the pelvis, which causes flattening of the lumbar curve. That's no good in the long run. If those hip flexors are your aim, keep in mind that they are rarely short to start with, so eking out a few more centimeters of length ought to be very low on your list of priorities. What's high on that list?? Protecting and supporting the lumbar lordosis. Period.

The irony is that most students need to emphasize their lumbar curve, not diminish it. That means that instead of asking folks to tuck the tail, we should offer the opposite:

> "Please lift your tail/sacrum toward the back of the heart ... feel the low back muscles engage ... draw the low belly

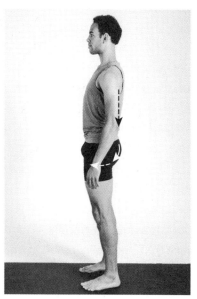 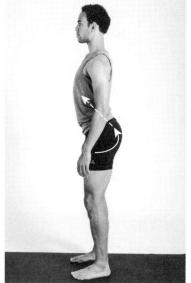 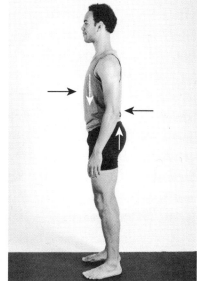

muscles back to support the organs, engage the pelvic floor, and stabilize this new forward curve of the lumbar spine."

Variations on these new instructions will help slowly build strength in the intrinsic muscles of the spine, reshape the lordotic curve, and generate deeper core stability over time. I've had numerous students relieve their chronic low-back pain by shifting this common but misguided paradigm.

Knee over the Ankle (Lunges, etc.)

This is a good one!! Well, most of the time. If you are in high lunges or any of the Warrior postures where the back leg is straight with the knee off the ground, it is integral to the long-term health of the knee ligaments to keep that front knee stacked over its ankle. What's interesting is many people won't

actually do this, even when told to, unless they know the consequences. Inform them of those!

"You may not feel pain now, but damage is being done. Stretching your ligaments, or even micro-tearing them as you can in that posture, will lead to major injury down the road. Keep it together, yogis!"

In high lunges, the weight of the body has forward momentum. If the front shin is upright, the physics of the pose very efficiently transfer that weight down the tibia and into the heel. Once the knee passes the ankle, however, the physics change, and most of the body's weight is projected along the femur and out through the knee. These forces are significant, and over time will stretch and even erode the fibers of the cruciate ligaments that are meant to stabilize against forward/backward stresses.

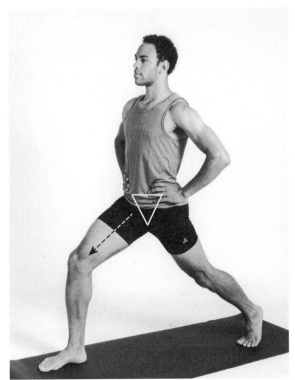
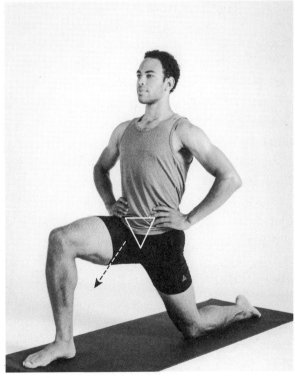

"Make sure that your front knee does not move past the ankle, the shin should be perfectly upright. Your ligaments are at risk here once the knee passes that point, no matter how strong you are … Let the heel take more weight than the forefoot—your glutes will do more work, and the forces will transfer efficiently from the thigh to the shin and into the heel, not out through your knee."

When you drop the back knee to the floor, however, the center of gravity shifts, and the onus of the body weight shifts to the hips, relieving the front knee ligaments of the burden of forward momentum. That knee is now perfectly safe to move past the plane of the ankle, as long as the ankle's bones and soft tissue allow it.

"Taking your back knee to the mat, make sure it lands at hip-width. Now the weight is centered in your hips, making it perfectly safe to let the front knee pass beyond the ankle, if your other soft tissue allows for it."

All of these instructions are even more important for those who have no ACL because of injury or surgical procedures. Not everyone actually gets that ligament replaced right away, so if you're aware of that condition for a particular student, emphasize these instructions for them before class and during these postures. They are at much higher risk for long-term injury to the menisci and strain in the quad tendon.

Weight Bearing in Standing Poses

There are some basic rules for the standing poses that apply some pretty basic physics to the system of bones and joints in the lower extremity. We want to harness the energy of gravity and use it to our advantage instead of addressing it as an adversary. Our aim is to create the most efficient track for the forces of gravity to follow, without losing any energy to "leaky" places like the ligaments of a locked or slack joint. These principles are outlined here.

Straight Leg Rules

When you are in a posture with straight legs, whether it's the leg in front or back, this principle applies: your weight bearing should originate in the root of the big toe, cross the foot to the outer heel, and travel in an external spiral of action up to the outer hip. This pattern will engage Pada Bandha, the front and back channels of the leg and thigh, and the external rotators of the hip. No one muscle group will

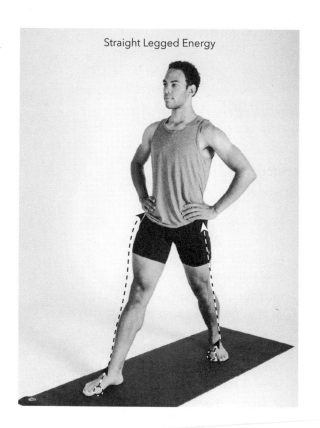

Straight Legged Energy

have to overwork, and you'll be less likely to lock out the knee or hyperextend.

Example: Triangle (Trikonasana), right leg forward:

> "Straight front leg, straight back leg. Press through the right big toe mound, let that be your anchor. Root as well through the outer heel, let that diagonal force support your arch and activate Pada Bandha. Let that spiral travel up the leg to the outer thigh and hip, pulling the sitting bone toward the back wall and activating the glutes. Anchor as well through the left big toe, then along the outer edge of the foot to the outer heel, grounding down that edge so the inner arch activates and rises. Make that energetic connection to the outer left hip, gently firing glutes to help you feel lift through the entire pelvis."

This rule is most noticeable in asymmetrical postures like the Warriors and Pyramid, where the straight leg is at a diagonal to the earth instead of upright, but it is absolutely necessary in standing forward folds as well. Remember, "forward folds have forward momentum," and the weight is always focused into the forefoot. This is true at neutral or in wide-leg variations.

> "As you fold forward, let the weight shift to the ball of the foot. The heels are light on the earth and the knees bend as needed to hinge deeply in the hips without dumping into the low back. The tips of the toes are light, the forefoot pressing down to maintain your balance. Even as the forefoot roots, the thighs and hips have upward momentum, they may or may not actually move higher, but the energy is there."

Bent-Knee Rules

In bent-kneed postures the weight is shifted into the heels. The big toe remains grounded via the muscular actions of the calf, but it does not take the burden of the body's weight, supporting our Pada Bandha. It is preferable that the knee stacks directly over the ankle, because in these poses the body weight tends to have forward momentum, which can drive a ton of force through the length of the femur and out through the cruciate ligaments of the knee. If the knee is stacked, however, and the heel bears the weight instead of the forefoot, and the large muscles of the hip engage fully (extensors and external rotators), relieving the quads of the full burden and preventing their fatigue, all while energy is translated efficiently from the femur to the tibia to the

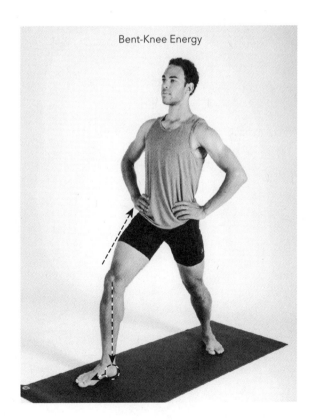

Bent-Knee Energy

calcaneus. Very little if any energy is lost to the ligaments because the muscles and fascial lines are engaged from the roots to the core.

Example: Warrior II (Virabhadrasana II), right leg forward:

"Bend right knee just over the ankle, not beyond. Let the heel take more weight than the forefoot. Feel the hips engage to take a little effort out of the knee. Imagine the hip crease pulling back toward the back wall, even as the shin presses forward. Try not to drop the hips too low, perhaps even pulling that right heel back to feel a little lift from underneath and buoyancy in the pelvis."

Balance Postures

These are a special category all their own. They are straight-leg postures, but they use the bent-knee principles. Just like in Mountain, balance postures rely on the most subtle zigzagging anterior/posterior counteractions, as well as the structural stability of the ankle joints, to ensure maximum efficiency in translating gravity through the upright system. If you put too much effort or weight into the forefoot in a balance posture, the arches collapse, you lose Pada Bandha, and the intrinsic muscles of the foot fatigue very quickly.

Example: Tree (Vrksasana), right leg up:

"Soften your left knee, and gently hinge in the left hip so you can sit back onto the left heel. Press down through that heel, then anchor the big toe root ... use the muscle of the leg, don't just lean forward again. There's a sense of sitting back ... Now push down through the heel to stand up tall, but keep the weight back. Resist the urge to thrust the pelvis forward. The arch is active, but the entire leg holds you up instead of just your foot."

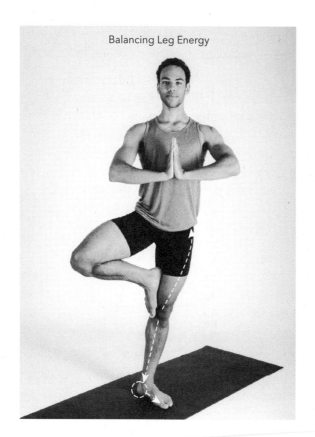

Balancing Leg Energy

The raised foot, whether rooted to the standing leg in Tree pose variations or hanging out in space as in the Extended Hand to Big Toe postures, also needs to be active and express Pada Bandha. This will help keep the pelvis balanced and the hip joints stabilized, as well as connecting both leg-roots into the core.

"As you place the right foot onto the inner thigh, press with the heel more than the forefoot, feel your right hip engage a bit. Now allow the forefoot to root as well, gently gripping the inner thigh with your arch, not just your toes. Keep the whole foot actively engaged; Pada Bandha. Press your standing leg into the foot as well, allow them to meet each other in the middle, one shouldn't overpower the other."

Lifting the Kneecap to Protect the Knee

This cue is most often heard in hot-yoga classes during balance postures, though I have heard it elsewhere. If you look at pictures of these admittedly extraordinary postures, they tend to have one thing in common: the knee of the standing leg is locked or even hyperextended. I mean, most of the body's weight is reaching forward in these poses, so that has to be countered somewhere, right? Well, in my opinion, the muscles of the leg and core need to find a different active equilibrium, not just rely on the knee's ligaments.

So here we have a muscular action cue to help ... Unfortunately, the act of "lifting the kneecap" is engaging the quadriceps, which are knee *extensors*. If you are doing this forcefully without any counteracting actions in the hamstrings, you are 100 percent going to lock out the knee joint, and most of the energy of the balance pose will be sent into the ligaments. It's doing exactly the opposite of supporting the

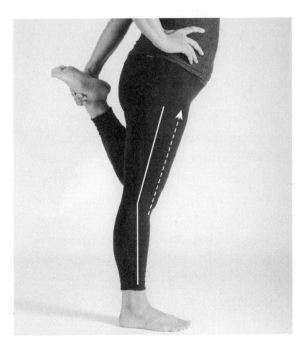

Lifting the kneecap only serves to reinforce hyperextension.

knee. In fact, that scenario leaves the joint at high risk for injury, either cataclysmic trauma at the time or accelerated wear and tear of the ACL/PCL, which will lead to increasing instability and degeneration of the joint overall.

It is imperative, then, that you always keep a slight bend in the knee when activating the quads with all you've got. This is the precise reason the rule of counteraction exists: you cannot muscularly stabilize any joint when you activate one of the muscle groups in isolation. You must use both opposing groups in equal measure to ensure the energy is shifted out of ligaments and into the myofascial tissues. In the case of balance postures, you bend the knee, take the weight into the heel, and slightly flex the hip. These actions combine to fire the glutes A LOT. Those glutes will get stronger over time, and THAT is what will end up countering the forward forces of poses like Extended Hand to Big Toe or Dancer.

Example: Extended Hand to Big Toe (Utthita Hasta Padangusthasana), right leg extended:

> "Keep the weight in that left heel, pressing down to lift the hips high. Resist the urge to clench the glutes or thrust the pelvis forward. Instead, soften the knee quite a bit, hinge a little in the hips, and draw the belly in deep. The glutes will work hard here, but avoid leaning the heart back and pitching the hips forward. That standing leg will work hard, but it will hold you up."

If you do all of this and still cue to "lift the kneecap," it won't typically seem to move a whole lot, even though the quads are working hard. So, students are likely to get very confused, or continue to try to work the quads harder to achieve this rather arbitrary instruction. Since neither of these outcomes is ideal, I suggest removing this particular rhetoric from your repertoire.

LEVERS AND TORSION ✺

The seated, externally rotated postures like Head to Knee (Janu Sirsasana), Figure 4, and Pigeon variations are a perfect storm of compensatory forces just waiting to tear apart your joints. Think that's an overstatement? It's not. The bones of the thigh, leg, and foot all act as levers to send movement one direction or another into the hip, knee, and ankle. If we use those levers to force movement instead of allowing resistance to be an active part of our postures, we will create compression and shear forces between bones, cartilage, and ligaments that those tissues are not built to absorb. Injury can result from either repetitive stresses or in a cataclysmic tearing. Neither is awesome.

Because these postures are reliant on mobility of the hip for the overall functioning of the foundation of the pose, if it is lacking there will be ramifications up- and downstream through the entire kinetic chain. If the stretch energy we put into the system can't translate evenly along the joints and out through the foot, then wherever it gets backed up will absorb a ton of rotational energy directly into the joint structures. This is compensation in action!

Let's examine the front leg of the typical Pigeon pose. What movements and forces are acting on the long bones of the leg and the joints from hip to ankle?

Your hip joint has moved on all three planes to set up the foundation of this pose:

- You have flexed the hip to bring the knee forward (quads face up).

- You have abducted the hip to bring the knee closer to the edge of the mat, wide of your hip joint (quads face up).

- You have externally rotated the hip to bring the ankle across your midline in front of you (quads face outward).

That means the hip joint is already near its end range in all of those actions (for many people). Because the thigh bone is stabilized by lying on the ground, the pelvis now moves around the head of the femur and places tension on all the tissues of the hip joint—that is, the femur has become a lever, and the hip joint is the fulcrum of movement. Resistance from ligaments and muscles determines how far the pelvis can move without compensatory rotations of the femur. If you move the pelvis past the hip's endpoint, the femur will roll inward again, the quads no longer pointing out to the side but more upright. (This is the femur compensating for lack of mobility in the hip joint.)

As long as the tibia is close to the femur—that is, a deeply bent knee, which keeps the two bones on relatively the same plane and moving more or less as a unit—the system remains relatively simple. If the knee is not bent deeply but goes closer to

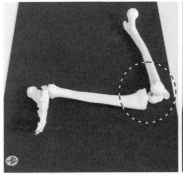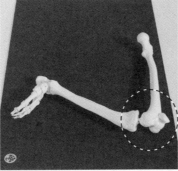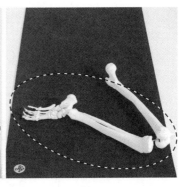

Only if the femur has sufficient external rotation can the knee be safely at 90 degrees. If the foot is flexed, this will encourage a dangerous torsion at the knee, potentially harming ligaments and then meniscus. If the foot is not flexed and the knee is not forced to remain at 90 degrees, the tibia can rotate naturally at the knee, preventing harmful torsion.

90 degrees, the shin bone becomes a lever as well, one that can impact the entire system in sinister ways. With the addition of this lever, the internal compensation of the femur is prevented and torsion energy either rebounds into the hip (over-stretching) and spine (side bending or twisting) or down to the knee joint.

Remember that the knee joint is built to rotate when it is bent—but not very much. In other words, it can absorb a finite amount of torsion energy before translating that to the next available mobile point, the tibia/shin. The larger the angle of the knee, the less compensation in the femur and the more rotation in the knee joint. The online video of Fred's lower extremity will help illustrate this process.

Consider the difference in sensation/resistance in a Pigeon with the front shin close to the pelvis versus pushed further away and more parallel to the front edge of your mat. You may notice that in the "close" version the front of the shin is rather close to the mat, indicating that the shin and thigh bones are on a similar plane, adjusting to the shifts in tension together. In the "far" version you'll see that the side of the leg, not the front, meets your mat, an indication that the shin has not rotated along with the femur.

Which one has more torque at the hip or knee (or both)? The deeply bent knee and closer heel provide less of a lever than the 90 degree version does.

One element yet to be examined in this model is the ankle joint. The foot is ultimately the end of this kinetic chain, the place where all the energy of movement will connect to Earth/Space or get jammed up. If we have a flexed ankle, we are essentially adding another lever to the system, another place where movement forces can get congested and create torsion in the knee. With a slack ankle, the foot and shin move together as a unit, allowing the entire system to absorb the rotational forces and saving the knee.

Flexing the Foot to Protect the Knee

This is a common cue offered in seated, externally rotated postures. It is rooted in the principle of counteraction, and while that is typically a good idea, it doesn't actually apply across the board to this entire family of poses. For full understanding, we'll need to break this one down a bit. In theory, this cue is trying to activate the calf muscles to stabilize the rotation of the tibia at the knee, while at the same time the pose is using that tibia as a lever to achieve rotation of the femur at the hip joint. This is a really complex system of movement that can put many different stresses on the knee joint, and we're attempting to control it by a very simple action.

Now, the breakdown. First, let's recognize that "flex the foot" is really an instruction to dorsiflex, which only fires the muscles on the front of the shin. For this cue to actually embody counteraction, both the dorsiflexors and plantarflexors need to engage simultaneously. That means you can't just "flex" the foot. You plantarflex the foot by activating the posterior compartment (gastroc/soleus), and then you can counter this action by dorsiflexing (pulling the foot and toes toward the shin), contracting the anterior compartment

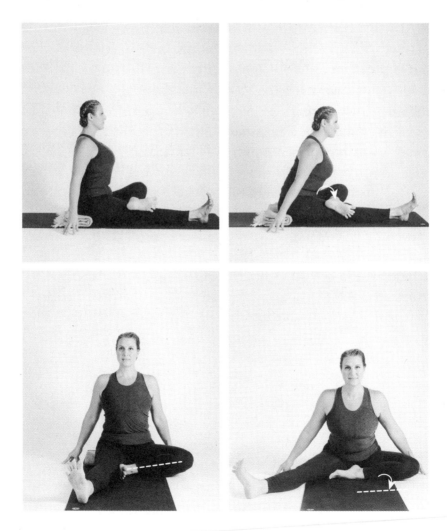

(tibialis anterior). That's an easy enough fix in terms of cueing, and I've always called it the "yogi toe-point" (I have subleased that from multiple teachers back in my early days of yoga ... it used to be quite ubiquitous). But we should acknowledge that this method is still only marginally effective at stabilizing rotation at the knee. Eh, maybe a little? The movement forces at play in these poses may be too much for the gastroc to overpower on its own. Here are the cues though, just in case.

> "Pull the toes toward your shin, flexing your foot actively. At the same time, press the ball of your foot away, like pushing on a gas pedal, firing the calf muscles and countering the dorsiflexion you began with."

Lastly, we should ask if this particular work is really what we want to do. Do we actually want to keep the tibia from rotating? The answer is "maybe." The thing is, you've gotta consider the pose you're trying to achieve, determine the position of the foot in question, and assess how you will shift your weight in the execution of the pose. These factors all contribute to the level of torsion through the knee as you attempt to increase the external rotation of the hip. Different postures call for different protections at the knee.

Ankle across Thigh Poses

If your ankle is across the opposite thigh (seated or standing), this cue applies. Go ahead and sit in this posture now so you can experience it. When you cross the ankle over the thigh, the knee will likely remain suspended at a plane above that of the hip. Notice that the flexed foot has room to rotate itself because it is not pinned against the floor. This freedom allows for energy to be dispersed through the system more evenly, so adjustments have very little impact on the knee. This would be applicable to prep poses for Lotus, like Fire Log (Agnistambhasana) and its variations.

> "Cross your right ankle over your left thigh. Make sure that the foot has passed the thigh completely. Now engage your yogi toe-point, pulling the toes back in flexion at the same time you press the ball of the foot forward. You'll feel the entire shin, front and back, engage muscularly."

Ankle on the Floor: Head to Knee Pose Family, Hero Variations, "Pigeon"

If your ankle is on the floor, however, you MUST let the anterior ankle lengthen and allow the plantarflexed position to occur. If you dorsiflex the foot here, as described in the sidebar, you are creating an extra lever that forces torsion energy into the knee joint instead of distributing it down the tibia. Your knee will absorb this force once the hip joint is maxed out, so you'll not only not accomplish your goal, you'll get injured in the process. These forces are amplified in forward folded postures, like the ubiquitous Pigeon pose (the "dead" version), so please do not flex your foot there.

There may be some wiggle room for a bit of dorsiflexion if you remain upright though, as in One-Legged King Pigeon, because you moderate your hip's external rotation by engaging adductors, extensors, and hip flexors on both sides to gain uplift—that uplift equals less external hip rotation force.

It's a good idea to feel these differentiations in your own body. Be very careful as you explore the flexed-foot versions.

In a Pigeon pose with right leg forward:

"Allow right knee to move toward edge of mat as needed to settle into the hip. Allow the right ankle to lengthen—then activate the foot with Pada Bandha. You might tuck your back toes and engage the length of the left leg, lifting the knee. Press with your hands, and if there's ample space, shift hips back an inch at a time, leaving right foot anchored, and finding a deeper rotation in the right hip. Stop moving back when you feel any resistance—don't move through it, just barely meet it. Untuck back toes. Allow hips to settle toward the floor, keeping them level and not collapsing onto right side. You may begin to fold forward, but please move very slowly, remaining aware of the right hip and the right knee; if you feel any torsion in the knee, allow the shin to roll slightly forward, the right foot tipping slightly toward its top side.

You may also feel the need to shift the hips forward once more. Be honest. There's no need to go forward too fast or dump into gravity. Remain active in the hips and belly, and long in the chest. Use your breath ..."

In a variation of Pigeon where it could be appropriate to keep the foot flexed:

"From your Pigeon-legs, roll fully onto right hip. Soften left knee a bit so you can find balance. Open the right knee joint to 90 degrees, flexing the foot fully. Turn chest to the left, aligning your right side-waist with the right inner thigh. Reach right arm overhead, lengthening right side—hinge in right hip, laying the ribs on the inner thigh, arm reaches out in front of heart along the floor, right temple rests on floor or on block. Left hand may reach out to meet the right hand at first. As you settle in ..."

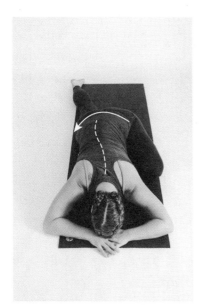 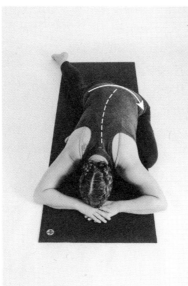 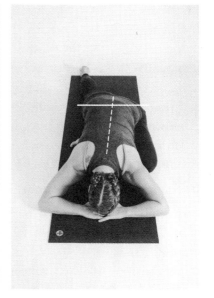

Many things can go wrong with this version of Pigeon. Be mindful of all the forces on the spine, hip, and knee. As the spine and pelvis shift, all the forward energy of the body will translate into the knee if the front foot is flexed.

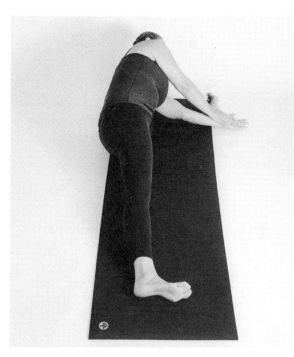
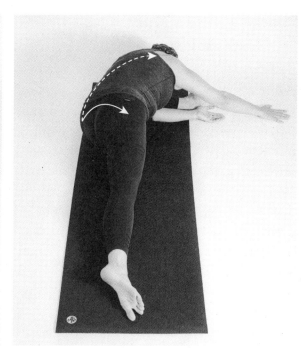

This version of Pigeon provides more inherent stability in the spine while reducing risk at the knee, even with the foot flexed. It also accesses attachments to the IT band that are difficult to address otherwise.

In One-Legged King Pigeon:

"Letting right knee move toward edge of mat as needed, find the appropriate bend in the right knee so no torsion is felt in the joint. Use blocks under hands as preferred to help heart feel light and lifted. Gather belly and rise through crown. Feel back knee pull forward, engaging the hip flexors. Pull right sitting bone back in space, activating deep hip and low back muscles. You'll feel some lift under the pelvis, keep belly firm. Breath is smooth. Right foot may flex into the floor to give extra activation to the entire right leg, but do not do this if the knee feels torqued; however the foot is aligned, press the ankle and shin into the earth while pulling back through hip crease ..."

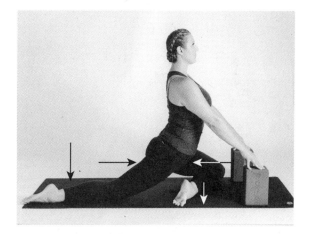

"Stacking" Hips in Open Standing Postures

There are ubiquitous cues throughout the Warrior II family of standing poses that encourage you to open the pelvis to make it parallel with the side edge of your mat. These are fairly traditional cues that may have worked themselves out in some communities, but I find that students still come to me with ingrained ideas that this is how it must be done in Warrior II, Triangle, and Side Angle (Parsvakonasana). What we know about the shape of the femur, however, and how range of motion varies significantly among people based on bony limitations and not muscular flexibility, suggests that this approach can have seriously ill effects, particularly on the SI and knee joints.

Instead, I suggest we work within the natural limits of the bony framework and then support that framework functionally by engaging the deep stabilizing muscles around the joints. For most people, their Warrior II pelvis will land somewhere between a traditional Warrior I and II alignment. The more we allow the pelvis some slack, the less torque will be translated into the knee or SI joint.

In Triangle, right leg forward:

"Make sure your right knee faces forward and doesn't buckle inward. Activate external rotation of the thigh. As you rotate the pelvis open, stop when you feel resistance in the right hip or SI joint. Don't force it. You may even allow the left hip to close slightly toward the earth (away from the 'stacking' action),

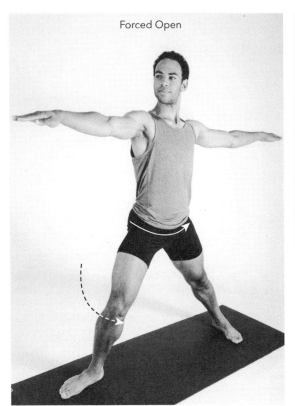

Forced Open

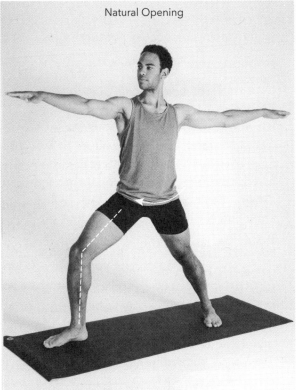

Natural Opening

A forced opening of the pelvis will pull the front knee off axis. Many times this is a condition of bony shape and ligaments, not short muscles, so we do not want to try to open more than is necessary.

making some space in the right hip joint. Now pull the right hip crease straight back to the back of the room and lengthen right side-waist. Root deeply through back (left) foot, big toe to outer heel, and feel that spiral continue up into the left hip, firing the glutes. You may feel more integrity from hip to core with that action."

All of the abducted standing poses will benefit from this approach. In the Warrior II and Side Angle variations, you'll know that the pelvis has opened too far if the front thigh and knee start to pull toward the center of the mat. This visual cue is harder to discern in Triangle pose, but similarly the thigh and knee will appear to "roll" toward that midline.

Practice Mechanics

Now that you have some principles of alignment and action to work with and some ways to approach your cueing, let's talk more specifically about the asanas of the lower extremity. In the following section I've outlined the primary alignment points for various posture categories. When appropriate, I've added notes for specific postures, but let's be honest, there's A TON of yoga postures! The lower extremity is integral to nearly every posture we do, so I've chosen to be somewhat judicious and limit the list by targeting them as categories.

To that end, we'll break down the postures to Standing, Seated Twists, Forward Folds, and Backbends. While this will not cover every single pose in its entirety, it will lay the groundwork for understanding these joints in gravity. That knowledge will provide you with blueprints for other, possibly more complicated postures by way of these basic components.

Standing Poses

In some styles of yoga, standing poses make up nearly the entire repertoire. They're kind of a big deal in the asana world. Since every individual on the mat has differently shaped bones, and their hip and knee and foot joints will move according to their own particular relationships to gravity, we need to establish some baseline instruction along with adaptations for those individual differences.

Admittedly, this could get both complicated and tedious. There are standing poses that are neutral or abducted, symmetrical or asymmetrical. Some are upright and some are forward folds and some are rotated. That's a ton of subcategories that begin to overlap. In order to avoid detailing each and every posture in yoga, I've chosen to list all the postures in a certain category but only outline one or two postures in detail. As you go down the list, hopefully it will become clear what alignment points apply to bent knees or straight legs, asymmetry, folds, and rotations.

There are some somewhat universal instructions that should become rote cueing for all of these poses. Actions at Pada Bandha will be necessary for every single one of them, though that applies beyond the Standing category too. You'll also need to be aware of the spine in these postures, so there will be a shorthand of sorts to remind you of the effort toward neutrality, without going into great detail as to those actions.

DEBUNKING TRADITIONAL STANDING ALIGNMENTS

The fundamental standing postures that make up the primary series of the Ashtanga lineage serve in many ways as a blueprint for most of the elemental Hatha and vinyasa practices in the West. B. K. S. Iyengar outlined some particular alignment points for these in *Light on Yoga*. Through those two channels, these poses have become mainstays in nearly every single yoga class I've attended. That said, I think there are still some mysteries of HOW to execute these ubiquitous postures and details that have been overlooked or misjudged until now. Of course, we'll completely eliminate cues to "tuck the tail." Hopefully by now that's a given. But there are other traditional shapes and instructions that continue to baffle me.

- For abducted postures, as noted in the "Stacking Hips in Open Standing Postures" section, I find it totally unnecessary to force the pelvis open to a full open alignment. Because of bony limitations, very few people will be able to find this opening in a safe way. To force it often means cranking in the knees, applying too much rotational force there. It will usually also result in compression in the SI and L5. Since none of these is remotely productive and will in fact cause injury down the line, I highly suggest forgetting that this alignment is any kind of goal. Be satisfied with an active and integral posture that aligns the spine as neutrally as possible, while accessing the most precise hinge that you can in that front hip.

- Another rather arbitrary measure of "fully expressing" the posture is the idea that our front thigh must be parallel with the floor. For many of us, this shape leaves us at a significant strength differential. Our front hip is unlikely to be in its midrange here, leaving that joint vulnerable to overstretching and instability. I suggest instead using knee-over-ankle as your benchmark alignment point in the legs and over time playing with how far apart the feet may go. Maintaining stability, uplift, and buoyancy is much more important than getting super-long and really low.

- In traditional lineages, the Warrior I postures encourage a heel-to-heel alignment of the feet on the mat. Again, this feels arbitrary. Because of the mobility limitations in the hips, this position is far too narrow for most people. With your heels essentially on a balance beam, it will be impossible to square your hips at all. Trying to achieve this will impose actions that create a great amount of torsion on the back knee and the low back. Instead, if we allow the heels to remain at our own hips' width, the pelvis meets far less rotational resistance, with less compensation stress at the other joints.

- Similarly, the heel-to-arch alignment prescribed for Warrior II postures is still too narrow for the average practitioner. I prefer to allow students to find their hip-width foundation here as well. This alignment creates space for the pelvis to open sufficiently, without the compressions in the lumbar spine that can accompany the traditional foot placement. There is ample space to find supportive counteractions in the hips and ankles instead of just leaning into stretch resistance. In addition, there is more ease in keeping the pelvis under the ribs, adding lift and buoyancy to the upper body.

Neutral Group

This is fundamentally the Warrior I family of poses. It includes Chair, Warrior I, Warrior III (though we'll cover that more specifically in the Balance Group), Pyramid, Revolved Side Angle, and Revolved Triangle. Note that Chair pose is the only symmetrical pose; all the others have one leg forward and the other one back. Fundamentally, you'll need to practice teaching those straight and bent-knee rules, then work on getting the pelvis balanced.

Warrior I (Virabhadrasana I)

Most people will not be able to fully square their pelvis to the front wall. Effort should be there, but compensating in order to achieve this isn't advisable.

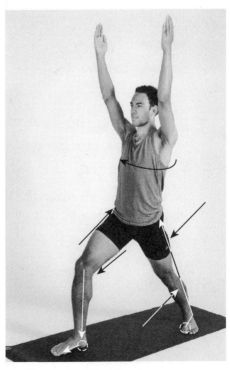

- Neutral spinal curves, active bandhas.

- Feet hip-width.

- Slight turn-out off back foot, accommodate ankle limitations, but avoid cranking in knee—sometimes more turn-out helps, but this is individual.

- Straight back leg—no locking knee, weight rooted from big-toe mound to pinky, to outer heel, spiraling to outer hip.

- Bent front leg—weight grounded through center of heel, then muscular anchor of big-toe mound.

- Knee aligned directly over ankle.

- Hip aligned directly behind knee—foot turn-out as needed.

- Back leg bears more weight, pressing foot through floor to urge that femur/hip forward; effort toward squaring hips to front wall.

Revolved Side Angle (Pariurtta Parsvakonasana)

(Left leg forward). This posture is named after an abducted pose, but its alignment is actually neutral to accommodate the twist. The arms and shoulder girdle are integral pieces of this puzzle, but we'll refrain here from detailing them too much. For now, please just acknowledge that we ought to avoid using the arms to leverage us into the twist.

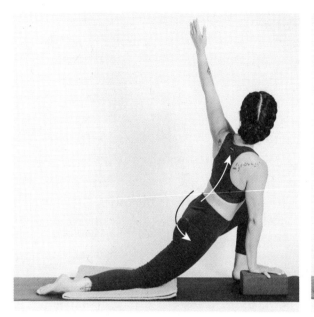 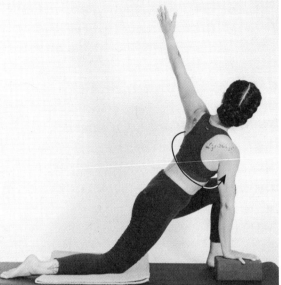

- Neutral spinal curves, active bandhas.
- Feet hip-width.
- Left knee directly over ankle.
- Right knee planted on mat, hip-width. (Alternative keeps knee lifted in Full Lunge.)
- Bent left knee—weight grounded through heel, then muscular anchor of big-toe mound.
- Grounded right shin presses down, external spiral to outer hip.
- Right knee pulls forward, left shin/heel pull back (scissor legs to stabilize pelvis).
- Hands in Anjali Mudra (palms meet at heart-center), rotate heart to right, thoracic twist; stable lumbar spine.
- Hinge deeply in hips, maintaining balanced pelvis; avoid dropping left hip/thigh.
- Right hand to block under right shoulder, or (advanced) left elbow rests on top of right knee/thigh.
- Core remains light.
- Over time, twist may deepen to allow elbows to extend, but do not force twist deeper using arms and levers.

Abducted Group

Extended Triangle (Utthita Trikonasana)

(Right leg forward). You'll notice that this pose is kind of a forward fold, and also a thoracic twist. This spinal rotation is how we allow the pelvis to remain less open and still create the "flat" or "pane of glass" feel of the posture, preventing the hips from swinging back and the torso forward. The same thing will occur in Side Angle.

- Neutral spinal curves, active bandhas.

- Feet hip-width.

- Straight legs—weight anchored in big-toe mound, translated to outer heel, spiral around outer thigh.

- Open pelvis—only to resistance point, don't torque knee or SI by forcing too far.

- Hinge deeply in right hip.

- Pull right sitting bone/hip crease to back wall.

- Lengthen heart/crown to front wall.

- Gather belly, spiral heart/ribs open to side wall.

- Keep right side-waist very active, equally long as right. Resist the side bend.

- Gather ribs; resist backbend.

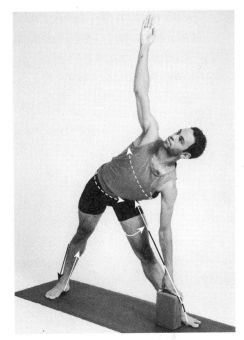

Be cautious with the front knee—ensure no hyperextension occurs.

Balance Group

Tree (Vrksasana)

(Right knee bent and lifted). Keeping in mind that balance poses use bent-knee principles in the standing leg. Also, don't force the opening of the pelvis here, it will only cause spinal compensations and throw the frame off its axis.

- Neutral spinal curves; active bandhas.

- Hands in Anjali Mudra (palms meet at heart-center).

- Left foot bears weight through heel, then muscularly anchors to big-toe mound. Some slight turn-out may be appropriate in some bodies.

- Left knee remains slightly bent; all leg muscles are activated and stabilizing for joints.

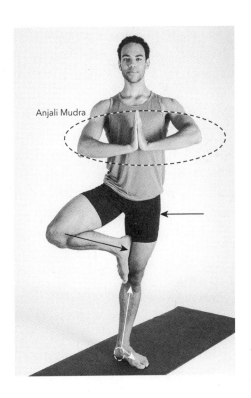

Anjali Mudra

- Hug left hip toward midline; resist letting hip jut out to the left.

- Right thigh opens to point of resistance, avoid forcing it wider; pelvis is likely to compensate if you force knee to point to side wall.

- Right foot activates Pada Bandha and anchors to left ankle, calf, or thigh. (Each level offers different stabilizing work in different areas of left extremity; they are not representative of beginning to advanced.)

- Hands may press up over head, may stay linked or reach out to shoulder-width.

- Maintain bandhas; don't let breaking points collapse.

Seated Twists

This group offers us many variations of spinal rotation with myriad leg orientations. There are traditional versions that are called twists, but for all but the very most flexible folks out there are executed as side bends. Revolved Head to Knee (Parivrrta Janu Sirsasana) is one of these. It requires specific opening in the hip, deep abduction to get the ribs out over the thigh, and incorporates significant side bending before you can access the rib rotation. Once all the parts are super-pliable, then it starts to resemble a twist. ✹

Other postures in this group are far more obvious: Lord of the Fishes (Matsyendrasana), Marichi's Pose (Marichyasana) variations, Bharadvaja's Twist (Bharadvajasana), and Revolved Squat (Parivrtta Malasana).

In virtually any twist, the pelvis needs to remain stable so the thoracic spine can activate fully in rotation. But it's tremendously easy to let those hips go while trying to get deep in our twists, using arms as levers and cranking ourselves around. In seated postures, it's integral to remain mindful of potential hip compensations and use our deep core to help maintain stability in our seat. It is common for the extended-leg hip to creep forward in asymmetrical versions, but most times we ought to avoid this compensatory movement. The obliques become stabilizers to the pelvis, core, and base-ribs, allowing the higher thoracic paraspinals and intercostal muscles to perform the rotation.

Typically, we want the arms to act only as supports or guides, rather than active cranks leveraging us deeper into the twist. Fingers can land on the ground to act as a kickstand. Hands or elbows can lightly cross thighs. We can use arms to create compression/tension between leg and core that promotes an upright axis. What can't happen is the hand grasping another body part and forcing the spine into a twist or bend. Once we engage the arms this way, we eliminate the deep contractions at the spine and lose all purposeful integrity.

Lord of the Fishes (Matsyendrasana)

(Right knee bent and crossed). This posture has multiple options for the bottom leg. Consider that the bent-knee option creates more torque on the pelvis and hips, resulting in more work to maintain a stable spine. Choosing which option is appropriate is not only about assessing the openness of the hip joints but the strength and awareness in the axis of the spine. Options also exist for the arms, but avoid cranking into the twist using their leverage.

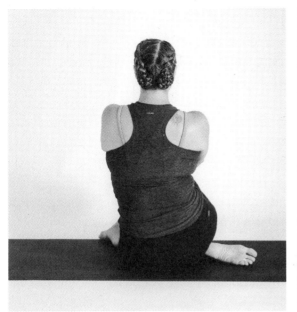 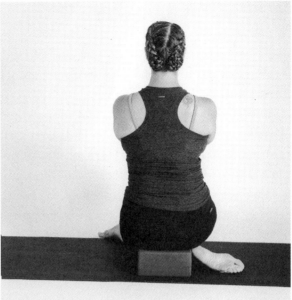

If using a blanket instead of a block, it can be helpful to lift only the bottom leg's hip, allowing the top leg's hip to drop slightly. Core must remain active.

- Left leg is either straight out in front of you (Half Lord of the Fishes) or knee is bent so heel is near right hip; bent-knee version may result in elevated right hip and tilted pelvis.
- Both feet active with Pada Bandha.
- Right foot may turn to face any direction that relieves torque from the knee.
- Right big-toe mound rooted.
- Neutral spinal curves, active bandhas.
- Right hand reaches outside of and behind right hip; light on the fingers, arm acts as a tactile cue to keep heart light and upright; no essential weight bearing in hand.
- Firm belly, stable lumbar. Navel remains aligned with pubic bone.
- Heart spiral to right; thoracic twist.
- Remain on axis; avoid side bends and backbends. Heart over hips, head directly over heart.
- Left arm options:
    - Left hand/fist rests on front of right shin, pulling straight back to activate through upper back and belly, lifting ribs up toward thigh.
    - Left elbow crosses the right thigh without cranking spine. Fingers point up to sky.
    - Left arm crosses right thigh deeply, internally rotating for the reverse bind, right arm reaching around back. Avoid cranking. (Very advanced; difficult to maintain spinal axis.)

Forward Folds

This is an interesting group to consider, because if we define a forward fold as a flexion in the hip, well ... let's just say that we do that a whole lot in our asana practice. Essentially every time we do any posture other than backbends, Mountain, or Corpse, one or both of our hips is in flexion. Consider that for just a moment.

If, however, we try to build a category where the forward fold is the primary element of the posture, we can narrow down the field slightly. If we eliminate the obvious twists and the standing postures where being upright is favored over bowing down, then we have sets of postures where the hip flexion and the forward momentum are the driving forces of the pose. Whether we're standing or seated, forward reach of the heart and crown is paramount to maintaining spinal stability and length. Gravity can be our friend or foe in this process, providing traction in standing poses (past a certain point, at least) but promoting collapse in seated variations. This means that while we are isolating movement to the hip we must also remain consistently aware of the actions of the deep core to decompress the lumbar region of the spine. We are acting to maintain lumbar lordosis as much as possible.

As always, Pada Bandha is a given here. The feet must remain active whether they are rooted to the earth or not. Neutral spinal curves will be impossible to maintain completely, but the effort is there to keep the back-channel muscles active unless traction comes into play. Ultimately, we must always have in mind the mantra "forward folds have forward momentum." This simple phrase will guide us into sure, clear hip folds regardless of our individual limitations.

Standing Folds

Standing folds use the feet and legs actively in order to relieve the spine of its work. If we use the legs effectively, the spine will be able to release itself to the pull of gravity, even if the weight of the torso partially rests on the thighs. Those with particularly short or stuck hamstrings and calves will find some extra slack in the back channel by bending the knees deeper, but they cannot allow that weight to shift too far back in space. Even with deeply bent knees, students will need to lean far forward into the forefoot to maintain muscular effort in the legs and allow the spine to surrender.

This group is represented by postures such as Wide-Legged Forward Fold (Prasarita Padottanasana), Standing Forward Fold (Uttanasana), Standing Half Forward Fold, Pyramid (Parsvottanasana), Big Toe pose (Padangustasana), Hands Under Feet (Padahastasana), and Downward Facing Dog (Adho Mukha Svanasana). These are all symmetrical postures, so the two hips will be endeavoring to find a balance of range of motion. Pada Bandha is critical in all of these postures, bearing weight in the ball of the foot without gripping the toes into the mat. In addition, the feet should be aligned individually to ensure neutral hip alignment. Some traditional alignment patterns ask that the big toes turn in slightly, but this causes added stresses on the knees and hip joints in the majority of bodies.

Standing Forward Fold (Uttanasana)

This posture is the blueprint for pretty much all of the standing folds, except Half Forward Fold. The effort is maximized in the legs so the spine can release into the traction of gravity.

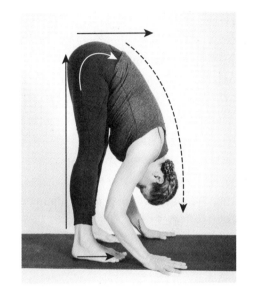

- Feet hip-width.
- Neutral hip rotation.
- Weight shifted forward to the forefoot, toes light.
- Knees soft, slightly bent or deeply bent depending on tension in hamstrings.
- Feet press down, hips and posterior thighs have upward momentum.
- Slight action in glutes; "squeeze sitting bones together slightly" or "open thighs/knees slightly away from midline until they align over ankles."
- Belly gathers deeply to spine, releasing guarding in lumbar and ribs.
- Face soft, breath smooth, and crown releasing to Earth.

Half Forward Fold (Ardha Uttanasana)

This pose is differentiated from the previous by the neutrality of the spinal curves. The actions in the legs are the same, but they tend to be more vigorous in order to counter the leverage weight of the torso hanging in space. It is common to see students rise from Uttanasana only using their mid-back and not reaching full height; the head, heart, and sacrum should be on one plane, parallel to the floor. That angle may change to look more upright if the knees are bent deeply to accommodate short hamstrings.

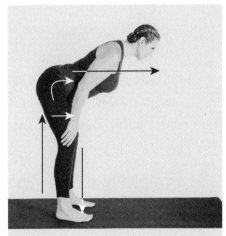

- Feet hip-width.
- Neutral hip rotation.
- Weight shifted forward to the forefoot, toes light.
- Knees soft, slightly bent or deeply bent depending on tension in hamstrings.
- Feet press down, hips and posterior thighs have upward momentum.
- Slight action in glutes; "squeeze sitting bones together slightly" or "open thighs/knees slightly away from midline until they align over ankles."

- Hands come to land lightly above the knees on the thighs.
- Hinge in hips is sharp, belly lifting to support lumbar spine. Tail tilts upward slightly like Cow pose (Mula Bandha).
- Front ribs gather upward toward spine, supportive of heart like Cat pose (Uddiyana Bandha).
- Chest open, collarbones broad like Cow pose.
- Vocal cords lift to support long back-neck (Jalandhara Bandha).
- Tail has energy toward back wall, crown has energy toward front wall.

Pyramid (Parsvottanasana)

This posture is distinguished by the asymmetrical legs. Because the front-foot side requires a much deeper flexion than the back-foot side, compensations are common and complex. Just getting your weight to balance evenly forward/back between the two feet is a challenge. Then getting the pelvis and spine to remain centered without any side-to-side shifts, which sometimes they do as a unit, and sometimes as rogue separatists. Blocks under the hands are a necessary tool at first for nearly everyone, taking some of the weight out of the heart and removing some of the stretch so that the details can be addressed with slightly more ease.

- Right foot forward, left foot back, hands on blocks framing the front foot at shoulder-width.
- Feet turned out as needed to accommodate neutral hip alignment.
- Shift forward and back to assess and find the center of gravity. (Students tend to have too much weight forward, compensation for hip tension/short hamstrings, and this is indicated by the right hip being too high. Shifting back will raise the left hip, shifting forward will raise the right hip.)
- Shorten stance as needed to accommodate level pelvis.
- Subtle external rotation of both thighs, softness in knees, no locking out.
- Heart is centered and light, not leaning over right leg.
- Pelvis is centered, weight balanced to keep the tail pointing straight back.
- Tilt tail upward, sharp crease in right hip, belly lifting to support lumbar spine (Mula + Uddiyana Bandha).
- Chest open, collar bones broad like Cow pose.
- Vocal cords lift to support long back-neck (Jalandhara Bandha).
- Tail has energy toward back wall, crown has energy toward front wall.

Seated Folds

This family of postures has so many variations, so many options, that it's mind-boggling to consider outlining all of them! Thankfully we've already addressed the twisting versions, so we really only need to contemplate the difference between folds with either symmetrical or asymmetrical legs. Symmetrical folds include Prayer/Child's Pose, Yogi Staff (Dandasana), Seated Forward Fold (Paschimottanasana), Boat, Bound Angle (Badha Konasana), and Seated Wide-Legged Forward Fold (Upavistha Konasana). The primary consideration in these postures is whether the lumbar spine is supported or collapsed. We need to be willing to maintain our spinal neutrality and muscular action indefinitely in order to decompress the low back. If passivity is a goal, such as in a Yin class, then we MUST be willing to use props to prevent compression and collapse. As teachers, it's perfectly okay to *insist* that props be used.

The asymmetrical group includes variations on Head to Knee, Marichi's Pose, and One-Legged King Pigeon. In addition to the neutral and active spinal considerations, we must also be mindful of the tendency for the pelvis to compensate. This is especially true in any folds that also involve a twist, because all of these movements will add complex tensions across the hips and pelvis.

I suggest that ALL seated forward folds use a double-folded blanket edge to elevate the tailbone. Catch that? For many people with long or supple hamstrings, they'll avoid sitting up on elevation—they believe that the blanket is only for people with short or tight hamstrings. I disagree. While lifting the whole pelvis will certainly help folks with too much back-channel tension, this technique of wedging the glutes and tailbone instead will help keep the pelvis and lumbar spine in neutral alignment with less effort or clenching. All of the forward folds should begin in Yogi Staff:

Seated Forward Fold (Paschimottanasana)

This fold, like many in this family, has a tendency to have too much downward momentum, collapsing the heart toward the thighs. Ideally, the spine will remain in neutral curves for as long as possible, lengthening the sternum forward toward the feet instead. If you can reach your feet, avoid using the arms to physically pull on the spine. Instead, build a subtle tension in the shoulders that helps engage the back muscles as a counter to gravity.

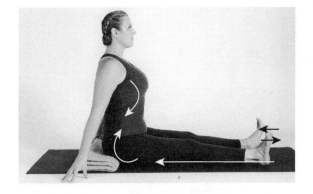

- Active Pada Bandha.
- Lifted tail, gathered belly; neutral spinal curves maintained as far as possible.
- Hinge deeply in hips, fire hip flexors and quads.

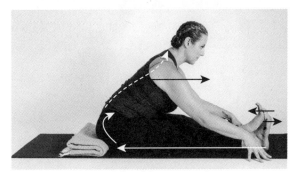

- Consider slight external rotation in hips, especially if there is a "pinching" sensation in hip crease.

- Heart lengthens toward front wall; do not collapse toward thighs.

- Once maximum flexion is reached in hips, active form maintains back-channel muscle contraction; restorative form uses props to support chest/head; continue to find lengthening energy without downward collapse.

- Arms may prop up behind you at first, assisting forward pelvic tilt; may reach forward to floor, shins, or feet as appropriate, keeping very subtle pulling for latissimus engagement.

Head to Knee (Janu Sirsasana)

In the asymmetrical folds, one must ask the question "What am I trying to achieve?" In the case of Head to Knee, traditional alignment has the knee bent deeply, placing the foot close to the groin, which has the effect for most people of opening the pelvis so it's no longer neutral. You'd then align the chest over the "long" thigh, making for a distinctively one-sided low back stretch. That's totally fine if what you intend for this posture is a spine stretch.

But if your intention is aimed at affecting the hip joints, then you'll need to make adjustments to that alignment so the spine doesn't steal your thunder. The alternative is offered here. I think this is an excellent example of how subtle compensations can significantly alter the outcome of any pose. You'll need to remain hyperaware of this pelvic compensation for all asymmetrical seated postures.

- Right knee bent out to right, aligning foot around left knee instead of pulling fully to groin.

- Pada Bandha active; right foot may plantar flex slightly as needed when folding.

- Keep pelvis square to front of mat.

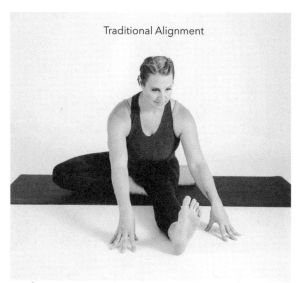 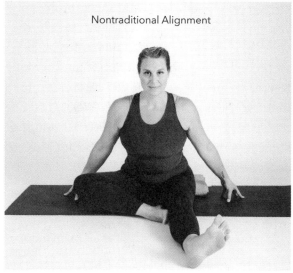

Traditional Alignment   Nontraditional Alignment

Traditional alignment includes a slight spinal side bend, creating a unilateral low back stretch. If the intention is to focus movement and stretch into the hips only, consider keeping the heart centered instead of taking it over the thigh.

- Neutral spinal curves; tail uplifted, belly gathered, neck long.

- Maintain axis; navel and heart in line with pubic bone; avoid veering off toward left thigh.

- Hinge deeply in hips, fire hip flexors and quads.

- Pull backward through left hip crease; avoid tendency for pelvis to shift open.

- Heart lengthens toward front wall; do not collapse toward thighs.

- In deep folds, left shoulder will land on leg, heart remains on line with midline.

- Once maximum flexion is reached in hips, active form maintains back-channel muscle contraction; restorative form uses props to support chest/head; continue to find lengthening energy without downward collapse.

- Arms may prop you up from behind at first, assisting forward pelvic tilt; may reach forward to floor, shins, or feet as appropriate, keeping very subtle pulling for latissimus engagement.

Externally Rotated Seated Postures

Externally rotated poses may include a forward fold, as in Bound Angle, but that isn't always the case. Again, one could get very technical and say that any time you're seated on the floor, by necessity the hip is flexed and therefore you are in a fold, but for now we'll assume that folds require the heart to actually move out over the legs when seated. With that in mind, this group consists of Bound Angle, Fire Log, Lotus and Half Lotus (Ardha Padmasana), Yogi Staff, and the Pigeon variations on your back or seat, sometimes referred to as Figure 4.

Please remain conscientious of the "flexing of the foot to protect the knee." This is not as useful a cue as many think, as outlined earlier in this chapter. If the foot is rooted on the floor, it is usually inappropriate for most people.

Fire Log (Agnistambhasana)

Fire Log pose is a tough posture for me. In fact, I find it far more challenging than a full Lotus. Since there is less bend in the knees, the shins are further out from the pelvis, creating a more profound lever on the hip. If the hip lacks sufficient external rotation range of motion, that lever has the potential to create far more torque on the knee joints. Be cautious. Move slowly. Be mindful of the forces at play in YOUR body, and offer it sufficient support where necessary.

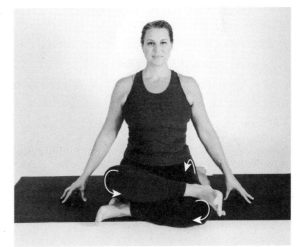

Never force the knees to go lower. If they are remarkably high, elevate the hips on blankets or block instead.

- Right knee bent, shin roughly parallel to the front of mat. Pada Bandha active, but ankle only flexed if no "tweaking" in the knee.

- Left knee stacks on right ankle (not foot), bent so shins stack like logs, foot past the right thigh. Pada Bandha active.

- No need to press knees down; let the hips open slowly. Forcing downward will only torque the knees. Sit up high on blankets or bolster if the knees are awkwardly high.

- Lift tail, gather belly.

- Align heart directly over pelvis, head over heart.

- Hands at Anjali Mudra or Reverse Anjali Mudra.

- If folding forward:

  - Let right ankle go slack to allow any necessary rotation in the tibia. Pada Bandha remains active.

  - Left ankle can remain flexed or not. Pada Bandha active.

  - Hinge deep in hips, moving slowly.

  - Belly lifts, heart lengthens.

  - Hands can reach forward to support upper body as needed.

Backbends

There is a propensity in backbends to release completely at the anterior hip and go into hyperextension there, jutting the pubic bone forward (or into the ground for prone poses, or up into the air in supine postures), but ideally we'd avoid this. For one thing, the hyperextension usually adds to the prototypical jamming up in the L5/S1 level. For another, if the hip flexors are stretched to their maximum, they have a nearly impossible time offering any counteractive force to the deep core. Ideally, we'd maintain a subtle flexion in the hip in order to have maximal control over the finer movements of the pelvis, so we can activate the posterior lumbar muscles and keep the lordosis active and long instead of compressed.

I recognize that it's totally counterintuitive to try to keep flexion in the hip, especially in deep bends like Upward Facing Bow or Camel, but believe me when I tell you that the deep extension will certainly result in compressive forces taking over the low back. Or don't believe me—just try the two versions for yourself and see what I mean.

Generally, backbends fall into three categories: prone, supine, or drop backs. Prone postures are the Cobra family: Cobra (and Baby), Upward Facing Dog, Sphinx (Salamba Bhujangasana), Bow (Dhanurasana) variations, and Frog. Supine backbends are the Bridge family: Bridge, Pigeon (Kapotasana, not the Dead Pigeon you envision), and Upward Facing Bow. The drop backs are the Camel family: Camel, Standing Backbend, and the drop back to Upward Facing Bow.

Bridge (Setu Bandha Sarvangasana)

This might be my favorite backbend to actually practice. It has elements of inversion; my whole body is active and also grounded. It is supremely calming for me ... but that wasn't always how it was. For a long time I succumbed to the common cueing, and I got all whacked out at L5, and my knees got fatigued from overworking in my quads. The key here is to maintain lumbar and core contractions that create decompressive forces—and avoiding the habit of shortening the front belly and hyperextending the hip.

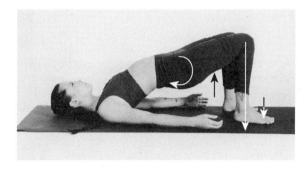

- Press elbows into the floor. (Bending elbows to 90 degrees can help build good acuity here.)

- Pull shoulder blades together toward spine. You should feel very little if any pressure on the upper spine; it should be mostly suspended off the floor between the shoulder blades.

- Pull tail toward back of heart; you should feel entire back-spine activating and extending into a backbend from tail to nape. (No pressing low back to the floor.)

- Head gently heavy to activate back-neck; avoid jutting shin to sky or scrunching it down to chest, throat collapsing.

- Root through big-toe mound and inner heel, balancing effort in adductor/abductor counteractions.

- There is a subtle hinge in the front of the hip, a sense of the pelvis tilting forward as the thigh bones rise.

- As tail pulls into extension, the back-heart coils and lifts the sternum toward the chin.

- Avoid binding hands beneath you, so you can remain active in muscles and not depend on the mechanical advantage that the bind affords you.

Cobra (Bhujangasana)

Until one is adept at utilizing the work of the arms in an efficient way, I HIGHLY recommend practicing Baby Cobra only. If you use your arms to lever you up, rolling through the spinal joints with little or no muscular support, you're not actually doing a backbend ... you're kind of just doing a really lazy push-up. Your arms need to work in extension at the shoulder, so the act of pulling against the mat alongside your torso can activate latissimus. This is key to making sure the posterior spine is both active and decompressive, not just jamming up at the breaking points.

- Press down with knees to activate hip flexors and release any clenching in the glutes.

- Gather belly to spine; lift organs firmly away from the floor.

- Hands aligned under elbows, not too narrow; follow your hand-width blueprint.

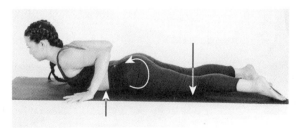

Pressing through the knees activates the hip flexors, helping stabilize the lumbar spine as the belly lifts.

- Pull hands back against the friction of the mat; do not press down, just pull back to activate the lats and mid- to low-back.

- Squeeze shoulders gently together, hug elbows slightly in toward midline.

- Lengthen sternum toward front wall, lifting subtly; let the length guide the lifting of the heart, avoid forcing ribs upward with the arms.

- Gather vocal cords to keep back-neck long (Jalandhara Bandha).

Camel (Ustrasana)

So many people hate this pose. Personally, I think it's because of the compression in the low back due to a thrusted pelvis. The tendency to reach back and down while also jutting the pelvis forward sets you up in gravity to crush the lumbar tissue. That is never ever gonna feel good.

Instead, offer yourself more sustainability in this posture: focus on uplift of the ribs and thoracic extension, while maintaining core compression and pelvic neutrality, and build strength slowly. Variations in hand placement will help you build up slowly and allow you to focus on activating the thoracic extension with less risk of lumbar compression. Keeping the hands on the sacrum is NOT an easier version; there is still plenty of work to be done there, IF you are actually doing the work.

- Press down through shins and tops of feet to activate Pada Bandha and firm quads.

- Palms align on the sacrum, very low, not touching the lumbar spine at all; pinky fingers will touch the coccyx. (Variations include hands reaching down the thighs, reaching back for high blocks, and reaching back for heels. Please master this primary version first.)

- Press sacrum into palms, lift tail toward back of heart, gather low belly gently toward sacrum; DO NOT lift the pubic bone (Mula Bandha).

- Thighs maintain backward momentum, slight hinge in front of hip to avoid collapse at L5; subtle forward tilt action in pelvis.

- Draw the solar plexus deeply in toward spine, pulling front ribs in (Uddiyana Bandha).

- Gather vocal cords into neck-spine; look straight ahead. (In deeper variations, the head may tilt back to look at sky or back wall, but ONLY if the movement originates at base of neck, not base of skull.)

- Squeeze elbows together slightly, sliding shoulder blades toward spine.

- Scapulae help propel sternum upward toward chin.

- Keep upper belly active, don't allow ribs to pop out and collapse in T10. (Maintain Uddiyana Bandha.)

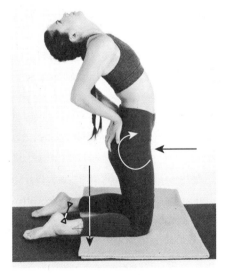

Thighs have backward momentum, creating a stable foundation from which the heart can rise.

Practice Teaching
Adjustments

The hips and lower extremity vary so much from person to person that each body will have its own happy place in space. Yet we have pretty clear visual cues all over the yoga culture to tell us what our poses are "supposed" to look like, and those examples are often performed by the "ideal" body for each particular pose ... because, well, Consumer Culture. In class we try to do what our teachers tell us to do. We try to move our body into those shapes. And frankly, we think we're doing a good job of it. Unfortunately, our own proprioception is usually not accurate, so our best efforts may still be a bit wonky or imbalanced.

As teachers we must remember that we're working with individuals who need personalized alignment, and that means we're gonna help each student battle between what they think they're doing and what is actually happening in their body. Gravity is an ever-present curmudgeon that wreaks havoc on the balance of the hips, especially in asymmetrical postures. The back-leg hip generally wants to drop in lunges, and stability seems impossible in twists. Students rarely know where they're actually bearing weight in the feet, and therefore they have a hard time adjusting it if asked to change it.

Since proprioception is so altered for most of us, this is the place where hands-on adjustments make the most sense. Using our words is still important, but we will certainly need to use our hands more often here than in the spine.

You'll still want to make sure that you let the student actually perform the movements, let your hands or fingers (or knees or hips or feet, as the case may be) act as guides for them. Make them push their knee into your hand, or trace the external rotation on their thigh; try not to force any movements, since this is likely to throw them completely off balance or add too much torque to joints.

Standing Postures

Whether you are in Lunge, Warrior I, or Warrior II family postures, with a straight leg or a bent knee, it's likely that you'll need to make adjustments to the front knee and to that side's hip, which oftentimes shifts out toward the edge of the mat. It is a ubiquitous misalignment precipitated by students not knowing how to place or engage their feet on the mat. If they don't understand their own bony shape, if they have no knowledge of the torsions of their femur or tibia, they'll likely have a tough time finding their accurate blueprint. Since tradition still insists on the toes pointing straight ahead, many students will find themselves fighting their own anatomy while trying to meet this rather arbitrary alignment. You now have the opportunity to not only offer them some ease in these poses but also teach them something about their structure that they didn't know before.

First, you'll want to make sure that their feet are really hip-width (or back knee in the case of the low lunges). Stepping the front foot out toward the edge of the mat is often the most stable of the adjustments, but sometimes moving the back foot is unavoidable. In those low lunges, I often ask them to move the dropped knee so they become aware of it, since many times they began with hip-width feet but brought the knee down at the midline. They need to learn to shift it out as they kneel down every time.

Sometimes adjusting just the width will be plenty to shift the front knee into alignment. However, if you see that the big-toe root has a tough time grounding even while the knee is collapsing toward the midline, this is a clear indication that their bone structure is asking for some external rotation.

"Let your foot rotate out just a bit. Now root through the heel and press down gently with the big-toe mound."

Typically, that shift will realign the knee over the ankle and allow them to find Pada Bandha all in one go.

Again, when the knee drops in toward midline, there is an associated misalignment in the hips. So the next thing you want to check in on is whether the hip has hugged in to midline. Sometimes the adjustment to the foot and knee will fix this, but if not, you may need to offer one last cue:

Stand outside the opposite hip and ask them to move into you.

"Bring your whole pelvis toward me. Press your hip into my leg ... now root through your front heel. Let your back leg support you, lift your back thigh, lift your tail ..."

As for that back leg, I often use my feet to make subtle adjustments, helping bring attention to the pinky-edge of the foot, since it has a habit of lifting up. I'll lightly press my toes along the edge so they root down firmly. Sometimes I will place my hands on the floor to indicate that they need to alter their placement or rotation somewhat, often asking them to step forward or take their heel closer to the end of the mat. If they have a hard time getting the knee straight, it's possible that muscle tension is the culprit, so you'll need them to shorten their stance slightly.

If you are teaching a twisting pose, all but the most advanced yogis will have the back heel up in a lunge position instead of rooted flat to the floor. If they are compensating for the twist by allowing the hips to rotate, I strongly suggest coming at this adjustment in a subtle way that helps them access Pada Bandha and maintain balance. If you try to rotate the pelvis itself, they are likely to be thrown off balance and lose their core. Instead, I make sure they

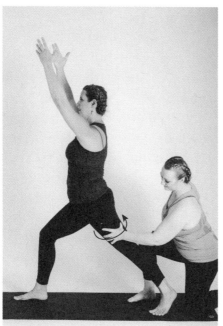 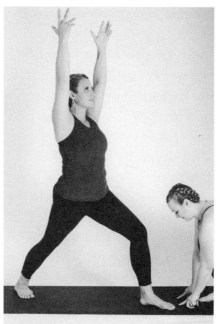

are using their foot and engaging rotational stability through the leg:

Place one hand on their toes and press back lightly, encouraging the ball of the foot to press back, while the other hand is on their heel, suggesting uplift. Then I trace my fingers on the back of the leg from outer thigh to inner thigh or, with a light grip, "twist" the thigh open (external rotation) by a degree or two.

"Very slightly rotate externally in this thigh, that will fire the glute a bit. Press back more with the big toe instead of pinky toe ... this will pull the hip back into balance so you have more access to the stability of the deep core, freeing up the heart for genuine rotation."

In Pyramid, the pelvis can go off course in so many directions. This is actually true of all of the asymmetrical standing postures, but it can be seen most profoundly in this straight-legged version. Very often we'll see the tail janked off to one side, one hip significantly lower than the other, and the low back rounded with a dropped tail.

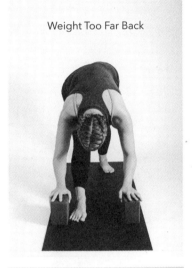

Weight Too Far Back

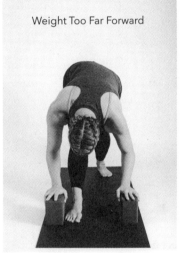

Weight Too Far Forward

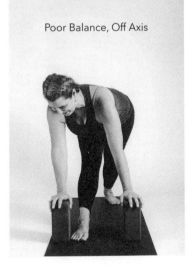

Poor Balance, Off Axis

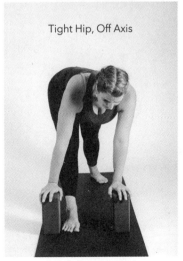

Tight Hip, Off Axis

The first thing you need to observe is that dropped tail. Offer blocks to lighten the heart and give them access to their core stability. If that isn't sufficient, a shorter stance may be needed. Then have them shift their entire weight forward and back; with this movement you'll see the hips change elevation in relation to one another. Those with particularly short hammies will usually bear too much weight in the back foot, trying to "run away" from the tension in the front leg, leaving that front-leg hip lower in space. As the weight shifts back, that low hip will rise and the pelvis will level out. Once that level is met, address the direction of the tailbone by placing hands on both sides of the hips and steering the tail toward the back wall. Lastly, ask for the tail to tilt up, activating the low back muscles and finding full stretch in the hamstrings. (This will suck. For most folks, that sensation they just found is exactly what they were running from in the first place.)

There are other pelvic adjustments to consider, especially in the Warrior II "open hip" poses. Considering that few of us have bones that allow a very clear and unrestricted abduction or horizontal abduction, very few of us will be able to fully open the pelvis until it's parallel with the side of the mat. To do this would mean cranking knees and ankles, compressing hip tissues and SI joints. In bodies on the mat, those who try to do this will exhibit internally rotated thighs and knees that struggle to neutralize. You'll see the whole pelvis shift back in space, trying to compensate for the compression in the hip joint. In postures like Side Angle and Triangle, the heart will swing forward and the hips will shift opposite. We can use our words and our hands to help correct these compensations, but we first need to understand that the over-opening is often the culprit.

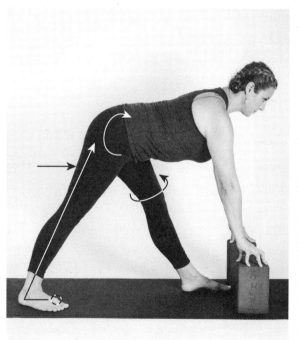
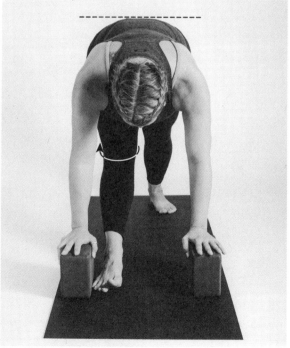

Weight is balanced front to back and side to side. Spine is active so hands are light.

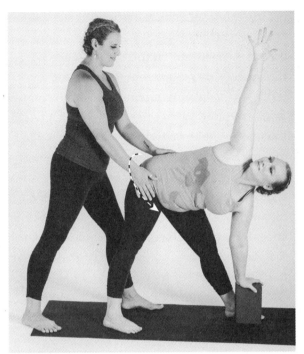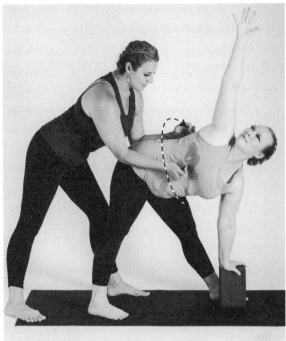

Allowing for less forced opening in the pelvis frees the hips and provides more space for genuine thoracic rotation to expand the heart.

In Triangle with right foot forward:

"Allow the left hip to turn back down toward the floor slightly, softening into the right hip crease. There is no need to stack the left hip over the right, allow the right hip to support you from underneath, and hug left hip into its socket. Root through right big-toe mound, and pull right sitting bone toward back of mat. Maintain softness in the knee. Pull tail toward back of heart, gather ribs like Cat, rotate heart open from the point between the shoulder blades, lengthen through the base of the skull."

You may need to use your hands to guide the pelvis into less rotation while you explain the movements. Help suggest the softer pelvic rotation, and then guide the thoracic twist so they can acknowledge that this action is what allows the joints to feel stacked.

But if you make all of these adjustments and then cue the "opening of the hips," you'll see the right SI joint collapse and most of the lumbar stability disintegrate. This opening will result in SI pain and dysfunction over time. Ick.

Seated Postures

Misalignments in seated postures are often collapses in the spine due to tension in the hips, so your adjustments may either be to the spine itself, or they'll be aimed at creating slack in the lower extremity so the spine can correct itself. Whether the hips are "open" or not, I highly recommend sitting EVERYONE up on a blanket so the pelvis can be supported in a neutral tilt before anything else occurs. There's a sidebar about this business of blankets back in chapter 8 (p. 95).

You can change the angle of the hip flexion by elevating the hips on a block, bolster, or blankets. This relieves some tension in the extensors. You can also prop up the knees into a slight flexion to create slack in hamstrings. If none of this helps the spinal neutrality, it may simply be a weakness in the spinal muscles, and that needs to be addressed directly.

In seated twists, there can be a knee pulled up to the chest, as in Lord of the Fishes or Marichi's Pose. In these cases, it's important that the shin bone remains upright and the sole of the foot rooted evenly. It's very common that the bent leg gets pulled in toward midline (Lord of the Fishes) or out to the side (Marichi's). Make sure you use verbal cues to ensure that the leg is stable without compensation.

> "In Lord of the Fishes, pull straight back on the shin bone. Avoid pulling it across the body in favor of a deeper twist. Press into the outer heel to activate the outer hip, and then root down with the big-toe mound for counteraction. Don't allow the arms to crank you into the twist; use your firm base and stable core to support a rotation in the ribs."

Since Marichi's Pose is an open twist, it's more common for the thigh to drop out to the side. You can minimize this by ensuring that the foot is not on the midline but at hip-width. Then allow any appropriate turn-out of the foot and find an active Pada Bandha. These adjustments will help guide the shin and thigh to a more stable upright form.

A less noticeable alignment adjustment may be needed if folks feel a bit tweaked in the knee or unable to get the hips equally weighted in Lord of the Fishes. Once the foot has crossed the opposite thigh, there is a tendency to want the toes to point straight ahead. I think it's pretty arbitrary, so try different alignments until less stress is felt in the other joints. My own toes point out to the side in these poses, but my big-toe mound remains the root.

In externally rotated poses like Bound Angle, remember that the depth of the bend in the knee will alter how the hip rotates. Adjustments to how near the heels are to the pelvis can have significant effects on a student's ability to access spinal neutrality or forward folding variations. Some folks will have their knees nearly touching the ground when their feet are pulled into the pelvis, but they rise up the further out the feet go.

Backbends

As we touched on earlier, this particular group of postures engages the lower extremity in some counterintuitive ways. Because extension in the hip can lead to extension in the spine due to compensation, there is a standing belief that the two belong together. I'm not so sure that's the case. Hyperextension in the hips prevents deep core engagement and therefore breaks down our ability to effectively employ the stabilizing effects of counteraction in the lumbar spine. Instead, activation of the hip flexors is paramount.

The adjustments we can offer our students in backbends are usually gentle admonitions to soften the glutes, to press knees into the mat in prone backbends, to activate both internal and external rotation in supine backbends, and to commit to backward momentum in the thighs in drop-backs.

In Cobra: "Unwind the tailbone; let it breathe." Sometimes soft fists pressed gently into the sides of the sacrum can help bring attention and release to clenched gluteals.

In Cobra: "Press the knees into the floor instead of the pubic bone. Don't lift the pelvis completely off the floor, but let it be light ..." Two hands on the back of the thighs just above the knees can help indicate exactly where the weight should be. You can also take the ankle into your hands, bend the knees to 90 degrees, and press down gently through the leg toward the floor.

In Bridge: "Press down through the outer heel and big-toe mound at once, this will draw the thighs into neutral alignment and activate glutes without clenching." Direct any applicable turn-out to help the student access Pada Bandha, then press your fingers into the top of the toe mound. If they need more help, foot width may also need an adjust. Your last move should be to have them actively move thighs toward midline—the other adjustments should accomplish this unless there is a significant weakness in the adductors.

In Camel: "Do not let the thighs press toward front wall. With hands on sacrum, push back into the hands and lift toward the back of the heart. A slight hinge will develop in the front of the hip. Allow this, encourage it, let the lifting tail support the coiling of the heart and the rise of the sternum toward the chin ..." Squat behind the student and with one hand pull back on the hip-hinge while pinching slightly between the scapulae with the fingers of the other hand. You may also, or instead, place hands on both sides of the pelvis, middle finger in hip-hinge and thumb on posterior ilium. Simultaneously press with thumbs and pull with the fingers to encourage forward tilt in the pelvis. A hand on the belly after one or both of these moves will remind them to gather the transverse abdominis for compressive support and traction.

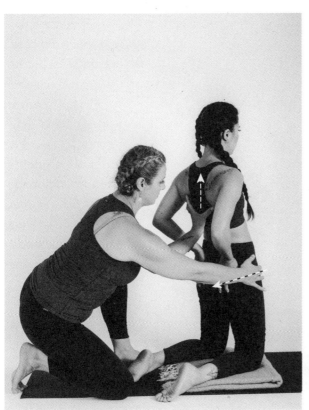
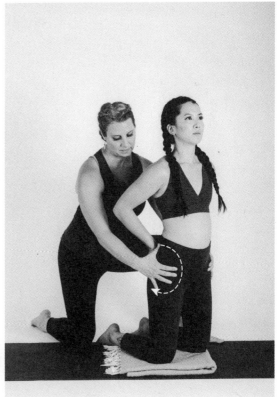

Downward Facing Dog
(Adho Mukha Svanasana)

This pose gets a section all its own. It's an inversion, it's a forward fold, it's ever-so-slightly a standing pose. The lower extremity is integral to this posture, and yet we can very easily overpower the remainder of the body by overemphasizing the efforts of the heels to reach the mat. Most people, even those of us who can reach the mat with ease, need to collapse their Pada Bandha to do it. Collapsed feet = collapsed legs and pelvis = collapsed spine and shoulders. Observe and adjust all the bandhas from the ground up. We'll cover upper body adjustments in a later chapter.

Begin with the feet. They should be hips-width. Big toe heavier than pinky, and Pada Bandha in full effect. Now look at the knees ... do they knock into the midline? Are they locked out? Both of these are very common, and they typically accompany an inactive foot.

"Soften the knees, look at them, rotate them outward until they make relatively straight lines instead of pointing in toward the center." From behind your student, hands or fingers may trace external rotation along the back of the thigh or knee. I will also stand with my own knees just outside of theirs and ask that they press them out into mine. Asking them to press heels together, touching the inner ankles as you do, can also achieve this if the misalignment is slight. "Hug an imaginary block with your ankles" is an appropriate cue here too.

The knock-kneed alignment is likely habitual because many students have been taught to roll inner thighs back in forward folds ... a despicable but ubiquitous cue. Showing them how much more prana can flow through these actively aligned legs can change how

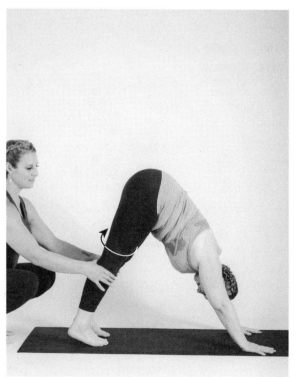

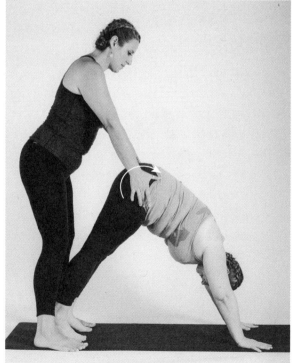

they perceive their practice. That's powerful medicine.

Lastly, consider the tilt of their pelvis. Even those with long hammies can exhibit a tucked-tail shape simply because they associate that action with a strong core. You'll need to both verbally and tactilely adjust the tilt to lift the sitting bones while maintaining a gathered belly.

"Make sure the tail tilts up to the sky. You may need to bend knees quite a bit for this. Find the backbending nature of Cow pose in the hips while continuing to gather the ribs like Cat." Make sure that their legs are aligned and properly rotated, then assist in settling weight back into the legs. The last thing you'll do is place hands on the pelvis itself to increase the tilt and lift the sitting bones.

Modifications

Modifications differ from adjustments. These are ways to change a pose specifically to accommodate an individual limitation. It may be a bony limitation in the hip. It may be that their hamstrings or entire back channel is tight and rigid. It may be that the ankles don't have full range of motion. Perhaps one leg is significantly longer than the other. All of these differences will alter their posture. They will definitely compensate elsewhere if we can't offer them relief in realignment.

Modification could be the use of props to help support the body in gravity. Blocks, bolsters, straps, blankets ... all of these can be used to offer ease to the body, but that isn't to say that the body won't still work hard. Effort is an integral part of every posture; props just help make our arms a little longer, our hips feel a little less strained, our spine less fatigued. In the lower extremity, we're usually trying to relieve the spinal compensations due to short hamstrings or relieve pressure in the knee or spine due to restrictions to external rotation in the hip.

Standing Postures

The modifications I use most in standing poses are blocks. Blocks under your hands make your arms longer, so your heart can be higher and lighter. When the heart is lighter, the deep core can activate with more ease and less strain, and you can then focus more on building a stable foundation in your legs. Lunges, Side Angle, Revolved Side Angle, Triangle, Pyramid ... all of these postures could use a block to help lighten the load of the heart.

When teaching to use blocks, I highly recommend that you have EVERYONE grab two blocks for EVERY class. It's not a choice, it's just how the pose is done. Then have them set up the blocks near the top of their mat, every time. Now they'll be in reach whenever you tell them to grab them. Again, it's not an option. Even other yoga teachers in your class will use them if you tell them to grab them and then offer instructions to the deep core. If you say, "Use a block if it helps ... ," no one is going to grab them. Most folks think about those blocks as crutches, but you're not gonna let them bear much weight on them, so crutches they are not.

A block is also a useful tool to help support a straight front leg that is prone to hyperextension. Postures like Triangle and Pyramid are a perfect place for this trick. On its highest setting, place a block behind the front calf. Have your student bend their knee ever so slightly, and tilt the block so the top side is flush with their calf muscle and the bottom edge is wedged into the mat. As they straighten their knee, the block will offer resistance, they won't be able to lock out, and they will be able to build better strength, stability, and awareness around the knee joint.

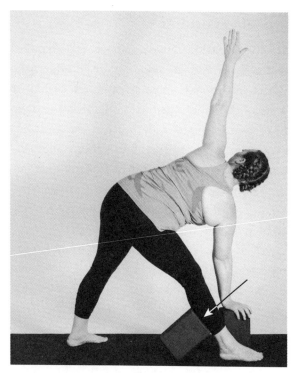

The block prevents hyperextension in the front knee, which allows Ka Shawna to build strength over time without further compromising her knee.

Seated Postures

We've already touched on elevation of the hips, but please please please don't be shy about this!! Insist that everybody elevate a bit so that those who need to elevate more don't feel like they are ostracized and faulty. The truth is, we ALL would benefit from a little support. For some of us it may be a temporary state on the way to more opening and strength, but for most of us it is just the way our practice will always look.

So, blocks. They aren't always the most comfortable to sit on, but they are high AND firm, which is exactly what is needed in twisting postures. If you have ever tried to do a Lord of the Fishes D (or 4, depending on your lineage), you'll probably have laughed your head off or burst into frustrated tears. It's a ridiculous pose that seems accessible only to cooked spaghetti noodles ... but even a busty, curvy girl like me can attempt it if I sit up on a block. If the requisite range of motion is there in the shoulders and hips, then lifting the pelvis so the thigh can drop out of your way a little will offer you more room for the spinal rotation. Just sayin'.

Other modifications may be appropriate for more mundane seated poses and twists. In abducted/external poses, Fire Log in particular, the bottom leg is subject to a tremendous amount of rotational force that can be translated directly to the knee. Because both hips are rotating simultaneously, the torsion on the pelvis can be extreme, and that can affect the spine or knees in significant ways. You need to be open to the option of straightening out the bottom leg to relieve some of this stress. This is the same modification that we see in Half Lord of the Fishes; this modification results in the same spinal twist without the bent bottom leg.

Backbends

Lower extremity modifications for the backbend family are few. These postures are more apt to be modified in terms of limiting extreme movements in the spine or upper extremity. Generally speaking, we would make small adjustments to ensure that the legs are in the correct place to support their joints sufficiently. For example, in the Bridge family, we'd make sure that the heels are directly under the knees and the hip doesn't overly extend. In the Cobra family, we'd ensure that the hip flexors are firing to prevent clenching in the glutes (some folks will need to bend knees to 90 degrees to feel this at first). In the Camel family, we'd help keep the hip extension in check by encouraging the thighs back over the knees instead of thrusting forward. We'd also ask for the feet to engage downward and inward energy, perhaps offering a block between the ankles.

I don't really think of any of these as modifications though. These are simply the activations needed to find integrity in the pose. If you think of any I am blanking on, please let me know!!

Practice

Now that we've covered both cueing and alignment points, it's time to teach some of these principles in context. This is not the time for brevity. This is an opportunity to use particular cues, explore your active vocabulary, and observe in real time the effects it has on the bodies in front of you. There are a million ways to explain the same movement, and this is your chance to see what works for whom. Take your time. Talk too much! Tell them what to move, where to move it, and how to get it there. Don't rush, take your time, and make changes as you go.

Again, it will be helpful to gather a couple of your book-group peers for this exercise, but friends or family members will work too. Three is ideal, one teacher to two students.

You'll now teach a simple lunge with the knee lifted. Start in Mountain and transition to Lunge. Teach the pose in as much detail as possible, highlighting the alignment areas we have discussed throughout the chapter, and then return to Mountain. While cueing, consider observations like:

- Foot placement
- Weight distribution

- Counteractions
- Hands on or off of blocks
- Spinal stability and alignment
- Planes of the pelvis

If you're working with peers, rotate through the group until everyone has had a chance to teach. The point of this exercise is to be able to adapt our language to what we see in front of us and not get caught up in more rhetoric.

Teachers

Use the new terminology we've worked on throughout this chapter. Be precise, don't worry about your students holding the pose too long, this is an exercise in excess. Get detailed and ensure they do what you ask. You'll need to teach the same detail two or three different ways to get the desired result. One person may get it the first time, while the other can't translate your instruction into action.

Use your words first, trying to offer each cue in more than one way, perhaps using different terminology to emphasize something different on each side. Consider using the hands-on adjustment models we have discussed only if words aren't working for a particular movement.

Students

This exercise is aimed at offering feedback for our verbal cues. Your teacher needs honest practical experience muddling through what works and what doesn't. Do only what you are told. Make adjustments based on what you actually hear, not what you are expecting to hear. Lunge as if it is your first time, listen intently, and move as you are told to. If their words are particularly confusing, kindly point it out and allow them the chance to adjust their perspective. It's not necessary to be intentionally difficult, but starting in a perfect pose or guiding them with your own adjustments won't help them in the long run. They need to build up a rich repertoire in order to reach all levels of students.

Once you have explored the options for observing and adjusting Lunge, try a couple of other fundamental postures. Remember to consider whether the spine needs to be stable or mobile, and include appropriate cues. Poses to consider:

- Down Dog
- Warrior II
- Plank
- Seated Forward Fold

11

The Upper Extremity: Structure and Nature

The practice of yoga incorporates all that the upper extremity can do and along the way asks much from it that it wasn't particularly designed to do. From the most subtle of mudras in the hands to the gravity-defying strength and balance present in arm balance and inversion practice, the upper extremity offers us perhaps the most dynamic range of strength and mobility possible in the body.

Because of this outstanding range, we must be more thoughtful of just *how* we employ these structures in our yoga practice in order to build strength without compromising the health of our tissues. It is integral that we understand the engineering of these parts and their relationship to the entire body, or else we risk serious and likely permanent injury. The risks are as high as the rewards when we engage in elaborate upper-body yoga asana. In these chapters, we will explore the anatomy from top to bottom and examine the ways we use the upper extremity in practice. As always, we'll pay close attention to inherent risks to the physical body and discuss skills we can develop to help ourselves and individual students find their own ideal alignments. We'll debunk some outdated cueing and redesign our practice and instruction based on the fundamental biomechanics of the shoulder, arm, and wrist.

Bones

The upper extremity is a complex set of multiple joints that work in dynamically different ways to move the arm through space. It is only in combination of these various joints that we can enjoy the full range of motion of the upper extremity without injuring our soft tissues.

The bones of the upper extremity are made for movement; that means many muscles, which means lots of attachment points, which means lots of hard, pokey bits. If we move in a way that gets these bits out of each other's way, no problem. But when we let gravity and poor mechanics rule, our tender tissues are at high risk for strain, impingement, and friction injuries, all of which lead to chronic pain or worse. The scapula and the humerus both have a number of bony outcroppings just waiting to pinch your squishy bits. Specific movements need to be made to create the widest berth between these bones; otherwise you risk injury to numerous tendons, bursae, neurovascular bundles, and cartilage.

Always keep in mind that the shape of our bones defines our range of motion. The upper extremity exemplifies this beautifully. The way the bones relate to one another, as well as how soft tissues attach to, cross, and manipulate the bones, creates a truly miraculous combination of possible movement—and possible mishaps. Be mindful of the intricate architecture as we add layers of tissue, section by section.

The bones of the upper extremity are as follows:

- **Clavicle** = collarbone. This long bone, along with the shoulder blade, creates the framework for the shoulder girdle. Its proximal end also articulates with the sternum to build the only true joint that attaches the upper extremity to the axial skeleton. (Translation: This is where your arm attaches to your body.) Because of its position across the upper chest and its relationship to the upper ribs, it offers surface area for large-muscle attachments, but it also creates the potential for soft tissue impingements. In reality, gravity pulls down on our arms with constant pressure. Most of us don't know any

better, so we allow the collarbones to press down on our ribs, an act that results in adhesions and impingements in the soft tissues of the neck and chest. The clavicle is meant to be suspended just above the ribs, which requires some conscious effort at first, or forever, depending on how toned you can get those shoulder-elevating muscles.

- **Scapula** = shoulder blade. One of the more irregular bones in the body, the scapula provides tons of surface area for muscular attachment. Both broad surfaces and pokey protrusions offer places for secure attachments while creating multiple leverage points to increase potential range of motion. Some pokey bits to notice:

  - Acromion Process. This ledge of bone reaches out as an extension of the spine of the scapula and creates the attachment point for the distal end of the clavicle. It also creates

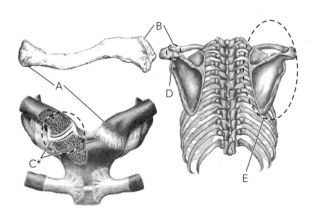

(A) Proximal clavicle (sternal end), (B) Distal clavicle (acromial end), (C) Sternoclavicular joint (*cut-away portion shows articular disc), (D) Acromioclavicular joint, (E) Shoulder girdle

surface area for the attachments of trapezius and deltoid muscles.

- Coracoid Process. A crooked little horn of bone that juts off the front of the scapula to protrude out from under the distal curve of the collarbone. This fixture has a number of ligaments that will secure it to the clavicle, but it also serves as the insertion for pectoralis minor.

The other thing to note about the shoulder blade is that it doesn't form a true joint to the torso. Instead, it is supported by a complex sling of muscles, so it kind of floats on the back of the ribs.

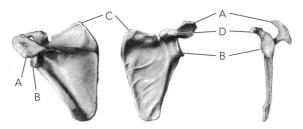

(A) Acromion process, (B) Glenoid fossa, (C) Superior angle, (D) Coracoid process

- **Humerus** = arm. Leverage is the name of this bone's game. For a single long bone, this one has a ton of potential for range of motion through space, but because of the knobby and ridged structures near its head (the greater and lesser tubercles, which resemble the greater trochanter of the femur), there is a high potential for soft tissue impingement. Its relationship with the scapula is dynamic and requires more conscious movement than most of us actually offer it. Pay attention to the tiny space above the head of the humerus, because through that space

runs a great deal of soft tissue, just waiting to be squished between those bony surfaces.

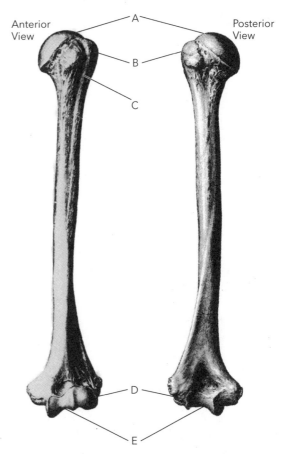

(A) Head, (B) Tubercles, (C) Bicipital groove, (D) Articulation with radius, (E) Articulation with ulna

- **Ulna/Radius** = forearm. These two bones offer multiple joint arrangements at both the elbow and the wrist. Intricate shapes fit together in precise ways to limit range of motion in one place while maximizing it in others. These two bones quite literally dance with each other as we move our arms and hands! Precisely shaped grooves allow for and protect the delicate nerves that need to get from the chest to the hand.

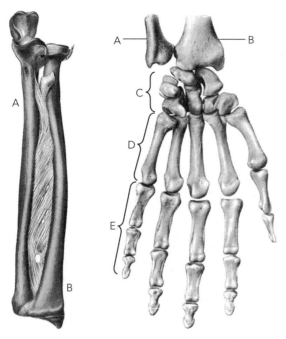

(A) Ulna (creates "point" of the elbow), (B) Radius,
(C) Carpals (wrist), (D) Metacarpals (hand),
(E) Phalanges (fingers)

- **Carpals** = wrist. This set of eight short bones fit together like a 3D puzzle, similar to the structure of the mid-foot. When perfectly aligned and well supported by their ligaments, these bones form the "carpal tunnel" and provide a very mobile joint system that allows our hands to be so expressive. This tunnel, in association with the long bones of the hand, also offers the structural framework that supports Hasta Bandha.

- **Metacarpals** = hand. Because of the mobility of the carpals and precise alignments of the metacarpals, we have the ability to grip with dexterity and strength. The opposable thumbs we humans are so famous for are actually

possible because of the relationship of the metacarpals to one another, not the fingers and thumb.

- **Phalanges** = fingers. My hope is that these are self-explanatory. We need to learn to use them as an integral part of the upper extremity—not just for powerful energetic mudra, but as an extension of Hasta Bandha, and an important tool in supporting us in weight-bearing postures, especially our inversions and arm balances.

Soft Tissues

These structures are integral to the working of the shoulder complex but are at high risk if we don't move intelligently. Again, because of the inherent mobility of the shoulder and arm, these tissues can easily be pinched between bones if we aren't moving thoughtfully and using our muscular system intentionally. In the shoulder complex, compression is the most likely mechanism of injury, since we're moving in the extremes of range of motion and bearing weight in ways that we aren't actually designed for.

- **Labrum**: This is the cartilage rim around the edge of the glenoid fossa of the scapulae. It gives the sense that there's a "socket" there, rather than just a flat bone, which in fact it is. Because it doesn't get good circulation, any injury to this cartilage is permanent, and so far only surgery can fix it.

- **Joint Capsule**: The fibrous encasement of the joint that essentially holds it all together. The shoulder's joint capsule is thicker than most and functionally acts in lieu of separate ligaments connecting the humerus to the scapula. To ensure maximal range of motion, the joint capsule has slack on its inferior aspect, slack that can bunch up and stick to itself if mobility is compromised for an extended time. This slack also means that there is little to no tension support under the ball and socket joint, leaving it vulnerable to *dislocation*.

- **Ligaments**: Because the joint capsule really does the heavy lifting at the glenohumeral joint, the ligaments we refer to here connect the clavicle to the scapula. First you have ligaments attaching the clavicle to the acromion process, forming the **acromioclavicular (AC) joint**, which when stretched results in a shoulder *separation*. Next we have a series of short ligaments that connect the clavicle to the coracoid process of the scapula, the little horn of bone that protrudes awkwardly underneath the clavicle and doubles as an attachment point for shoulder muscles.

- **Tendons**: Lots of muscles means lots of tendons. One to be ultra-aware of is the **biceps tendon**, which is at high risk for impingement, tendinitis, and rupture due to its path under the acromion process and fusion through the labrum. Its

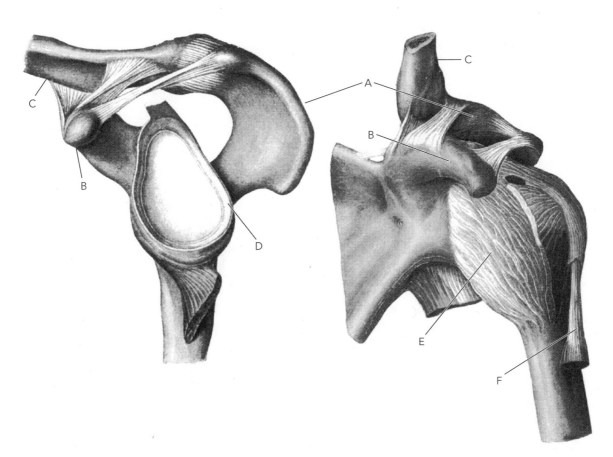

(A) Acromion process, (B) Coracoid process, (C) Clavicle, (D) Labrum (on glenoid fossa), (E) Joint capsule, (F) Biceps tendon (long head)

path to that attachment travels through a bony groove (called the *bicipital groove*, conveniently) on the humerus. Another tendon of note: supraspinatus ... it also travels under the acromion process to attach to the humerus, so it's prone to compression injury as well.

Since the remaining muscles of the arm and forearm are mostly long and thin for optimal leverage, there are many stringy tendons that form attachments at the elbow, wrist, and hand. Some of these tendons are encased in *tendon sheaths*, extra layers of slick connective tissue, to keep them moving with less friction. But every system can break down, and many of these tendons are prone to inflammation, especially in yogis who use our hands and arms to bear weight in novel ways.

- **Bursae**: These little synovial fluid–filled sacs reduce friction between bones and soft tissue. They are ideal in a place where tendons run over the edges of rough bones, but the ones in the shoulder joint take up valuable space between the humerus and the acromion process and therefore are themselves at risk for impingement and friction injury if we don't move intelligently.

- **Neurovascular Bundles**: Veins, arteries, and nerves travel together in packs. Where there is one, you'll usually find the others. Those that serve the arm begin in the cervical spine as the *brachial plexus*, and they unite and split in various patterns to enervate the shoulder complex and beyond. Some travel under the clavicle, through the armpit, and down the arm to the hand. Anywhere along that path, there is risk of impingement by soft tissues, usually due to spastic or adhered muscles and fascia.

- **Retinaculum**: This is a thin band of connective tissue that holds tendons in place around bendy bits, so they don't bulge out during movement. In this case, there is one on both the front and back of the wrist. The anterior one helps form the carpal tunnel.

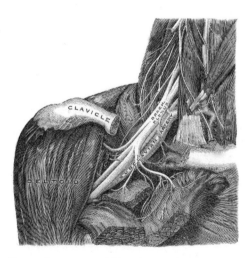

Tons of nerves and blood vessels travel through this congested area. If the clavicle isn't actively lifted off the upper ribs, these tissues get compressed.

Joints

As mentioned earlier, the upper extremity is a complex system of many joints. All of them are small compared to similar joints in the lower extremity and, with only a couple exceptions, have substantial range of motion for their size. Here they are in order from proximal to distal.

- **Sternoclavicular** (SC) = sternum + clavicle
- **Acromioclavicular** (AC) = clavicle + scapula
- **Glenohumeral** (GH) = scapula + humerus
- **Humeroulnar** = humerus + ulna (elbow)
- **Radioulnar** = radius + ulna (elbow and wrist, for rotation)
- **Radiocarpal** = radius + carpals (wrist)
- **Carpal Tunnel** = carpals + retinaculum (connective tissue)
- **Carpometacarpal** = carpals + hand bones (saddle joint = thumb's carpometacarpal joint.)
- **Metacarpophalangeal** = hand bones + fingers

Most of these joints don't require a long-winded description beyond just identifying the articulating pieces, but a few will be better served by some functional elaboration. All of the above-mentioned joints are mobile synovial joints, *except for the AC joint*. This is a ligamentous joint that honestly shouldn't move much, if at all, unless it's already been injured. All of the other joints have pretty remarkable range. After all, the upper extremity is built to reach around in our world, so range of motion is the name of the game.

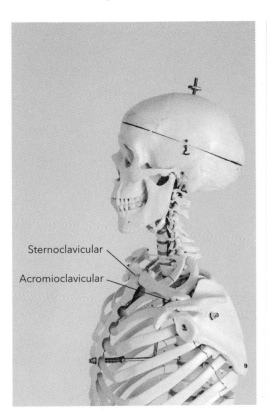

Sternoclavicular
Acromioclavicular

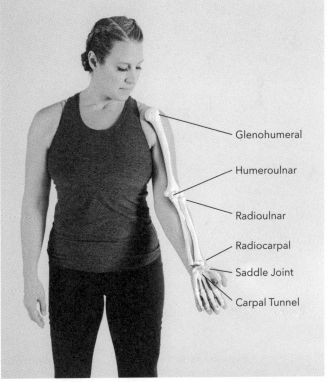

Glenohumeral
Humeroulnar
Radioulnar
Radiocarpal
Saddle Joint
Carpal Tunnel

The Shoulder Girdle vs. the Shoulder Joint

To understand the complex nature of the upper extremity, we must first break down the components of the shoulder. The first piece is the combo-pack of the clavicle and the scapulae plus all of the small joints holding those bones together and attaching them to the body. Be clear that the upper extremity is articulated to the torso at just one small true joint: the *sternoclavicular joint*. This articulation—along with the *scapulothoracic joint*, which is not really a joint at all—holds our upper extremity onto our body. Since the scapulothoracic joint is not the articulation of two bones connecting at a synovial joint but rather a muscular relationship between the ribs, shoulder blade, and clavicle, we call it a *false joint*. So, the collarbone, scapula, and all associated joints and muscles create the *shoulder girdle*.

The second component is the ball and socket joint, the *glenohumeral (GH) joint*, or *shoulder joint*. This is the ball and socket connection of the humerus to the shoulder blade. This is the home of the rotator cuff muscles, whose common function is to hold the joint together.

From here forward we'll refer to these two primary sections as the **shoulder girdle** and

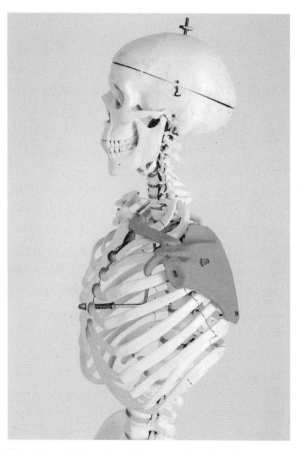 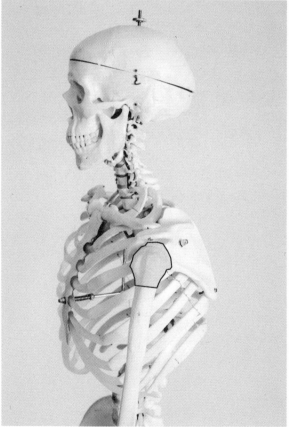

Shoulder girdle = clavicle + scapula. Glenohumeral joint (shoulder joint) = scapula + humerus.

the **shoulder joint** and use these terms interchangeably with their technical names.

- **Shoulder Girdle** = clavicle + scapula (+ the sternoclavicular joint that attaches them to the body) + muscles that move them (scapulothoracic)
- **Shoulder Joint (GH)** = scapula + humerus + muscles that move them (rotator cuff)

This complex is engineered to work as a fluid unit, each component moving within a prescribed range to achieve an overall dynamic and large reach in nearly any direction. Just as the spine is capable of moving in infinite directions because of its multiple facet joints, the upper extremity requires a concert of movements from each of its many articulations to achieve full range of motion. Understanding these joint structures and their particular individual range is integral to moving with intention, in a manner that both prevents injury and engages our muscular support.

Although the ball and socket joint is generally thought of as a joint with limitless movement possibilities, the bony structure of the GH joint limits its potential. The combination of bony prominences and soft tissues packed into small spaces creates a high risk for impingement in nearly every direction. It's important to note that the majority of movement in our shoulder complex actually comes from the shoulder girdle. If your scapula is adhered to your ribs, or your clavicle can't move freely due to spasm or lack of strength in the appropriate muscles, you will inevitably move more in the GH joint, wearing on those tissues and promoting degeneration. It's fundamental that we work to maximize the potential for both strength and mobility in the shoulder girdle for healthy function of the upper extremity overall.

Elbow

At first glance, the elbow seems pretty straightforward: it bends and straightens. When you look closer, however, there are multiple joints at play here as well. You have the articulation between the humerus and ulna, a hinge joint that operates only on the sagittal plane for flexion and extension. Another joint nearby, the proximal connection of the ulna and radius, is a pivot joint that works in concert with its distal partner to allow for the pronation and supination of the forearm.

It's important to examine these joints closely in terms of function and alignment, because as we bear weight throughout an average yoga asana practice, the physics of our individual bony shapes and angles define how and where we place our hands for optimal efficiency. Once we understand the structural facts, we can better employ our muscular support, using counteracting rotations of the shoulder and the forearm to create very strong frameworks for all of our weight-bearing postures.

The most profound individual difference to be aware of is the lateral deviation of the elbow common to just about every one of us: the **carrying angle**. The angle varies individually from mild to extreme and will be the primary determiner of where you place your hands while bearing weight. If you don't heed this differentiation, the wrists, elbows, and shoulders are all at risk. Because of this angle, our optimal alignment is to set our elbows at shoulder-width, not our hands. With even a slight carrying angle, the physics of weight bearing are most efficient with our hands wider than our shoulders. Just like a pyramid being broader at its base, this wider setup allows for greater stability and more efficient translation of gravity through the upper extremity to the core, with far less risk of injury to the joints along the way.

Wrist

The wrist is a devil. It has intricate relationships with both the forearm and the hand that are engineered for maximum fluidity and dexterity for reaching and gripping. It offers mobility on multiple planes but unfortunately has very little direct muscular support. All of

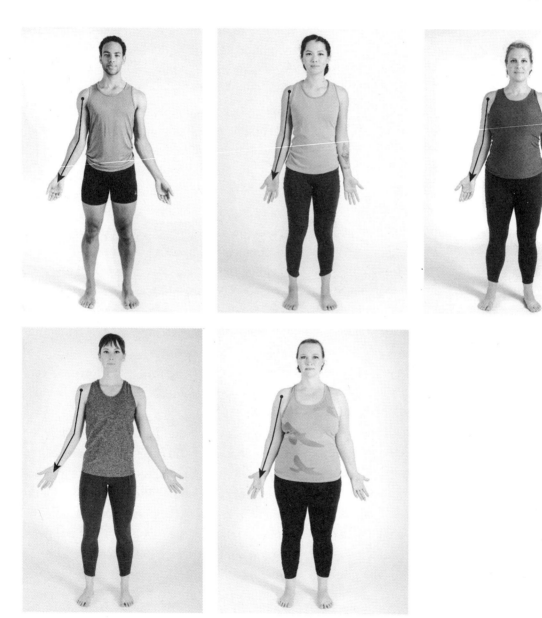

Carrying angles vary greatly from person to person, meaning we each have a very distinct personal alignment when our hands move through space or meet the earth.

its articulations rely on ligamentous support to keep the bones in place, and since we use it in our yoga practice for more weight bearing than it is really designed for, we have to be incredibly thoughtful about how we employ it when we place our hands on the earth. The blood flow and nervous support to our hand have to travel through this very bony region, so if we use it haphazardly, we will surely compromise the health and function of these structures.

One specific joint stands out here in the wrist. It is the articulation of the wrist with the first metacarpal, or thumb. We call this the **saddle joint**. I point it out intentionally because it is a very fragile, precise joint that tends to deteriorate faster than other joints in the wrist or hand. In weight-bearing postures it's easy to misalign this joint and then put too much weight into it. These actions work together to twist and grind the bones, which leads to degeneration and arthritis. Ideally, we learn to place our hands appropriately for our own individual alignment, and we engage our muscles so there's very little or no weight in our thumb pad, relieving pressure from the saddle joint, and instead focus our effort to the index- and middle-finger knuckles. We'll discuss this in detail later.

Range of Motion

The range of motion of the upper extremity is dependent upon the unified relationship between the shoulder girdle and shoulder joint. If you reach your arm to its maximum in any direction, combining all the movements into one sweeping arc, you can typically come pretty close to 360 degrees of range. If you are engaging with optimal efficiency, only 30 degrees of this is actually coming from the GH joint; the remainder comes from the dynamic mobility of the shoulder girdle.

To be clear, if the scapula isn't moving in its full range of motion, the GH *will* compensate and damage the tendons, bursae, and neurovascular bundles that travel through the joint. These systems are designed to work together using *intentional compensatory movement* to achieve the full range of motion of the upper extremity. Here compensation is actually a good thing, built into the system strategically to allow for more efficient movement. If your intention is to reach overhead, you MUST move from the scapula as well as the GH.

Shoulder Girdle (SG)

Because the scapula isn't attached to the ribs at a synovial joint and moves via the lever that is the clavicle, the SG's range of motion is defined very differently from the traditional range of the shoulder joint. Please note that different textbooks define movement of the shoulder in different ways. I have studied many of these, and the descriptions here allow for the most specific definitions of its total range of motion. I suggest you stick with these to avoid confusion later.

- **Elevation/Depression** = straight up and down
- **Abduction/Adduction** = around the ribs, away from the spine/toward the spine (pinching scapulae together)
- **Rotation Up/Down** = pivot on a central point; acromion process moves up/down
- **Protraction/Retraction** = tilting over the ribs; superior angle moves forward/back

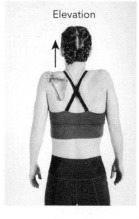
Elevation

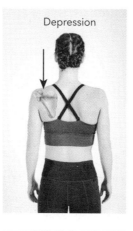
Depression

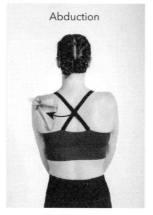
Abduction

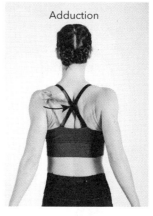
Adduction

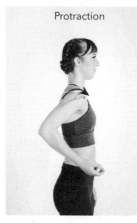
Protraction

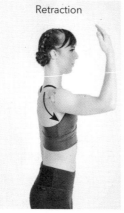
Retraction

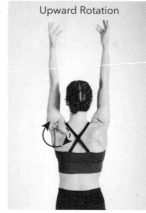
Upward Rotation

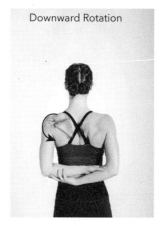
Downward Rotation

When we move through our full-reaching range of motion, we must combine some of these actions in order to keep the GH joint safe. Remember that the shoulder girdle moves in concert with the shoulder joint. Compound actions are integral to the proper working of the upper extremity. Be aware that there is a gentle balance to be achieved between stability and mobility at the SG in order to move safely and efficiently through weight bearing, reaching, and binding.

Shoulder Joint (GH)

Consider carefully that each of the GH movements listed here can only go about 30 degrees. The remainder of our movement should come from the shoulder girdle. Even that 30 degrees comes with some risk of soft tissue impingement, so move intentionally. You can create a little extra space in flexion or abduction by first *externally rotating* the humerus to get the bony tubercles out of the way of the acromion process.

- **Flexion/Extension** = reaching forward/back

- **Abduction/Adduction** = reaching out to the side/back into the body (midline)

- **Rotation Internal/External (medial/lateral)** = biceps turns in toward the midline/out away from the midline

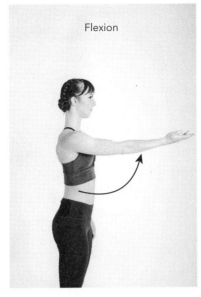

Flexion

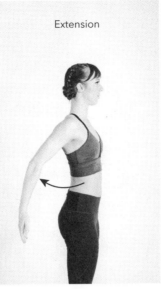

Extension

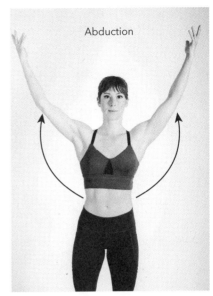

Abduction

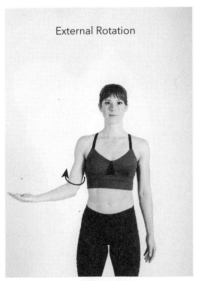

External Rotation

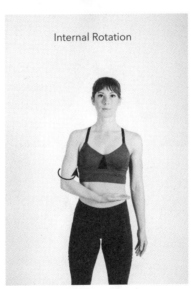

Internal Rotation

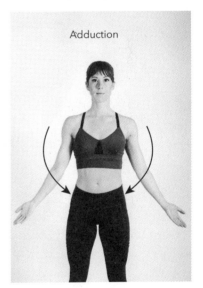

Adduction

Compensatory Movement by Design

"Compensation" has usually been treated as a negative thing up until now. In many regions of our anatomy, compensation in our joints can cause wear and tear on tissues that otherwise would be protected by good biomechanics. In the upper extremity, however, we need to think about compensation in a slightly different way. It's important to acknowledge that certain actions of the shoulder girdle and shoulder joint are designed to work together, that the compound movements are integral to maximizing safe movement in our full range of motion. Counteracting or avoiding these compound movements can cause damage. In order to reach maximum range in the movements below, you must combine the movements of the GH and shoulder girdle.

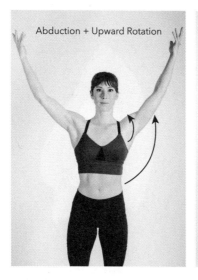

Abduction + Upward Rotation

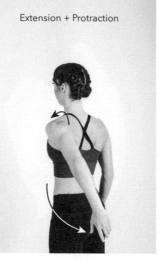

Extension + Protraction

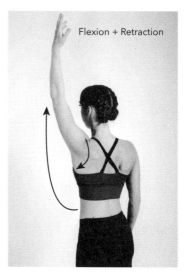

Flexion + Retraction

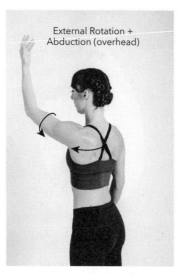

External Rotation + Abduction (overhead)

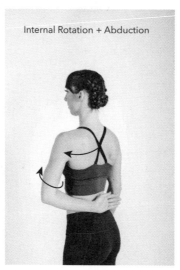

Internal Rotation + Abduction

- Abduction at GH *requires* UPward rotation at SG.

- Extension at GH *requires* PROtraction at SG.

- Flexion at GH *requires* REtraction at SG.

- Internal rotation at GH *requires* ABduction at SG.

- External rotation at GH *requires* ADduction at SG. *(This is reversed when reaching overhead.)*

These compensations are engineered into the system for optimal efficiency. When we use the entire system as a unit, work and stress are distributed across many muscles instead of overloading just one. We use energy more efficiently as well as decrease wear and tear on any one particular point, reducing risk of injury.

COUNTERACTION IN THE UPPER EXTREMITY

If counteracting within the shoulder is ill-advised, then how do we stabilize this part of the body? When considering the shoulder, we need to observe the strong connection of the rib-spine and the shoulder girdle. Stabilization actually occurs here, where the scapula attaches to the ribs and spine. When you reach or bear weight, the entire shoulder girdle/shoulder joint system must work together, so the core actions come into play to resist the movements of the scapula. This is apparent when we reach overhead (flexion + retraction at the shoulder): the ribs have to press back into the scapula by using Uddiyana Bandha (deep core activation) and subtle flexion in the rib-spine. I'll often describe this as your Cat action—the ribs pressing into the scapulae even as the scapulae press into the ribs. Any posture where the arms reach out or up without the ribs blowing out is achieved through counteraction at the shoulder girdle.

The arm and elbow counteract in a different way, especially for bearing weight. In this part of the upper extremity, rotations become the primary supporting actions. When our hands are on the ground, we need to stabilize the wrist, elbow, and shoulder joint. The wrist is pretty easy, since we really only need to press into the mat, which by its nature resists us perfectly well. The elbow and shoulder, however, require a bit more internal resistance. Since we already know that external rotation sets up the shoulder joint for more success, we activate that here too. The counteraction occurs when we use internal rotation of the forearm, or pronation. We can affect this relationship by simultaneously pressing the root of the index finger into the ground (internal rotation) while also wrapping our elbows to point back toward our thighs (external rotation).

Elbow

Because the elbow has two separate joints, its range is more dynamic than it may first appear. The *humeroulnar joint* allows for **flexion and extension**. Depending on the shape of this joint in the individual, hypo- or hyperextension may be available here. Even though the joint is mostly stable, any exploitation of hyperextension will lead to joint degeneration and dysfunction over time.

The second joint, the *proximal radioulnar joint*, works in conjunction with its distal partner to allow rotation of the forearm: **pronation and supination**.

Wrist/Hand/Fingers

The carpal joints articulate with the radius at an elliptical joint that allows for **flexion/extension and adduction/abduction**. The carpals themselves meet at relatively flat surfaces

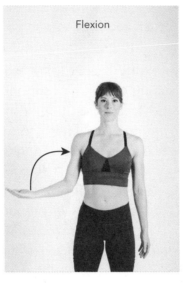
Flexion

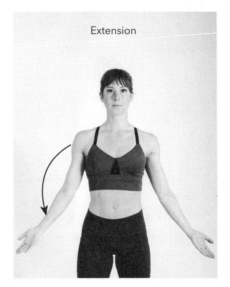
Extension

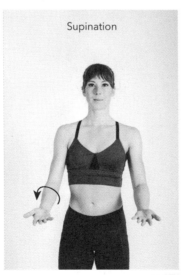
Supination

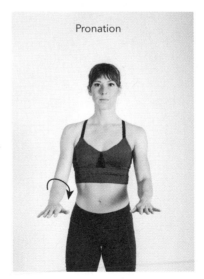
Pronation

that are limited only by their ligamentous support. The nature of these joints is that they can move in virtually any direction, and as a system they allow for the movement that approximates circumduction.

The hand's range of motion is limited, except for at the thumb. Because of the saddle joints, we can create **opposition**, or reaching the thumb across the palm. Some range is available in the remaining carpometacarpal joints, allowing the long bones of the hand to kind of cup themselves around the palm. These movements are supported by small intrinsic muscles as well as the more powerful thenar muscles, which move the thumb in opposition.

The strength of the palm and fingers is really controlled by muscles in the forearms, but the fingers also have tiny intrinsic muscles that allow for fine dexterity. All of these play a role in our yoga practice as we grip the mat and find Hasta Bandha.

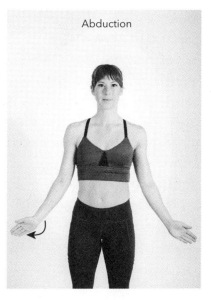
Abduction

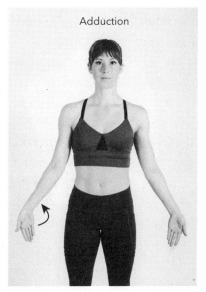
Adduction

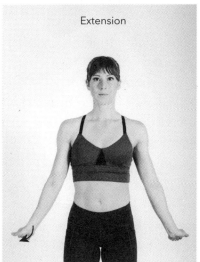
Extension

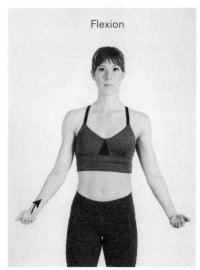
Flexion

Muscles

Since the shoulder alone is a combination of many small joints, the musculature to move all this gets pretty complicated. It's not nearly as straightforward as the spine or even the hip. In those sections we could make some generalities: muscles on the back create extension, muscles on the front create flexion … While those statements may be true about the muscles of the arm and forearm, any muscles that cross the shoulder or shoulder girdle have more complex roles to play. So, we'll be organizing these muscles in a slightly different manner than we did in previous chapters.

As you study the lists below, it is important to recognize that an individual muscle can do more than one action. Many of these muscles have multiple fiber directions, so different parts of the belly may create different movements at the same joint. It's possible then that some of these act as *stabilizers for themselves*, such as deltoid, whose anterior and posterior fibers oppose one another, stabilizing the rotational range of motion.

It can also get complicated when considering counteraction relationships. Because both direct and indirect relationships form between the movers of the shoulder girdle and shoulder joint, defining true counteractions can feel confusing. These complex slings of muscle work together and against each other in pretty remarkable ways. It will take a long time to become totally familiar with all the layers and their actions. Trust me when I say that you'll be referring to muscle charts and flashcards for a while to come. Repetition is certainly the key to learning this particular system.

For now, focus on the concept that the upper extremity is dependent on a very complex muscular system that both stabilizes and mobilizes it. In class, the names and functions of these muscles will be lost on your students anyway, so it's much more important to offer simple actions instead of muscle names. This provides them experiential learning and increases sensational awareness instead of just spewing big Latin words at them.

THE ARM AS A LEVER

To complicate matters just a little more, we should note that the upper extremity, in its complexity, also uses leverage to a great degree. Consider this: in a Cobra setup, pulling your elbows together (movement at the shoulder joint) also broadens the collarbones (movement at the shoulder girdle). That movement is really initiated by shoulder joint muscles, but it levers the collarbones as well. This relationship is different from the built-in compensations described earlier—and can be the cause of injury if we aren't aware of it.

As you apply the principles of combined movements, counteractions, and mobilizations in your yoga asana practice, you need to understand that the arm bone acts as a lever for the shoulder girdle. You'll see muscles that are arm movers at the shoulder joint—chest muscles like pectoralis major and back muscles like latissimus—and even though they aren't shoulder girdle muscles, the forces they exert on the arm bone may translate to secondary movements at the shoulder girdle.

The reverse can also occur, where the scapular movements shift the alignment of the arm bone. A common place for this phenomenon is in Low Plank, when the pectoralis major can overcompensate for lack of strength in the upper back and core and pull the SG into abduction. Pectoralis minor contributes here as well, protracting the scapula to create a very hunched posture with a collapsed chest. These SG positions create an internal rotation in the arm and shoulder joint, as well as send the elbows pointing out to the sides. All of this puts immense pressure on the biceps tendon and labrum, and it leaves the triceps with the brunt of the work of actually keeping you from doing a face-plant.

If Low Plank is done like this as a matter of course, repeated pressure is applied to the soft tissues of the shoulder joint, and injury over time is inevitable. Unlike the compensations-by-design, these secondary movements require active counteractions to keep the shoulder safe when bearing weight. In this case, the upper back must activate to balance out the contractions of the chest, the arms need to be pulled back into their alignment with the ribs, and the core needs to activate to take weight-bearing pressure off the triceps.

Shoulder Girdle

In this section we'll cover the muscles that directly move the scapula and collarbone. Remember, these two bones move as a single unit. If the shoulder blade goes up, so does the clavicle. Recall as well that range of motion is defined differently here than elsewhere. We reference the movements of the scapulae to describe the movement of the shoulder girdle as a whole.

Trapezius. Oh, trapezius. This may be one of the most recognizable muscles to the layperson, but only by name. Functionally, it's a mystery to most. It's a very large, flat, superficial muscle that spans the space from the base of our skull to the base of our ribs. In weightlifting circles it's considered a back muscle ... but

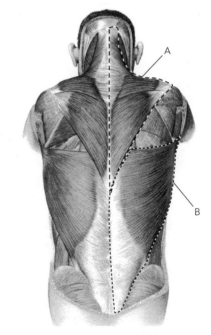

(A) Trapezius (note three separate fiber directions: upper, middle, and lower), (B) Latissimus dorsi

in anatomical terms it moves our scapula as part of the upper extremity.

Often referred to in lay terms as "traps," it has three fiber directions. The upper fibers run from the skull to the acromion process *and* the distal clavicle. Because of this insertion design, the flat fabric of muscle wraps over the top of the shoulder blade and kind of encases the smaller levator scapula muscle underneath it. This alignment leaves these muscle bellies very vulnerable to adhesion to one another. When the spine is stable, these muscle fibers will elevate, upwardly rotate, and/or adduct the shoulder blade. If the scapulae are stable though, then the upper fibers can mobilize the spine—as in lifting the head off the ground in prone positions like Cobra.

The middle fibers are mostly horizontal in alignment from the thoracic spine to the spine of the scapula. This fiber direction sets them up as strong adductors. Some studies have shown that because of the nature of the insertion angles on the shoulder blade, these fibers can also assist in upward rotation of the scapula.

The lower fibers of traps run up from their spinal attachments to insert on the "root of the spine" of the scapula. This is the most medial point on the scapular spine, meaning that the medial portion of the scap will draw down when these fibers fire. This results in the acromion process rising, and by definition this is upward rotation. These fibers also have the capacity to draw the entire scapula straight down in depression. **(elevation [upper fibers], depression [lower fibers], adduction, upward rotation)**

Levator Scapula. This little muscle runs from the lateral neck bones to the superior angle of the scapula. It's the one that gets hugged by the upper fibers of traps. Its action is to assist traps in elevation. Most often targeted in bodywork instead of strength training, since it is notorious for forming adhesions and trigger points. **(elevation)**

Rhomboid. Rhomboids are sometimes separated into Major and Minor divisions, but since the bellies have no separation and perform identical actions, I lump 'em together. This muscle is deep to middle traps and assists in its function of adducting the shoulder blade. Because rhomboids are at an oblique angle downward from the spinous processes of the vertebrae to the medial border of the scapula, they also create a bit of downward rotation, so they can counter (stabilize against) the upward rotation created by traps. This is one of those interesting relationships I mentioned earlier, where two muscles can both support and resist one another in different actions. **(adduction, downward rotation)**

Serratus Anterior. I love this muscle. I love it in the only way you can love something that pains you repeatedly and often, something that seems to be always at odds with you on some level! I genuinely hated this muscle until I was able to get it legitimately strong and long, which took some doing. Serratus is a multi-bellied muscle that originates on the lateral rib cage and follows the ribs back under the scapula, to its insertion on the medial edge of the scapula. Because of this position and path, serratus has a high potential for adhesion to the front side of the shoulder blade. It commonly goes into spasm when being challenged with work that it's not accustomed to, and it has trigger points that refer pain patterns to the neck, chest, and shoulder. Why, then, do I love it so much??

When it's not totally dysfunctional, serratus helps form the sling that makes it possible for us yogis to hold ourselves up in gravity with our hands. Down Dog, Plank, Low Plank, all the arm balances, and most inversions—none of these would be conceivable without a strong serratus anterior. It pulls the shoulder blade around the ribs in adduction. When utilized properly, this action is responsible for assisting our abdominals with Cat pose, and for not allowing our ribs to collapse to the earth in inversions. For a relatively small range of movement, this action is integral to many of the most simple postures we take for granted in our practice. **(abduction, retraction [low fibers])**

Pectoralis Minor. On the front side of the ribs, we find this small muscle that packs a punch. It doesn't look like much, but it's aided in part by

gravity and the general shape of our rib cage. If we aren't incredibly conscious of our posture, our shoulders droop down and forward, passively shortening pec minor. Once this muscle memorizes this length and shape, it's a helluva job getting it long and strong again. Pectoralis minor is a major contributor to poor alignment in weight-bearing postures like Plank (and all the other associated poses). If you see the scapulae "wing out" in these postures, it's an indicator that pec minor is short and serratus is weak. If the bottom tips of the shoulder blades poke out when just standing, then pec minor is usually the primary culprit. **(protraction)**

Glenohumeral (Shoulder) Joint

The muscles that move and support the GH joint are varied in their design and purpose. Recall that small or short muscles close to a joint are usually responsible primarily for stabilization, and only secondarily to move the limb. You'll notice that there is a diverse combination of these shorter muscles and others with long, lanky bellies here. Pay attention to how intricately the ends of these muscles interweave to find their destinations—it's remarkable that anything can move in there at all!! Once you see how packed-in these structures are, it becomes pretty easy to understand how much potential exists for dysfunction to arise due to adhesion, spasm, or strain.

Rotator Cuff. The primary function of this group of four muscles is to hold the head of the humerus in its joint. Collectively, these muscles create the active sling that secures the head of the humerus in the "socket." Notice, though, that there is no significant support underneath the joint. Just like the connective tissue layers, the underside of the GH is

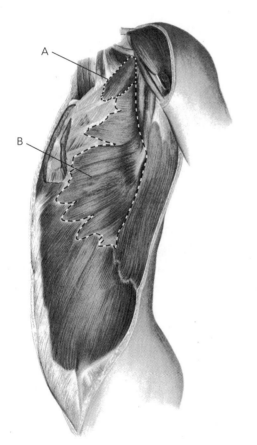

(A) Pectoralis minor, (B) Serratus anterior

free to fall apart if exposed to the right forces. These muscles are small compared to some of the other shoulder joint muscles, yet they are responsible for creating stabilizing resistance against the actions of those larger contributors. This is a tall order, and one that can only be filled if we act thoughtfully and intently to keep the whole shoulder active in gravity.

Supraspinatus. "Supra" is the thin muscle that lies in the groove above the spine of the scapula. Its tendon is one that travels under the acromion process to attach to the head of the humerus. This puts it at risk of impingement if we move too much in the GH and not enough in the shoulder girdle. When irritated, this little belly can send all sorts of referral pain to the shoulder and neck. Because of its size, it doesn't act as a powerful mobilizer, but it will assist a little bit when the deltoid abducts the arm. **(abduction)**

Infraspinatus. "Infra" fills in the whole dish of bone under the spine of the scapula. Its broad origin coalesces into a thin strip that wraps around the back of the head of the humerus on its way to its insertion on the pokey bits on the lateral side (the *greater tubercle*, if you really want to know). You may notice in images of this muscle that it appears to almost twist on itself near the top. You are not imagining that. If you were to feel it on a body, you would notice a palpable ridge where it kind of turns on itself. This area is ripe for stickiness and can cause limitations in infra's ability to contract fully or at full strength.

Considering that it is one of only a few rather small muscles that perform external rotation, its health and vigor are rather important to supporting the stability of the GH. In the following chapter, you'll see that this action is an integral part of keeping our postures safe and

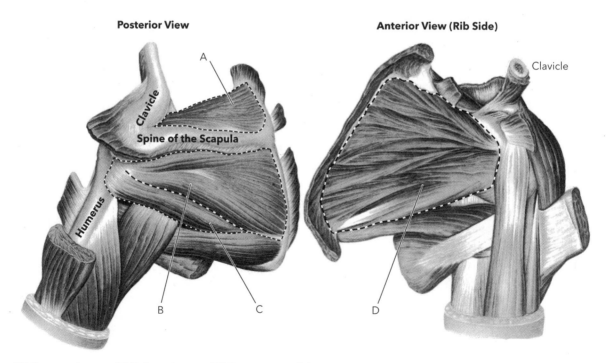

(A) Supraspinatus, (B) Infraspinatus, (C) Teres minor, (D) Subscapularis

well-aligned. It will also assist a bit in adduct-ing the arm. **(external rotation, adduction)**

Subscapularis. Ahhh ... sub-scap, such a schemer. It hides under the scapula and, for its small size, can cause big problems. In a way, this muscle is the mirror image of infraspinatus, fill-ing the entire front aspect of the scapula (the surface that faces the ribs) and then traveling under the armpit to attach to those pokey bits near the head of the humerus (this time it's the *lesser tubercle*). This pathway under the joint means that sub-scap will actually create *inter-nal rotation*, because it will pull that front side of the humerus toward the midline in rotation. It will also add an assist to adduction of the arm.

Because of that circuitous path, it has a high risk for adhesion to surrounding tissues on the ribs and through the armpit. Since internal rotation tends to be the passive posi-tion for many of us at any given time, it also develops trigger points that cause pain within the muscle belly as well as referral pain into the shoulder, chest, and neck areas. **(internal rotation, adduction)**

Teres Minor. As the name suggests, this is the smaller cousin of teres major, which we will address in a moment. Minor begins on the lat-eral border of the scapula, about halfway up, and travels along with infra (as if they were one belly, honestly) to the insertion on the greater tubercle of the humerus. Because of this path, it will mimic all the same actions as infra. **(external rotation, adduction)**

Latissimus Dorsi. "Lats" is huge. It is big. Like traps is bigger than you think it is, lats is even bigger. From the middle of your ribs all the way down to your tailbone, it attaches to the spine and out onto the top ridge of the pelvis (see posterior view illustrated on p. 245), inte-grating into the thick connective tissue sheet

at your low back (the thoracolumbar aponeu-rosis, as discussed in the spine chapter). It travels like wings wrapping around the torso, narrowing to thin straps that sweep under the armpit to attach near the front of the humerus on the lesser tubercles (right along with sub-scap). Again, because of this path under the joint, contraction of lats will pull the front of the humerus in toward the midline, internally rotating the arm. Due to lats' position on the back body, the arm will also be pulled into extension, and will do this very powerfully if the arm was flexed to begin with. Let's be honest, the extension of the upper extremity is pretty limited in most bodies, so lats will be used most often in pulling the arm back down from a flexed position. It will also pull the arm down (adduction) from an abducted position. **(internal rotation, extension, adduction)**

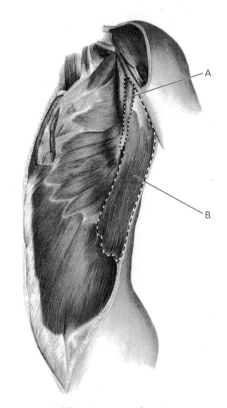

(A) Teres major, (B) Latissimus dorsi

TRAPS AND LATS ARE ALSO SPINAL MUSCLES

A principle in kinesiology states that a muscle will move either of the bones that it attaches to. While principally the trapezius and latissimus move the upper extremity, their origins on the spine inform us of their secondary function: to act on the spine. Depending on where you are in space and what movements you are trying to achieve, these two muscles are likely to play a role in stability of the spine, not only the arm.

When you look at these two muscles' spinal attachments, you'll see that they cover four-thirds of the back spine. No, that's not a typo. Traps attaches to the top two-thirds, from the skull to T12, while lats attaches from T8 to the tailbone, the bottom two-thirds. They overlap in the middle, conveniently in that bottom-rib area we've already designated as a potential hazardous weak point. They are, in anatomical lingo, some big-ass back muscles.

When the scapula is stable, the upper fibers of traps will work directly on the neck to move it in both lateral flexion and rotation. Especially in weight-bearing postures, this function works to stabilize the neck when the arm is working to hold us up.

When the arms are stable, let's say in a pose like Baby Cobra, the lats will help engage the low-back extension that protects the low back in backbends. It will literally assist in preventing the typical breaking points of L5 or T10 by distributing tension across the entire length of the lumbar system. We can use all the help we can get there!

With this information in mind, we can better access our support systems to hold us in gravity instead of relying on just a few intrinsic muscles to do the heavy lifting. The more muscles we use, the less each of those muscles has to work.

Teres Major. This little synergist (literally referred to as "Lats' Little Helper") attaches to the shoulder blade and then fluidly joins up with lats as it travels under the armpit to its insertion on the humerus. It's too small to help much with extension behind the back but will assist in all the other actions. Even though it attaches to the scapula, for some reason it isn't lumped in with the other rotator cuff muscles. Go figure. **(internal rotation, extension to neutral)**

Pectoralis Major. This is familiar to most of us, whether or not we sport a strong one ourselves. The major muscle of the chest, pec major will be short in most bodies due to gravity and our seemingly universal commitment to allow it to pull our shoulders down and forward. See the sidebar offering a little enlightenment on the details of this predicament.

Pec major is large, even when not particularly toned up. It originates along the entire

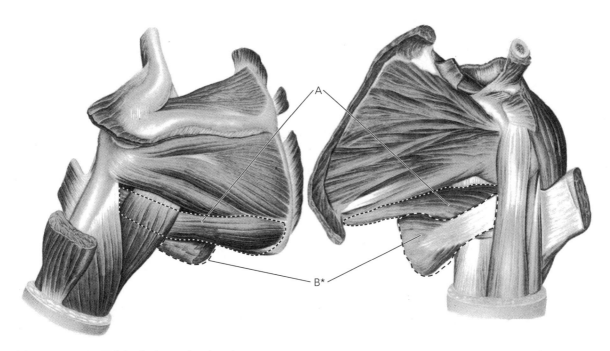

(A) Teres major, (B*) Latissimus dorsi, cut

length of the sternum and rib cartilage. It also begins in a broad attachment that narrows to a rather small inserting tendon, but this one also rolls on itself, similar to the design of the infra. Here though, it's more profound—the lowest originating fibers actually attach higher on the humerus than do the upper originating fibers. It quite literally flips over itself to attach to the arm bone. From the standpoint of leverage, this is a sweet and incredibly efficient design. Now those upper fibers have a better angle to flex the arm from, while the lower fibers now have better leverage to pull that flexed arm back down (extension to neutral). Genius. Thumbs up to whoever did that, 'cause it helps us functionally ... but also sets me up in my bodywork practice for job security—because that little flip creates tons of potential for adhesion and spasticity. Prime bits for massage and manual therapy! **(internal rotation, flexion, extension to neutral)**

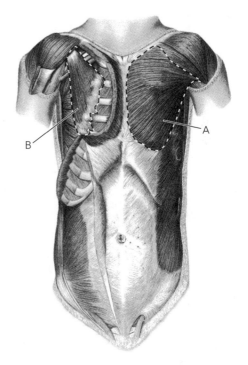

(A) Pectoralis major, (B) Pectoralis minor

Biceps Brachii. The biceps muscle is thus named for the two bellies (*bi* = two, *ceps* = bellies) that run the length of the arm from elbow to shoulder on the anterior side. The muscle's long head has a long tendon that sits in the bicipital groove and attaches to the top edge of the glenoid fossa of the shoulder blade. Many times the tendon's attachment is also fibrously interwoven with the labrum that rims that fossa, so if any damage occurs to that cartilage, the biceps may be affected. The short head diverts a bit from the path of the humerus to attach to the coracoid process, that little horn of bone poking out from under the clavicle, that same place where pec minor inserts. In combination, these two heads give good leverage to help flex the arm at the GH joint.

It's important to note that the origin of this muscle is on the distal side of the elbow, so biceps will also flex the elbow joint. This muscular relationship of elbow and shoulder means that when we do things like bear weight in the hands, we need to be particularly aware of how these two joints move together. If we aren't particularly stable in one, the other will have a tough time moving with integrity. **(flexion)**

Triceps Brachii. Triceps is the opposing muscle to biceps and runs along the posterior arm. There are three bellies, but two of them terminate on the humerus itself, with only the long head spanning the posterior/inferior shoulder joint to attach to the scapula. This position offers it some leverage for extension on the shoulder.

Like its antagonist, the triceps also originates on the forearm, crossing both the elbow and the shoulder. This muscle is capable of extension at both joints, meaning it is integral

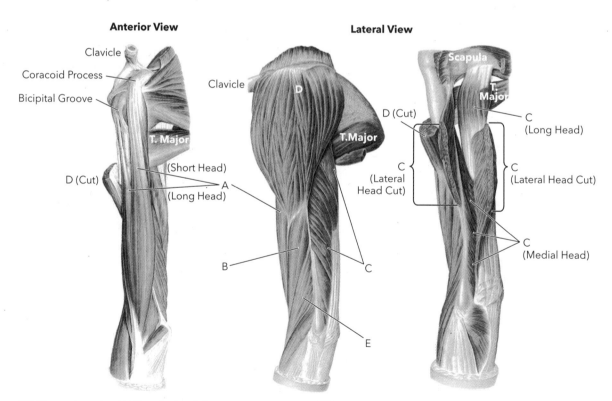

(A) Biceps brachii, (B) Brachialis, (C) Triceps brachii, (D) Deltoid, (E) Brachioradialis

to the stabilization of both in counteraction when bearing weight in the hands. **(extension)**

Deltoid. This is the most superficial of the GH muscles, recognizable even when it isn't particularly toned. Deltoid has three fiber directions—posterior, middle, and anterior—in one belly that "caps" the shoulder and upper arm. The posterior fibers originate on the spine of the scapula, creating an oblique angle toward their insertion point at the middle of the lateral humerus. Because of this position and angle, deltoid will both extend and externally rotate the arm at the GH joint. This is the only other muscle that does that external rotation, along with the infra/teres pair in the rotator cuff. It's a big job for relatively small muscles.

The middle fibers begin on the lateral acromion process and run down to that same midpoint of the lateral humerus. Together with supra, these fibers are the prime mover of the shoulder joint in abduction. Again, little muscle bits doing a big job.

PEC MAJOR TAKES OVER THE WORLD!!

If you look at anyone, and I mean nearly everyone, you'll see that they stand with their shoulders pulled down and protracted and arms internally rotated. Mostly we don't even notice we're doing it; in fact, many folks will tell you they are all scrunched up around the upper shoulders and neck instead of pulled downward. This perception is not accurate to reality. Consider for just a moment that the way we move our body through the world is really conducive to downward and forward posture, not upward pull. I mean, which direction does gravity go?

In addition, we're built with our eyes on the front of our head, built to move forward through space—life happens in front of us, so that's where our arms are reaching most of the time. In addition, the majority of us don't actively control our posture in gravity, dropping the collarbones and shoulders heavily onto the ribs, leaving our spine to collapse into its curves in imbalanced ways, seeking some center of gravity that is held up by our ligaments instead of our muscles. All this leads to one very common condition: shortened pectoralis major.

Because pec major is such a large chest muscle, it can pack a punch, but that also means there are a lot of fibers to get stuck together and get habituated to certain postures. That means when we try to reverse our forward-reaching trend and open our chest, we are likely to meet hefty resistance. It also means that when we attempt to bear weight in our arms, pec is likely to act first and ask questions later. As the largest of the arm flexors and abductors, it wants to take over the task of holding us up, even when it's not in our best interest functionally.

We really need to balance that chest work by activating the upper back muscles. We need to give pec major something to work against other than gravity—that will mean less work overall, and more buoyancy to boot.

Lastly, the anterior fibers originate on the distal clavicle and run at an oblique angle to the insertion on the arm bone. This angle creates internal rotation. This opposition to the posterior fibers sets up the two parts of the muscle to stabilize against one another. I like to think of deltoid as the glute medius of the shoulder—an abductor that can act as a stabilizer to itself in rotation, flexion, and extension. **(abduction, flexion, extension, internal rotation, external rotation)**

Elbow

As mentioned in "Range of Motion," the elbow actually consists of two separate joints that move on different planes: a hinge joint for flexion and extension, plus a pivot joint for rotation. Depending on their attachment points, the muscles listed here may do more than one action, working at both joints simultaneously. What is key to keep in mind is that with compound joints such as the elbow, there are typically many muscles working at the same time in an intricate dance of stabilization and mobilization. The closer we get to the hand, the more dexterous we need our movements to be, so the more muscles will work together in both opposition and symbiosis to achieve finer and finer control.

Biceps. Here we are again. Biceps brachii crosses both the shoulder and the elbow, so it will move both joints. Because of the distal tendon's attachment on the radius, it can perform supination (internal rotation) as well as simple flexion. **(flexion, supination)**

Brachialis. Though biceps is generally given credit for the bulky nature of a toned upper arm, it is usually brachialis that actually provides that ubiquitous profile. Because brachialis only

crosses the elbow, it is responsible for flexion alone and doesn't get sidetracked with other joints or actions. **(flexion)**

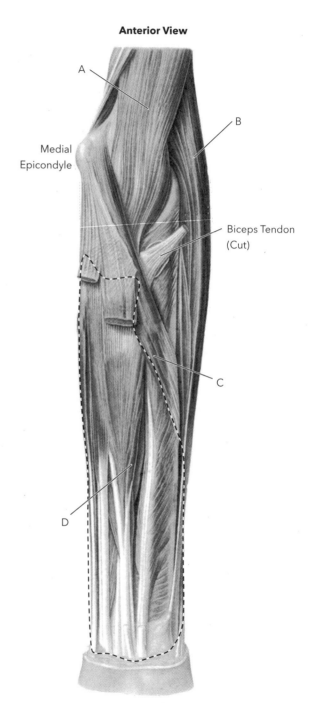

Anterior View

A

B

Medial Epicondyle

Biceps Tendon (Cut)

C

D

(A) Brachialis, (B) Brachioradialis, (C) Pronator teres, (D) Wrist flexors (middle layer)

Triceps. Just as in the shoulder, triceps acts as the antagonist to biceps at the elbow. This time, however, it's only in the act of extension. The distal tendon secures to the pokey end of the ulna (the point of the elbow) on the posterior side, which provides profound leverage for extension. **(extension)**

Brachioradialis. This muscle is smaller than its proximal allies, and it only helps out a little bit when weight is added to the elbow-flexion scenario. You can see it pop up on the lateral forearm when you're in a handshake posture or holding a hand weight, meeting some resistance. **(flexion)**

Pronator Teres. This is not a large muscle either, but it has a pretty big job to do for us yogis in particular. With just a tiny bit of help from some other bits, this muscle is primarily responsible for the pronation (internal rotation) of the forearm. Why is this such a big deal?? Well, this action is what roots your index- and middle-finger knuckles down to your mat while the rest of the upper extremity is working to externally rotate the GH joint and hug the scapulae into the armpits. This pronation is the stabilizing force that protects the shoulder and the elbow and the wrist. It's also what helps us access our Hasta Bandha to feed our energetic upper body. That's no small task. **(pronation)**

Wrist/Hand/Fingers

We aren't going to dissect the many layers of the forearm and hand, since that's just too much detail at our level. For now, we'll just consider the fact that we know how much control is needed to do things like create a mudra, or hold a pencil, or type on a keyboard, or wield a knife in the kitchen while chopping garlic. Hopefully, at this point we can make the leap that all those fine actions require intrinsic hand muscles that work in concert with the mobilizers of the wrist and elbow and shoulder. Because we are talking about a number of separate muscle bellies, we also must consider all the layers of fascia in play—providing tons of potential for sticky adhesion and possible dysfunction.

Now we'll group those muscles together and make some generalizations about some of the movements they'd create in yoga asana practice.

Posterior View

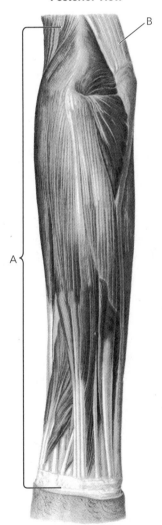

(A) Wrist extensors (superficial layer), (B) Triceps brachii

Flexors. There are a couple layers of these muscle bellies; some move only the wrist, while others span the hand and fingers. Most relevant to us as yogis is that these muscles help us engage our hand with the floor in weight-bearing postures. In many people these muscles aren't particularly strong, but they may be tight and stuck—the product of a life full of typing and gripping our phones! So, for many folks it will take a ton of effort to get these working in a way that promotes both the grounding and the lifting forces necessary to maintain our poses with ease instead of fatigue and pain.

This group runs the length of the anterior forearm, crosses the wrist through the carpal tunnel, and inserts at various points along the palm or fingers. In case you missed it, the whole group will work together or in part to flex the wrist, hand, and/or fingers.

Extensors. It's usually a surprise to people how very tight and cranky their forearm extensors are. We think more about the flexors because those are the muscles working to grip and hold all the things we use in our world. What we rarely consider is that if we spend a ton of time at a keyboard, it's the extensors that prevent our hand from collapsing fully onto the keys, and it's our extensors that lift and move our fingers around the keyboard and mouse. They're working an awful lot with relatively little credit.

So, once we make it to our mat, we have to acknowledge that these extensors may not be in optimal condition to provide the adequate oppositional forces for the flexors who are doing most of the heavy lifting. After all, these muscles will be the stabilizers if we intend to keep our wrist in a neutral position, or if we require the back of the wrist to not simply collapse. Counteraction is the key to safety, especially in joints that are supported mostly by ligaments and tendons ... those tendons have to maintain some active tension on both sides of the joint to truly support it.

Bandhas. Just as in the feet, the hands have a secondary bandha system. These bandhas connect the upper extremity to the core, weaving our hands into continuity with our solar plexus and throat. Besides the physical connections, we should also consider the Chinese meridians here because they connect our extremity directly to the heart, lung, small and large intestines, and pericardium. ✿ These are powerful organs/energies that interact as nervous system engines and act as the seat of our deeper body of awareness. Learning to activate Hasta Bandha can have a deeply profound effect on your practice, especially in weight-bearing postures. Just as you use Pada Bandha to anchor the lower body to the earth, offer the Mula Bandha a grounding force and buoyant uplift, and allow for pranic energy to flow from top to bottom, so too the Hasta Bandha acts on the upper body. Whether or not the hands touch the ground, activation of these muscles and energetic containers will help energize and integrate your extremity with your deeper core.

Experiential Learning

There is no doubt that by now you have come to recognize the very complex nature of the upper extremity. This stuff makes the spine seem downright simplistic! So in the long run, it will be important to have a clear understanding of the functional basics in place before you can start to integrate this into your teaching.

To that end, I highly recommend that you leave the muscles alone for a while. You've gotten an overview of them; you know they exist. Now leave 'em be for a bit.

Instead, I invite you to create some flashcards that help you discern the shoulder girdle from the shoulder joint. Perhaps you make a card for each bone in the system, and simply drill yourself on what belongs to which group. Become familiar with the pokey bits that muscles will eventually attach to. It doesn't matter what those are called, only that you are aware they exist.

Next, maybe you start connecting those bones into the joints that build the upper extremity.

- Is it a true joint?
- Does it have extensive range of motion, or is it limited?
- What are the actions and even the planes available at each joint?
- How do the actions at one joint affect the actions at the next?
- Can you begin to experientially map out those compensations-by-design?

To do this, you may ask a friend to act as a model so you can move their arm around both passively and actively to observe these relationships in real time, in real life. Watch what happens to the scapula and clavicle as their arm bone moves through space. Take notes on what you see, and then begin to translate those into the more technical terms we've learned along the way. This exercise will help you clarify your understanding of the movements while also beginning to lay in information that will help you in your cueing later.

Limitations

Though the entirety of the upper extremity is engineered for mobility, there are particular limitations we should be aware of. These limits may be met in either the bones or the soft tissues. Because of our broad range of motion, it can be easy to assume we get to move however we want and to the extremes, when in fact the shoulder complex is very susceptible to injury when improper alignment is employed. If we instead remain aware that our soft tissues have small spaces to travel through, or that pretty small muscles are being asked to do some pretty heavy lifting, we can much more mindfully approach our asana practice and remain safe as we do so.

Common Bony Limitations

The upper extremity has many joints and therefore an increased potential for a person's individual bony shape to influence the most healthy and efficient alignment for them in practice. The length and curvature of their clavicles and shape of their ribs may make them more or less prone to impingements to the soft tissues that run in between these structures. Arm length differences can have major impacts on shoulder and spinal alignment when bearing weight in the hands. The torsion of their humerus and shape of its distal end will influence their placement of hands on the mat for weight bearing, and also which direction their fingers will point. There are both gross observations to make and super-subtle clues to look for when helping your students find optimal shoulder/arm/hand alignments. For now, we'll discuss some of the biggest, boldest differences.

Head of the Humerus. First we should consider the shape of the humerus at the GH joint. It is very bumpy because there are many muscles that attach to it. Protuberances such as these are called *processes*, *tuberosities*, or *tubercles*. These bumps in particular are of importance because of the relationship of the acromion process to the humerus. In between these pokey bits are lots of squishy bits: soft tissue structures that are none too happy to get jammed up between the rock and the hard place. Whenever we reach, in either flexion or abduction, it's important to get the pokey bits out of the way as much as possible **by externally rotating the humerus**. Even then, once you get to around 90 degrees of abduction, the scapula must start moving or risk injury to the labrum, bursae, tendons, and neurovascular bundles that travel through this small space. **Upward rotation of the scapula** is integral to safely achieving the arm's full range of motion when reaching overhead. When moving into full extension of the humerus, the **scapula must tilt forward in protraction** to avoid shearing forces on the labrum. These are engineered compensations that must occur to keep the shoulder safe.

Elbow. Then there is the shape of the elbow. Most people have a lateral deviation of the elbow joint that is evident from Mountain pose. When you look at your student standing in Mountain with their arms active and straight, the elbows

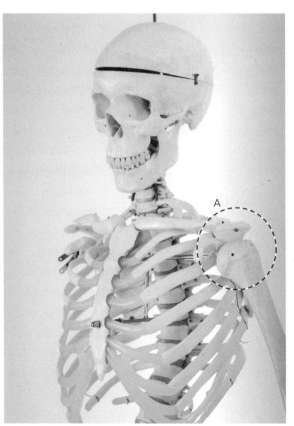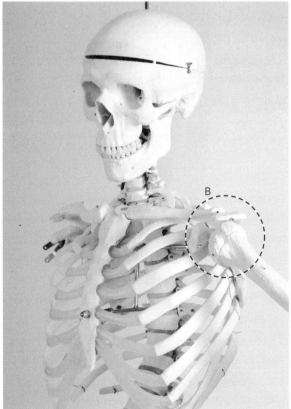

(A) Very little space between the acromion and the tubercles of the humerus. (B) When abduction occurs, there is almost immediate impingement of the soft tissues that travel through that space.

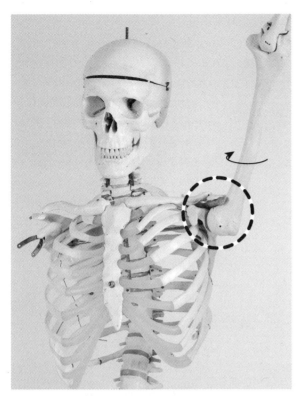

External rotation of the humerus will move the tubercles out of the way, providing a bit more space, but upward rotation of the scapula is still needed to reach fully overhead.

will hang directly down from the shoulder while the forearms jut out to the sides, making the hands hang wider than the shoulders. (As mentioned earlier, we call this a **carrying angle**.) So, the natural alignment of their hands should be wider than their shoulders when they place them on the mat for weight bearing, in order to offer the shoulder the best alignment and least risk of injury. Elbows will be shoulder-width, but hands will be wider.

The shape of the humerus and ulna will also determine the end-feel of extension at the elbow. Bone meets bone here by design, but the shape and size of this hinge will determine whether you can extend all the way to 180 degrees (some people can't get there), or go beyond that into

hyperextension. Even if your bones allow it, it's not a great idea to exploit hyperextension, because the ligaments can still stretch and you risk losing stability over time. My left elbow didn't always hyperextend, but it does now, after years of locking my elbows while weight bearing. Be careful. Be mindful. Save your bits.

Wrist and Hand. The *saddle joint*, the place where the thumb meets the wrist, is special, and also pretty fragile: it's the first place many people develop arthritis. In part this is because it does not exist on the same plane as the rest of the palm or fingers. Look at your own palms; it sits just anterior to the other metacarpals and rotates medially, so that the pad of the thumb points across the palm instead of on a plane with the other fingertips. In this position its shape allows for it to move very specifically: to stretch the thumb out to the side, to take it forward and back, and to reach across the palm to the pinky in opposition. But when we bear too much weight on the thumb side of the palm, we torque the metacarpal out of its alignment with the carpal and put an amazing amount of stress on the saddle joint, leading to damage, degeneration, and dysfunction. It

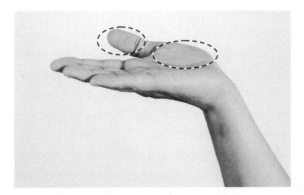

The thumb is not on the same plane as the hand. Notice that the pads of the fingers point up while the thumb faces across the palm. It's also set "above" the palm at the saddle joint.

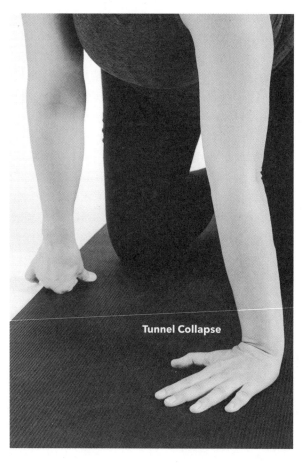

Tunnel Collapse

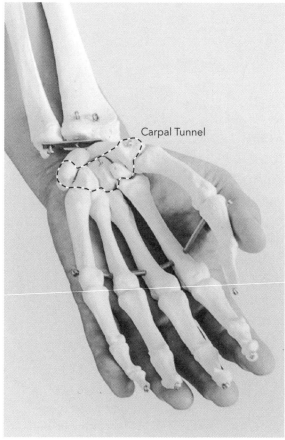

Carpal Tunnel

is vital that we align the bones of the hand to transfer our weight efficiently through the rest of the palm to avoid the saddle joint as much as possible. Arm turn-out and rooting through the index and middle finger joints are essential to building the necessary physical and energetic alignment to support our body weight.

One specific condition that can be caused by bones is **carpal tunnel syndrome**. You've probably heard of this one. It's a very specific impingement of the *median nerve* serving your hand. That pinch is usually in the actual carpal tunnel of the hand, often caused by a functional collapse of the bones that build the tunnel itself. It can cause numbness, tingling, aching, shooting pain, weakness, etc. There are

other impingement syndromes that can occur to other nerves, and these are often misidentified as carpal tunnel syndrome. If you have a student telling you they have this, make sure they have a clear diagnosis so you can give them proper instructions. If they lack one, you need to refer them to a physician.

Common Soft Tissue Limitations

Range of motion can and will be affected by soft tissue compression or tension. Muscles that are experiencing any of the following will have trouble reaching their full range:

- Too weak

- Short or spastic

- Significant fascial adhesion
- "Muscle-bound" (as can be found in people who overtrain and bulk up their muscle tissue significantly, thickening their fascia)

When muscle layers are adhered to one another, there can be a significant disruption to the leverage systems of the upper extremity. When you look at the crisscrossing and overlapping nature of this network, you can imagine how any sticky points will have an effect in both direct and indirect ways—at any of the joints of the upper extremity. Since this complex is designed for maximum range, with complementary and compensatory movements engineered into it, even minor disruptions to the pattern can have ripple effects throughout.

Shoulder Girdle and Joint. Let's start at the top of the system. In the shoulder girdle, it's typical that adhesions exist in the muscles that support the scapulae. Traps and rhomboids get stuck to deeper structures in the neck or the ribs. When this happens, the scapula can no longer slide easily over the ribs. Neck muscles go into spasm and have a difficult time contracting functionally, so fine movement of the scaps becomes nearly impossible. In the chest, tiny intrinsic muscles get hard and prevent the clavicle from elevating off the top ribs. Pectoralis minor gets short and spastic, which fixes the scapulae in a protracted position. Serratus anterior, underneath the scapulae, is nearly always short and weak and sticky, abducting the scaps and making it very difficult at first to mobilize them back into neutral. All of these combine to create a hunched shape to the upper body that places a ton of stress on the upper back and neck, and over time it will impede range at both the shoulder and the spine ... backbending becomes significantly limited.

When you consider the rotator cuff muscles, all of the above certainly play roles in the quality and quantity of movement of the GH joint. Considering that these muscles are very small in comparison to the muscles of the shoulder girdle, they already have a big hurdle to overcome in finding strength balance in a complex system. When they are weak, spastic, and/or stuck, they have an even tougher time doing the job of stabilizing the head of the humerus in its socket. Consider for just a moment how many muscles produce internal rotation of the GH:

- Pectoralis major
- Latissimus dorsi
- Anterior deltoid
- (plus a couple of rotator cuff muscles too)

Large, powerful muscles. And to counter them with external rotation, we have:

- Infraspinatus
- Posterior fibers of deltoid

This means we have to make sure that those large muscles are able to get long—but also that infraspinatus is healthy and strong in order to be an effective counteractor.

In addition, many bodies have trigger points that can create pain patterns that limit a student's inclination to move, even when a particular range would be physically possible. If you're not willing to move in a certain way, it really doesn't matter at all if the range is there or not. The thing about trigger points is that they create pain in an area different from where the actual dysfunction is. It makes pinpointing the issue more difficult—and can present a teacher with quite the mystery in making modifications or guiding them into solid alignment. This is an instance where we'd refer our student to bodywork to help them achieve some relief before coming back to the mat for reinforcement of better movement patterns.

Elbow. The elbow is one joint in the upper extremity where overworking a muscle group could create less range of motion. Biceps that are muscle-bound, or too bulky and fibrous to lengthen effectively, could restrict the extension that the bones would otherwise allow. Irritation or overwork in the triceps can have a similar effect.

Bursitis is also common in the elbow, presenting as a round swollen knob on the tip of the elbow, and typically it will arise out of the blue. It is usually benign and painless but can be quite painful and nervy, preventing any pressure on the forearm/elbow joint and limiting flexion/extension.

Because many of the forearm muscles cross the elbow, the condition of these muscles and their fascia can have an effect on how the forearm rotates. This effect could limit how a student finds the strong counteraction of external/internal rotation between the arm and forearm that creates a strong base for all our weight-bearing postures.

While this next condition is rare, it certainly does come up, especially if you're teaching athletes who throw things as part of their sport. Since the elbow nerves are so close to the surface, we need to be aware that the nerves themselves may get entrapped in the surrounding fascia, impinged in the hinge joint (especially in hyperextension), or, in extreme cases, may slip out of their groove completely. This may be a chronic condition they come to class with, and it may affect the quality of movement and strength available in their arms. Irritated nerves have a direct effect on one's ability to fire muscles, reducing overall strength.

Wrist and Hand. As noted in "Structure," the wrist in particular relies on the strength of the muscles above and below it to engage for stability. Since just the tendons actually cross the wrist joint, counteraction is key to keeping it from collapsing when bearing weight. If there is significant weakness, adhesion, spasm, or (usually) a combination of these in either the flexors or extensors, it's probable that your student will have a hard time in upper-body postures like Plank and its counterparts.

As mentioned in "Bony Limitations," the wrist can be compromised by carpal tunnel syndrome. While sometimes it is precipitated by a bony collapse, there are times when the tunnel is pressurized by a constriction/shortening/hardening of the retinaculum or intrinsic muscles of the palm. In this case, stretching the palm and actively contracting the muscles in weight-bearing postures will act as a relieving practice.

It's important to note that these symptoms may be mimicked by soft tissue impingements upstream. Anywhere along the path (neck, clavicle, pectoralis minor, rotator cuff, biceps, forearm...) muscles can squeeze the nerves and create pain, numbness, and/or weakness in the wrist and hand. The pattern is usually different from classic carpal tunnel syndrome, affecting the middle, ring, and pinky fingers instead of the thumb, index, and middle fingers. When it presents this way, it is called **thoracic outlet syndrome**, regardless of the actual point of impingement.

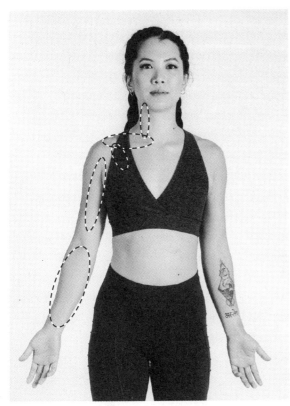

The nerves and blood vessels of the brachial plexus can be impinged by bones or soft tissues at any point along their path.

Risks

- **Impingements**: Compression of any soft tissue, commonly tendons or nerves—most likely to happen between the humerus and the acromion process, but may also occur at the ulnar nerve as it crosses the posterior elbow. We mostly think of this as a bone-on-soft-tissue condition, but it can happen when spastic or tight muscles compress nerves or blood vessels against a bone or other muscles; arm, forearm, and wrist.

- **Labrum tears and biceps tendon avulsion**: Cartilage/tendon torn and/or pulled away from the bone—GH joint injury. Surgical; there is no other rehab for this injury. That said, many people function at a high level with minor tears to their labrum and will likely come to class with this. Ensure you are teaching the best range of motion to protect that area, especially in these cases.

- **Rotator cuff strain/trigger point**: Muscular tears or connective tissue distortions. Typical in infraspinatus, teres major, and subscapularis, causing pain patterns in the neck, shoulder, arm.

- **Tendinitis, neuritis, bursitis**: Localized inflammation of the tissue. Common in the GH, elbow, and wrist.

- **Thoracic outlet syndrome**: Impingement of the brachial plexus nerves anywhere along their path by either bones or muscles. Typical locations include the cervical spine, clavicle, pec minor, biceps, and forearm muscles.

- **Saddle joint irritation, degeneration, and arthritic conditions**: Affecting wrist and hand. Often requires alternate/modified hand placement and bolstering heel of hand with cushioned wedge or folded mat.

- **Carpal tunnel syndrome**: Potential for pain, numbness, and weakness in the wrist/hand. Requires individual modifications to prevent further compression; depending on the case, it may be either aggravated or relieved by continued practice.

12

The Upper Extremity: Principles of Teaching and Practice Mechanics

From an anthropological perspective, the upper extremity is designed to reach. We had to reach up in the trees for fruit, dig in the earth for roots. Our hands had dexterity to build and use tools, we pulled ourselves up in tree limbs and scaled rock faces to gather eggs ... out of necessity our range of motion was expansive.

Our framework is engineered for reaching and gripping, pushing and pulling, but in our yoga practice we place our hands on the floor and bear the entire weight of the body. We wrap our arms around each other and our legs and our torso, using leverage to torque us this way and that. Even though we can make our arms and hands do these things, it is not what they are fundamentally designed to do. That means we must be incredibly thoughtful about teaching our students how to make these new movements and binds. If we engage haphazardly in this practice, we will surely injure ourselves.

Principles of Teaching

As both teachers and practitioners, we must begin to emphasize an awareness of the isolation or integration of the shoulder girdle and shoulder joint. Range of motion becomes a focal point—expanding or actively limiting it as appropriate to the individual. Because the shoulders and wrists in particular are prone to tendon and ligament injuries, our placement on the mat and how we support ourselves in gravity will have lasting impacts on the functioning of these joints and tissues. Working to find optimal alignment for both structural and functional efficiency will help prevent injury, build strength, and prolong our ability to practice in these exciting and enriching ways. We need to understand the extremity's interaction with the core to ensure that they work together and do not undermine one another. If we have a working model for the energetic systems at play here, we'll be able to greatly enhance our experience of asanas that we may have thought we were already deeply familiar with.

This section is dedicated to building an understanding of how the upper extremity works with the physics of gravity and integrates with the deeper core, balancing the principles of mobility and stability, and translating individual differences into modifications and personal alignment points. Of course, in order to do this, we need to explore those differences and how they impact our practice. We need to learn to see them in the bodies on the mats in front of us. We need to get comfortable with upending some long-held notions of traditional alignment and personalizing this practice for each student. By now, I'm sure it's no surprise that we'll be throwing out some outdated cues, or that we'll be looking at our body from its biomechanical imperatives. We will rework our teaching to guide students through more appropriate movements, to find their best alignment in every posture.

Observation Skills

As teachers, we must become adept at seeing the misalignments that are most risky—usually those at the wrist and shoulder joint. These tend to be more subtle than in the lower extremity, where generally we can see very clearly if major joints align atop one another. Joints being stacked in the upper extremity may not be the most efficient way of going about alignment, at least not once the hands meet the mat and we bear weight. When reaching out into space, joint alignment or stacking makes more sense. To that end, learning to let your gaze soften—so you see not only the bony alignment but the pranic flow through the structural system—will allow you to offer ever more individualized adjustment and help your students embody each posture fully.

Of course, you still want to look at the clothing (that faithful representative of our fascial patterns) and bony landmarks, but we'll need to find other ways to see misalignment or collapse:

- Looking at how the skin bunches and ripples at the wrist while we're bearing weight
- Assessing the space, or lack thereof, between the scapulae
- The direction the elbows point
- Whether or not the palm collapses inward onto the thumb
- Are students connecting to their core, and is their spine neutral?
- Are the ribs or hips dropping or blowing out?

You'll become adept at seeing the energetic lines *only if* you first learn to see the way the skeletal and fascial lines support one another. It's not the same as the hip-knee-ankle aligning on one plane—most times, the hands aren't directly under the shoulders. You'll need to be able to see the most efficient line through gravity to the core. Fingers, palm, wrist, elbow, shoulder, ribs ... it's not a straight line, but it is a continuum.

In the lower body we can see a pretty clear zigzag from front to back to front to back. But the upper body has a more subtle forward/backward interplay, reflected both in static postures and in transitions from one pose to the next. We'll see this reflected in Plank when held, but also as Plank transitions into Low Plank. Because of the movements available at the scapula and the GH, and the inherent risks of the movements there, we need to be able to quickly assess the complementary rotations that make reaching through space safe, fluid, and integrated with the core. When we combine reaching and weight bearing as we do in Downward Facing Dog and inversions, these observations become even more integral.

Reaching

The upper extremity is built for reaching around in our world. Unfortunately, we don't engage it the same way our ancestors did. On a daily basis they may have plucked fruit out of trees from overhead, or dug up roots, or climbed rocks and trees to plunder a bird's nest of eggs. They actively engaged all of the range of motion available to them and maintained strength in doing so. In our world today, we rarely even reach onto the top shelf of our cupboard for a snack. Most of how we engage our daily routines is conveniently right in front of us. We reach forward, but not too far. We have designed a physical world that readily accommodates all of our biomechanical inefficiencies, and also reinforces many of our bad postural habits.

And then we come to yoga!

In yoga asana practice, we reach overhead and we reach back; sometimes we even wrap our arms around other body parts at odd angles. Since we aren't inherently observant of our typical state, we don't have a good basis to assess how to engage in these more difficult movements with integrity. It's up to you as the teacher to see what students can't immediately feel.

External Rotation. Because of those bony processes that provide muscular attachment points, we need to move the humerus in specific ways to make space for the soft tissues of the GH joint. External rotation of the humerus is integral to maintaining safety while reaching overhead.

What you'll see: It's common for the elbows to point out to the sides and the scapulae to adduct toward the spine. Because the lats tend to be short, and because they are extensors, flexing the shoulder when reaching overhead will challenge them. Remember that lats are also internal rotators, so to compensate they'll attempt to gain slack by internally rotating the arm as it flexes. This leads to the compensation in the scaps too.

To counter this, externally rotate the arms, turning the triceps toward the midline and opening the biceps away from each other. The hands do not need to stay narrow, so let them go slightly wider than the shoulder joints.

Shoulder Girdle Shrug. So many people say they "carry their stress in their shoulders," and because they feel tension in the shoulder/neck area, they have a belief (as do many teachers) that the scaps are elevated up toward the ears all the time. If you actually observe your students, however, you'll see that maybe one in a hundred people truly hunches up around their neck. Look closely and you'll observe that most people actually drop their shoulders down onto the ribs and protract. This leaves the chest short and the neck overly long, overstretched. The sensation of this tautness is interpreted as tightness, but it's wholly inaccurate. Our teaching should reflect the reality, not the perception.

What you'll see (and hear): When students reach overhead, the experienced ones will start pulling the shoulder blades down their back almost automatically. The novices will usually not get their arms all the way overhead and will start looking around to see if they're doing it right. If you happen to be the student in class, there is a ubiquitous cue you'll hear, "Draw your shoulders down, away from your ears." I think you should ignore that.

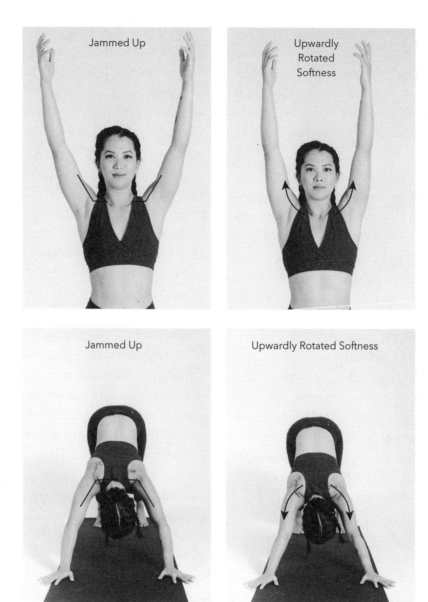

The sharp angles that occur when pulling the shoulder blades down create impingement at the shoulder joint.

Instead, employ that external rotation we discussed earlier: wrap the elbows in toward midline, and the scaps will settle into their proper position on the ribs. No need to drop them down, the neck has more than enough space. Remember from our range of motion discussion in the last chapter, upward rotation of the scapulae is a necessary movement when abducting or flexing the arm. So, let that happen—don't pull those bones down and compress the soft tissues of the GH joint.

Core Integration. When folks reach overhead, there is a nearly universal compensation in the T10 level of the spine. Because so many

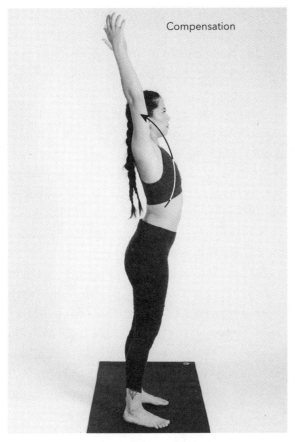

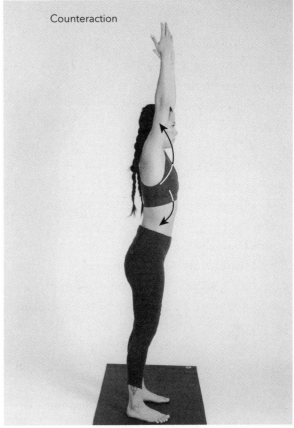

people suffer from short lats, as they reach overhead their spine compensates by breaking/collapsing at T10, blowing out the front ribs. Reaching overhead shouldn't automatically become a backbend. We ought to be able to maintain stability in our neutral spine even while challenging short lats. You'll need to rectify this at both the class and individual levels. Because students will be working on that stability FOREVER, you'll want to demonstrate this difference in front of class repeatedly, in pretty much every class you teach, from here to eternity.

Weight Bearing

Okay, here's the elephant in the room: we aren't actually engineered to bear weight in the hands as much as we do in our yoga practice. But because we do put our hands on the ground a lot, we need to build a structurally sound foundation. That means aligning our bones in such a way that gravity will translate through them as efficiently as possible. This IS NOT stacking the joints. Every single one of us is gonna need to get right with this concept. We need to understand our own bones, our own proportions, our own bends and torsions and strengths and weaknesses. As teachers, we need to acknowledge that this is one of the MOST important things we can teach our students, because no one else is going to see their body from this perspective, and no one else is in the position to offer them direct information that will keep them safe.

The other thing we are learning to see here is the energetic body. Just as in the lower extremity, how do we transfer the prana from the earth through the arms to the core? You should be able to see how the palms actually interact with the floor, how that transfers through the arms and into the heart/throat centers. Over time, these observations will allow us to offer ever more refined adjustments, subtle movements, and activations that help us feel more buoyant and graceful on the floor.

Are Hands Wide Enough? Traditional alignment asks that we align the hands "under the shoulders." But what the heck does that even mean? And why? Just as it seems to be an arbitrary directive to place feet together, this cue isn't rooted in any biomechanical truth. This alignment is unfortunately reinforced by the fact that it's pretty tough to have an accurate visual perspective on which direction our own arms go, because as we look down their length from our own viewpoint, a bunch of optical illusions occur, so we usually cheat inward a bit. So you'll need to be their eyes on this one, and you'll need to ask them repeatedly to trust you on this.

What you'll see: Students, whether newbie or old pro, will inevitably place their hands about eight to twelve inches apart under their chest. It won't matter if they are a lady who's five-foot-two or a gentleman at six-foot-four with shoulders as wide as his mat. This is a traditional way to see the hands, and many teachers will prompt this.

Instead, we need to encourage them to find a wider stance. I start by offering the width of their mat as a guideline, then start getting more personal and more technical. We'll go over this in detail later in "Cueing Practice," but for now you know that a person is too narrow if the inner edge of their thumb is aligned inside the crease of their armpit. That is a universal starting point.

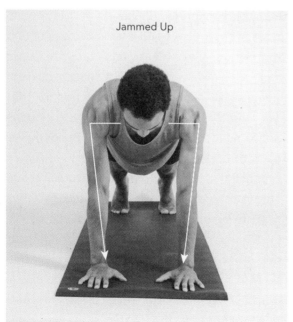
Jammed Up

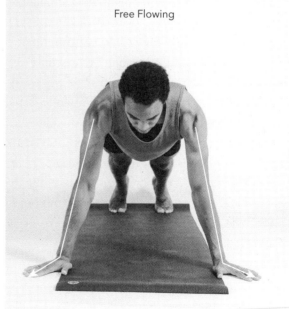
Free Flowing

Proper Turn-Out. In order to engage fully and safely with the floor—to ground down with strength and rise with levity instead of jamming down through the joints—you'll need to have balanced pressure through the palm. To be able to do that, the bones of the hand need to align with the arm and wrist so energy flows from the fingers to the shoulder. If the traditional alignment of "middle or index finger pointing forward" is employed, many if not most people will end up losing connection with the front of the palm and collapse into the heel of the hand, jamming the wrist and thumb. In this position, it's very difficult to root though the knuckles and even more difficult to align the arms correctly so the shoulder joint is protected.

What you'll see: The knuckles of index and middle finger will lift up, and a bowing of the palm will be present. The wrist wrinkles will be deeper and more numerous on the thumb-side. Oftentimes this is in conjunction with the elbows pointing out to the side, a little like a bulldog. If their hands are still too narrow, it will be even more exaggerated.

This indicates that the elbows are pointing back (rotation at the shoulder), but the hands haven't turned out sufficiently to find wrist-elbow-shoulder agreement. Turn the entire hand out until the index and middle fingers can lie flat on the mat and the wrist crease evens out.

Hands in Front of Shoulders. The final retuning of the arm alignment in weight bearing is the front to back alignment. If students are still adhering to "under the shoulder" alignment, even with the previous adjustments, it's likely that they will still place their hands too far back underneath their chest. This placement

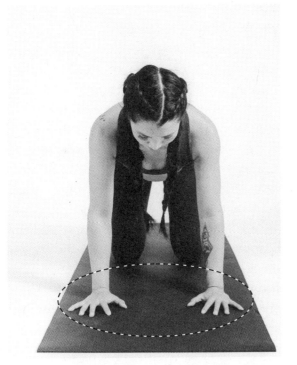 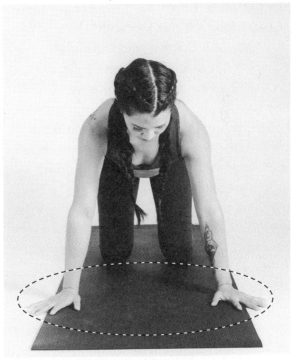

Notice that the knuckles of the index and middle fingers buckle in the first image. When the hands turn out, Elena can externally rotate her shoulders without her hands losing contact with the earth.

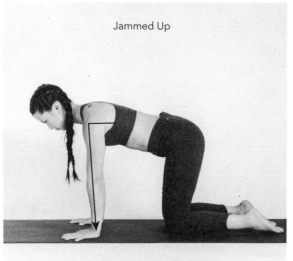

Jammed Up

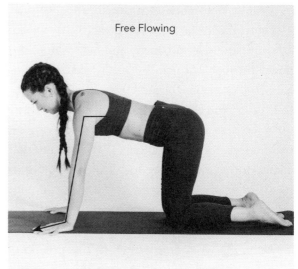

Free Flowing

Hyperextended wrists are not in midrange, so the flexors have a hard time activating sufficiently to support the wrist or hold up the weight of the chest.

puts the wrist in hyperextension and prevents them from engaging their full forearm strength. That is risky for the tendons and the wrist joints, and the whole system will fatigue much more quickly than it will in proper alignment.

What you'll see: The shoulders in Table or Plank will jut out over the hands, and the wrist joint will be in a deep hinge, sharper than 90 degrees. There will be deep wrinkles in the wrist crease, and the heel of the hand will jam into the mat. It will seem difficult to keep the finger-roots grounded, even with proper turn-out.

You'll want to encourage the entire front plane of the arm to align behind the wrist crease ... which may require an adjustment backward for the knees or feet as well.

Hyperextension vs. Carrying Angle. Being able to observe this distinction is very important. Hyperextension is *extra movement* on the sagittal plane in extension, so the elbow appears to bend too far backward. The carrying angle is a lateral *deviation in the shape* of the joint that results in the forearms jutting out

to the sides but does not affect mobility either way. Additionally, the carrying angle is engineered into the body on purpose; it's an actual evolutionary advantage so we can carry things more efficiently. Even though these two conditions are very different mechanically, they can be difficult to discern in asana practice.

What you'll see: It's possible to observe hyperextension any time the hands are on the ground and the elbows lock out. It is often exaggerated when a student follows your cue to "rotate the elbows to point back toward thighs." If they aren't particularly aware of muscular counteraction and they lock the joint, you'll see the "eye" of the elbow jut forward as the joint collapses. Severe cases will look like the elbow is actually bending fully the wrong direction when observed from the side. People with a profound carrying angle may present with elbows that appear to point in toward the midline, especially if their hands aren't wide enough.

You'll want to encourage external rotation only to the point of shoulder neutrality, not

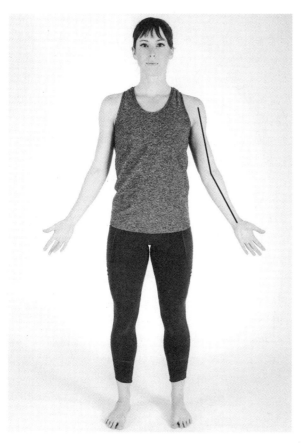

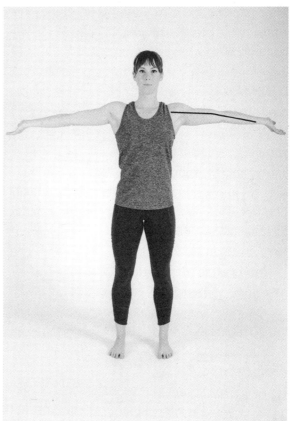

so the elbows point toward the midline. Adjust their hands wider on the mat, with appropriate turnout, so the elbow joint lines up under the shoulder instead of the wrist under the shoulder. This will create the geometry that supports the proper shoulder and elbow alignment too.

Now it gets complicated. In Downward Facing Dog, since we are bearing weight while also reaching overhead, even more forceful counteraction must be utilized. Someone with an exaggerated carrying angle, and who is effectively using counteraction, may *appear* to have a hyperextension. Although it is possible for a person to have both conditions simultaneously, there is some risk in adjusting them out of a presumed hyperextension if it doesn't actually exist.

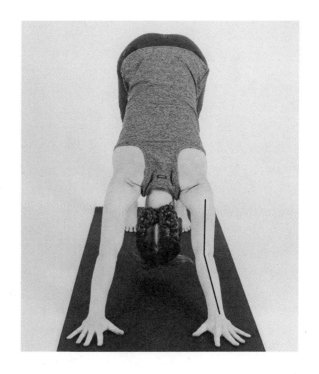

If you ask them to soften a bend into the elbow, and their only option seems to be elbows pointing out to the side or shoulders collapsing around their neck, then it's possible that the hyperextension you thought you saw is really their carrying angle presenting you with another optical illusion. You need to keep the shoulder safe first because it is at most risk of injury, and messing with the elbows can have a direct impact on the alignment of the shoulder. Use the technique outlined in the sidebar to assess whether the student has one condition or the other.

Integration with Core. Just as in the lower extremity, we need to be constantly on guard for the potential disconnect from the central core. This can happen both physiologically and energetically, and you'll develop the skills over time to see both.

What you'll see: The most pervasive collapse is between the shoulder girdle and the

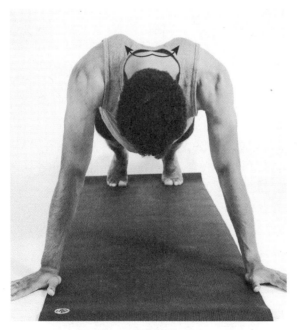

There is insufficient activation of serratus anterior, allowing the ribs to drop and the scapulae to wing out.

ribs. Especially for students just starting out, there tends to be very little acuity in the workings of the shoulder girdle. Weakness in muscles like serratus and trapezius, the abdominal core, and the arms results in gravity taking over completely. Some of the previous tell-tales will be present here too: elbows pointing outward, wrists collapsing, knuckles uprooted. But even if these items are fixed, there are other, more immediate clues to the specific dysfunction of the shoulder girdle.

In this case you'll also see the scapulae jutting out away from the ribs and spine. Sometimes this looks like a deep valley between the shoulder blades. Sometimes it looks like the top of the scapulae pour over the top of the ribs toward the chest, while the bottom tips wing out from the rib cage. In either situation, you are seeing the results of muscular imbalance wreaking havoc on our core functionality. Unfortunately, the fix that many teachers offer is to pull the scaps down the back, and that just creates other problems.

What we really need is external rotation of the arm, which will help realign the scapulae through compensatory movement. Then there is the matter of using both serratus and the abs to help lift the rib cage up to meet the shoulder blades. Specific cueing for this will be offered in the next section.

Binding

In a sense, binding in yoga is an extension of our reaching practice. But these reaches aren't exactly functional in our everyday lives, and therefore accessing these positions can be a confusing mess of tangled limbs. If we aren't clear about the compound movements of the shoulder, our binds will prove to be yet another source of trouble for this high-risk joint system.

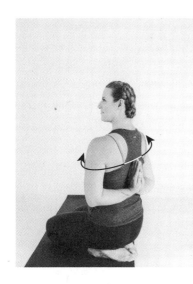
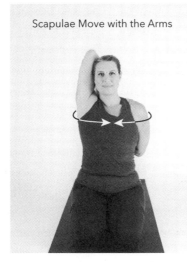
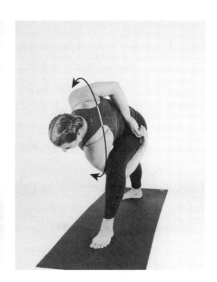

Scapulae Move with the Arms

We typically start practicing simple binds like hands clasped behind the back very early in our exploration of yoga. With a little practice under our belt, it's tempting to try to reach around our legs and twist things up just because it looks really cool. But even the simple bind is deceptive in how precise the combined movements of the arm and scapula must be to execute this posture safely. Getting fancy before you understand the subtleties of movement and stabilization is a sure path to injury.

CARRYING ANGLE OR HYPEREXTENSION?

So, to determine if your student has one or the other, first have them sit back and let their arms hang at their sides like in Mountain, elbows straight with a neutral shoulder joint. Ensure that their arm is hanging naturally without any abduction. With their palms facing forward, assess whether their hands are wider than their elbows in this position. If so, a carrying angle is present.

Now have them reach out to the side, elbows at shoulder height. Look at the elbows, and remember that they may not present the same way. I myself have a little hyperextension in one and not the other, so be clear about each. In this position, you'll be able to see if the forearm dips lower than the shoulder/elbow. If so, the elbow will appear to be bending backward, because, well, it is. And that's hyperextension.

Through this process, you will see a clear picture of whether your student has a carrying angle, a hyperextension, or some level of both. Armed with that information, you can offer more prescriptive instruction and adjustment in all of their weight-bearing poses, and they will be more knowledgeable about the how and why they should align their hands in specific ways (see images on p. 273).

What you'll see: There is a long history of miscuing the shoulders in our binds, so it's likely you'll witness students overcompensating for perceived compensations. In even a simple bind behind the back, folks will squeeze their palms tightly together and lock out their elbows. These actions lead to external rotation in the shoulder joint, adduction in the shoulder girdle, and a blown-out chest. This is a typical presentation, but it's not biomechanically sound.

Although we normally encourage external rotation to make space in the shoulder joint, in binds it actually works against us. This is how the mechanical advantage of the bones takes over for muscular intent. After all, to reach your hands behind the back requires *internal* rotation at the shoulder joint, plus some abduction of the shoulder girdle. We must allow these to happen to remain strong and aligned in the shoulder joint. We can still lift our chest up, avoiding the hunching that can accompany these shoulder actions; we just need to acknowledge that the spine can actually move independently from the shoulders. You need not sacrifice one for the other—they can and will support each other if we move with intelligent and active intent. For any bind, regardless of whether the arms are overhead (Cow Face) or behind the back, it's integral to the safety of our shoulder to honor the inherent combined efforts of the shoulder girdle and shoulder joint instead of opposing them.

We also need to ask whether the arm bind is actually an active or passive place to be. Consider your Bridge pose with hands bound underneath you. As soon as you join your hands, there is a release in the muscles and you begin to rely solely on the bones rolling toward each other to keep your ribs aloft. There

is less spinal action, less core activation, less overall control over how the spine moves into a backbend. But with the hands unbound and allowed to find alignment with the shoulders, you can once again actively engage the upper back muscles, connect them to the deep core, contract the full length of the spine, and extend into a well-rounded backbend from tail to neck.

When you bind your arms in Eagle, it's common to fling the arms quickly around one another to make the final grab. Instead, consider each separate movement that is needed to achieve the shape you are making: deep abduction of scaps, horizontal abduction of the arms, external rotation of the shoulder joints, deep internal rotation of the forearms. If you pause in between each of these movements, your brain has time to figure out which muscles to fire to refine these actions, building strength over time and refining the recruitment for best efficiency.

These points are true for all the binds: assess the combined actions of the joints, use your deep core and spine to create stabilizing counteractions, ensure that your muscles are active and not relying solely on the mechanical advantage of the connections. These efforts will lead to safe, strong, and more natural binds in the long run.

Experiential Learning

For this exercise, we will look at our colleagues' particular blueprint for their upper extremity. We'll look at examples in both reaching and weight bearing. You'll need to assess where they are in space compared to where they ought to be.

Begin by doing the carrying angle vs. hyperextension assessment. Observe them with their arms in front of them (parallel arms!!) and with their arms reaching out to the sides. Determine if they have specific alignment protocols to consider in practice.

Observation Exercise. Work with just one other person in the beginning. Get used to seeing and discussing the nuances of the upper body alignment before trying to assess multiple people at once. Starting in Table pose, look at where the hands land on the mat:

- Are they too narrow? How do you know?

- Are they rotated properly? How do you know?

- Are they too far forward or back in relation to their shoulder? How do you know?

Talk this out aloud with your partner. Make sure you understand the geometry of the upper extremity, so when you begin to make adjustments, you can be clear and concise. It may be helpful to mark their new width on the mat with pieces of tape, so they have a consistent visual cue to no longer go narrower than that.

Now practice the detailed way to explain their new blueprint. Begin by having them sit back on their heels and reach their arms forward. Help them align their elbows to actual shoulder-width. Once there, they'll flip their hands over to see how wide their hands will need to be once they meet the mat. Make sure they really look at that. They'll be tempted, even unconsciously, to bring their hands back in toward midline as they move them to the floor. Offer them a visual reference while their hands are still in the air, like, "Notice that right now your hands are wider than your elbows, they're closer to the mat's width, they might even be slightly wider than the mat. What if that's just okay? What if we're not worried about that? Let's just move the hands to the

floor without losing any of that space we've found between them."

Once they reach the floor and begin to bear weight, assess again. Ensure that they haven't changed the width. Notice the palms and how they meet the mat. Are the knuckles able to ground down evenly, or do the index- and middle-finger roots pop up? Is the wrist taking all the weight? Notice the elbows and where the tips point, outward or inward or straight back. What is the relationship between the hand, the wrist, and the elbow? What effect does this have at the shoulder, collarbone, and chest? Is there continuity from the hands all the way through to the rib cage? Notice how these things change if they alter their position, rotation, weight/balance.

Once you have repeatedly observed this person from their habitual placement through this newly blueprinted shape, switch partners, or find someone else in your household to examine. Repeat the previous steps with as many folks as you can over the next few days. The more bodies you look at, the better you will become at noticing more than just the gross misalignments of the bones; you'll begin to see how more minute engagements change the entire energy of the posture. You'll be able to see whether prana is flowing freely or jamming up, and this will serve you well as you begin to cue more elaborate postures. This principle is outlined in more detail in the "Cueing Principles" section coming up.

Vocabulary

The new Yoga Engineering perspectives on the upper extremity's movement will likely be some of the most difficult to process for your students. They have been taught to pull their shoulders down; they have been taught specif-ically to place their hands a certain way. They may resist your new language and direction at first, so you need to be able to communicate clearly *why* these changes are imperative to their long-term success. This is where individ-uality gets celebrated to its fullest.

Invariably, you will have new students who have yet to trust your words over their earlier guides; that's the natural way of things. Take this opportunity to explain to your entire class about their individual bony differences. Work-shopping the arm shapes and placements even in an everyday yoga class is a fantastic way to blow some minds and change their perspective on their upper body practice. To prepare for that, develop a clear understanding of the variance of carrying angles and individual differences, the risks to soft tissues from improper range-of-motion practices, the importance of Hasta Bandha to the activation of the core body, and the relationship between our upper extremity and gravity in weight-bearing postures.

The more readily you can discuss these principles in real time, the more your students will be open to the adaptations you recom-mend. *Why* you're asking them to move differ-ently is far more compelling in the long run. I assure you, this methodology will create buzz within the student body and get them sharing information throughout their yoga community.

Cueing Principles
Hasta Bandha

Some fundamental engineering principles come into play here. If the wrist is asked to bear weight in a hyperextended, deviated, or torqued position, it will not be happy. Not only are the muscles too long to be effectively strong, but the carpal joints are taking on enormous stress, which will result in inflam-mation, degeneration, and dysfunction. Earn the strength in your forearms by finding your best alignment then distributing weight from the outer edges of the palm, "up" through the center of the palm, like a little suction cup ... or like the arch of the foot. In the foot we call it *Pada Bandha*; in the hand it is *Hasta Bandha*.

Hasta Bandha is created muscularly when we arrange the hand bones in their appropriate alignment and use our muscles to support the uplift of the center arch. This cannot happen if our weight descends through the thumb and saddle joint. The most efficient energetic line from the ground to the chest runs through the space between the second and third metacar-pals (the index- and middle-finger hand bones). This space aligns with the ulna and radius when the forearm is pronated, as it is when we place our hands on the ground. So our most effective place to bear weight is in those bones.

If you soften your gaze and watch people in Table or Plank pose, you can see this ener-getic line, and you can also see whether it jams up in the wrist or flows freely through the hand. Practitioners whose hands are red or white with effort are usually allowing all of their weight to bear down through hands, without the benefit of rebounding. They are not making the connection between the earth and their core. By engaging the subtle work of the hands, they'll be able to feel an energetic component that will help them access and build their core body muscles. Once estab-lished and re-habituated, using Hasta Bandha will help you connect the earth directly to your chest, your heart, and the depth of Uddiyana Bandha. These are integral to the stability of all weight-bearing postures, but especially as you move into inversions and arm balances.

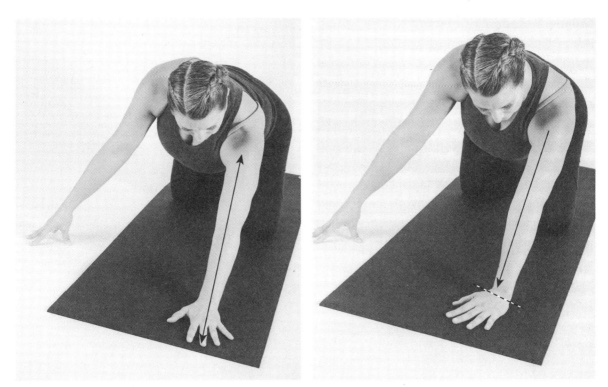

We want the bones of the hand, wrist, forearm, and arm to align in such a way that gravity-force can travel smoothly up and down, without jamming up in any one joint.

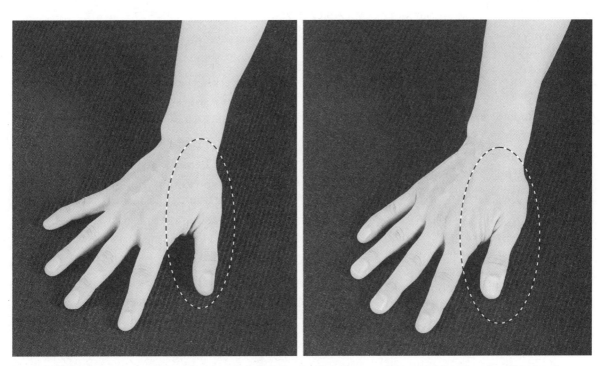

It's subtle, but you can see that the thumb is light in the first image, the pad of the thumb still turned slightly toward the palm. In the second, the thumb is pressed down, twisting it to flatten to the earth.

Cueing Practice

First, you need to find the proper width to place your hands, then your optimal turnout. This will help find the most efficient distribution of weight across the palm, without pressurizing the thumb or wrist. Next you'll need to shift the entire plane of the shoulder and arm to align behind the crease of the wrist joint (I like to suggest around a 95 degree bend in the wrist). Then notice if the palms can lie flat when rotating the points of the elbows to point back. If the index- and middle-finger knuckles lift up, some external rotation of the arm/hand is needed; pivot the bones of the hands to point outward slightly, until those knuckles can root down powerfully. This will offer the most efficient transfer of gravity through your joints and into the core. It will take time to build up the strength necessary to maintain these actions, but it is imperative that you do so in order to protect the wrist and thumb over time.

To access Hasta Bandha specifically, here are some sample cueing exercises: ❂

"Press down through the index- and middle-finger roots ... the knuckles where finger meets palm. Press so much that the heel of the hand begins to lift off the mat. Begin to alternate the left and right hands, kneading the mat a bit like a cat would use its paws to knead a blanket."

"Use your right index finger to trace the edges of your left palm. Become engrossed in the sensation of the edges of the palm, imagining that the center can become hollow. Place the palm lightly on the mat, allowing only those same edges to take any weight. Slowly add pressure while also engaging your muscles to keep the center of the palm up off the floor."

"Imagine you have a softball to wrap your fingers around, one in each hand. Grip that pretend softball with your whole hand and fingers, trying to make the most round shape you can. Repeat this action as if it were a basketball, trying to use the fingers a little less with each subtle squeeze. Enlarge the hands again as if holding a beach ball, pulling the fingers back little by little until you are mostly using your palms. You'll find an increasing acuity for making a 'fist' with just your palm, activating both the forearm muscles and the intrinsic muscles of the hand with subtlety."

Your Individual Blueprint on the Mat

As discussed in the sidebar on carrying angles, when you look at an individual in Mountain pose, arms hanging at their sides with palms open to face the front wall, you'll notice that the hands rarely hang directly down from the shoulders. This effect is masked in our common posture, with palms soft and turned toward our thighs, but in anatomical position, the nature of our carrying angle reveals itself. Because of this lateral deviation of the elbow, the hands naturally align wider than the hips, and generally wider even than the shoulders. When standing, if we adjusted our hands to shoulder-width, we would notice the awkward nature of this posture and might be more inclined to allow the hands to recover their more natural alignment. In fact, our elbows will fall in line with our shoulder joints, while our hands splay out to the sides a bit—or quite a bit, as certain cases may be. Following this lead, any time we reach overhead or down to the mat, the most efficient bony alignment will be with the elbows at shoulder-width and the hands as wide as they need to be to accommodate the carrying angle for the individual.

When we place our hands on the earth, the ramifications of this architecture are even more profound, because their alignment will translate through our bones to our shoulder girdle and into our core. How we place our hands not only impacts the health of our wrists and shoulder joints, but it significantly affects how efficiently we bear weight through our musculature. It's much more difficult to recruit all the muscles of the hands, forearms, arms, chest, back, and core if we aren't in optimal bony alignment. So I suggest that EVERY time we place our hands on the mat, we pay very close attention to how and where they land. Most yogis, even those petite folks who have shoulders narrower than their mat, will need to place hands wide enough that the pinky fingers touch the edges of their mat. Those of us with larger frames will very likely need to go even wider. On a standard-width mat, my own hands land so only the middle and index fingers are still on the mat ... the ring and pinky fingers (and the attached palm bits) land on the floor, wide of the mat. This is okay! Perfectly okay, in fact, because the places that need to bear the majority of our weight are the knuckles of the middle and index fingers, the roots just where finger meets palm.

Those who exhibit a profound carrying angle (and many who don't) are also likely to need a rotational adjustment to maintain good hand contact with the mat. In my observations, very few yogis exhibit healthy wrist or shoulder alignment when their fingers point forward. Many people will require more external rotation in order to align their bones correctly to avoid wrist impingement or saddle joint collapse. When you place your hands on the floor, if the roots of your index and middle finger lift off the mat, you are more likely to hyperextend the wrist, place too much weight in the carpal bones, and way too much weight into the base of the thumb (the saddle joint). None of those prospects will lead to good wrist/hand health down the line, nor will you be able to access the strength necessary to achieve the levity you'll need for inversions and arm balances.

Speaking of hyperextension, it's very important that you align your shoulders behind the crease of the wrist—otherwise you cannot access the full strength of the forearm muscles. According to the principle of midrange, you need to maintain a bend in the wrist that is larger than 90 degrees, or you risk straining the flexor tendons and muscles. This is true when you are setting up a Table pose, or Cow/Cat, or Plank ... any pose where you will bear weight in the hands.

Cueing Practice

Since this is really such an individual alignment practice, how do you cue effectively to an entire class? Can you offer a more generic blueprint that then gets subtle modification in more extreme cases? I think so.

Table is an ideal place to start for this. Just as Mountain is the blueprint for all standing postures, Table pose becomes the standard alignment for all postures on your hands. Here is a generic opening cueing example:

> "Make sure hands are wide enough to accommodate the full width of your shoulders. Your thumbs will be wider than the armpit ... all of us will touch the edge of the mat with our pinkies, but some of us will need to go even wider. To avoid hyperextension in the wrists, you need to shift your whole body back until the plane of the arm is behind the crease of the wrist. Turn elbows to point straight back.

When you do this, if the index- and middle finger-roots lift up, please turn your whole hand outward just a few degrees until those knuckles can root down firmly. It's unlikely that any of us will have our index or even our middle finger pointing straight ahead ... and that's okay!"

Integration with the Spine

It's important to note that the musculature of the shoulder girdle is functionally integrated with the central core. They cannot be separated. There are fascial continuities between the obliques, erector spinaes, serratus, rhomboids, pecs, and lats that create slings of support and stability. So any small imbalances in the shoulder girdle can have a functional effect on the spine/core, and vice versa. Some of these fascial patterns extend into the arm, and some all the way down the legs. It is too complex a system to go into detail here, but still very important to acknowledge that the connections exist. (If you're curious about these, I highly recommend diving into Thomas Myers's *Anatomy Trains*.)

Because of these relationships, our stabilizing counteractions aren't always the most obvious—because they don't exist solely in the extremity; they are a combination of actions at the shoulder and the spine/core. For every forward action, we'll need to incorporate a backward action. For example, as the scapulae retract into the ribs, we need to counteract by firing our upper abdominals in order to keep the front ribs from blowing out. The range of the scapula can be a bit deceptive here; the mechanics of protraction/retraction means that, functionally, serratus anterior pulls the inferior angle of the scapula *forward* into the ribs, even though we may focus on the visual action of the superior angle tipping back.

Cueing Practice

Movements need to occur at the hand, arm, chest, upper back, and abdomen. For weight bearing it may sound like this:

"Press into the knuckles of index and middle fingers, point the elbows straight back toward the thighs. Broaden the collarbones (pulling scaps toward the spine slightly), press the bottom tips of the scaps into the ribs. Finally, lift the solar plexus deeply, pulling the organs to the spine and preventing a backbend or collapse in the mid-back."

These principles of alignment work whether you are reaching or weight bearing. Take the upper arm in Side Angle for example, or any twisting posture with extended arms. It's very easy to let the top arm swing back behind our heart to feel like we are getting more heart-opening and more twist. This is, of course, an illusion, but it can feel so good on the inside! It lacks integrity though and adds nothing functional to the posture. Instead, we need to access our internal resistance to really embody the strength of our expansive heart. Pull back the ribs by firing the solar plexus, tap into Uddiyana Bandha, retract the scapula forward into the ribs, and press the palm forward as if pressing into the plane of your heart-center. This pressing is an added counter to the backward momentum of the ribs and gives integrity to the core continuum.

So if you are reaching, as in Side Angle, you may cue this way:

"Look up at your top hand. Notice if it's fallen back behind your heart-line. Pull your front ribs back with some Cat effort. Press your hand forward to meet that backward momentum ... they meet in the middle."

Integration with Lower Body and Core

This section describes the total integration of the regions of the body and may seem overwhelming in its nuanced connections. Before diving in here, be sure that you have a clear notion of how the spine integrates with the hips and how the shoulder integrates with the spine. If those principles are well-established in your understanding, the following information will satisfy some potentially nagging questions that have left you curious for more.

Standing postures and weight-bearing postures both benefit from an integration of the relationship between the core and the upper extremity. Thus, we need to effectively cue into the counteractions that stabilize them together into one unit. This includes the relationship between shoulder retraction and activation of the solar plexus (upper rectus abdominis and the deep core). This upper extremity portion of Uddiyana Bandha's muscular action assists the entire upper body integration.

In addition there is a subtle but potent connection to the lower body via psoas. To fully access the power of Uddiyana, psoas must fire to place just a little forward tension on the thoracolumbar junction; otherwise we go into a deep hunch instead of lengthening upward off the pelvis. This hip flexor action also counters the forward momentum many of us feel in the pelvis while standing, creating neutrality and stability through the hip, while offering resistance against the hamstrings and glutes that urge us into hip extension or pelvic thrust. We

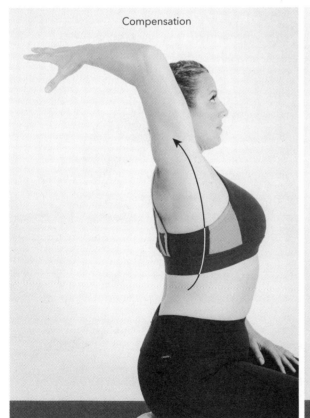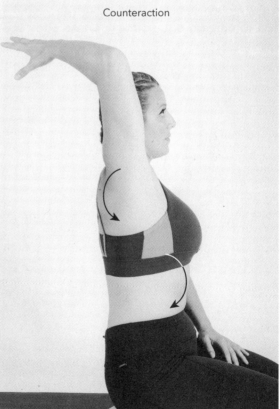

Compensation

Counteraction

The rib-spine is used to counteract and stabilize the movements of the upper extremity.

end up with a series of flexion/extension counteractions that zigzag up the body, all the way from the ankles and knees, through the tail and Mula Bandha, up through the middle-spine and shoulders, and finally through the throat pulling back to lengthen the back-neck (Jalandhara Bandha) and rise through the crown.

All of those counteraction points are necessary whether you are standing upright or working long on the earth in Plank family postures. Each of these hinges needs counteraction to prevent collapse and tie the entire body together. Think about the difference in stability walking across a rope bridge that is only anchored at its two ends versus a bridge with support both above and below along its entire length. The principle of tensegrity tells us that our feet are connected to our hands and our head, that work in one area will affect the other, and that the more we use the connections between each set of bones in between, the less effort any of those sections will need to work individually.

What if you're practicing with only one hand on the earth? In Side Plank variations, you must integrate the shoulder and arm with the obliques, paraspinals, and hip abductors in addition to all the anterior/posterior muscular work. Whether or not you have a supporting knee or foot on the ground, the lower extremity

must be working against the mat to propel the hips upward. The side-waistlines will contract to support the low back bones and integrate the work of lats, serratus, and the remaining SG and GH muscles to lift the ribs with a sling of muscles. If you disengage either the hand (Hasta Bandha) or the legs, this posture feels dense and heavy, drooping to the floor instead of floating light and high. The same front-to-back counteractions are in play, but here they are utilized to keep the body in balance on its side-edge, keeping you from tipping front or back. The side-body is acting as the engine of effort in gravity or in flow. The top arm will need to integrate with the spine as discussed earlier.

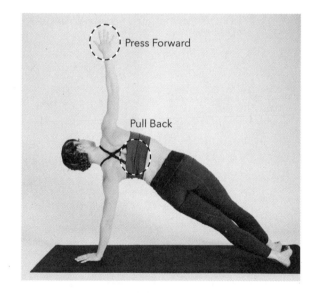
Press Forward
Pull Back

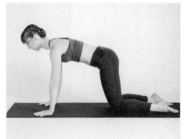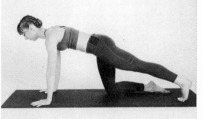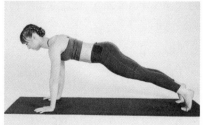

The upper extremity and core body remain stable as the legs move to assume the Plank position.

Cueing Practice

In a posture like Plank where you must integrate the work of the deep core with all of the extremities, it's important to remind students of the actions of the spine, and how to keep the curves neutral while the upper body gains strength. Engaging the legs and feet will help the core and upper body feel lighter over time. All of the following cues apply whether or not the knees come down to the ground.

> "Start in Table pose. Press into the knuckles of index and middle fingers, point the elbows straight back toward the thighs. Broaden the collarbones (pulling scaps toward the spine slightly), press the bottom tips of the scaps into the ribs. Lift the solar plexus deeply, pull the tail slightly toward the back of the heart; don't clench the glutes. Reach right foot back, tucking toes, then follow it with the left one. Step far enough back that the heel stacks just over the ball of the foot. Press through the ball of the foot instead of the heel to activate Pada Bandha ... you may feel a lift in the shins, then in the thighs. Lift the belly deep, open the front-heart, lengthen the back-neck. DO NOT lock out the elbows."

In the one-handed variation, Side Plank, integration is slightly different. Since that top hand can go rogue, sagging back behind the heart to give the sense of an open chest, we need to become mindful of its alignment directly over the heart.

> "Notice the top hand. Look at it. Is it flailing behind you or actually reaching for the sky? Integrate the whole arm by pulling back deeply in the ribs, like Cat. As the front ribs move back, press the hand slightly forward, let that action come from deep in the shoulder girdle.

Press until the hand aligns directly over the center of the heart—not over your face or waistline, but over the center of the ribs. You'll notice that it feels like the ribs and hand are opposing one another, meeting at the center plane and hugging into it. This counteraction builds stability in the upper core, and may even help you to feel lighter on your grounded hand."

Binds

Binds are an interesting and dynamic part of our yoga practice. Even the simplest binds can advance a posture to "the next level," adding both sensational and visual intensity. These movements incorporate the full range of the SG and GH. As introduced in the previous section, the problem is that traditional cueing has emphasized counteraction in a way that is likely to do harm to the GH. This is one area where we need to fully embrace the compensations of the scapula in order to reach our full range, and then be subtle and deliberate in our counteractions. These combined actions are necessary when binding, or else we will do damage to the labrum and tendons.

Cueing Practice

We'll begin with a simple bind in a standing or seated pose. This exercise is essential to assessing the mobility of the scapulae, the strength of the extensors, and the acuity of the student to access the unified movement of the shoulder joint and shoulder girdle.

> "With your hands in a simple bind behind your back, fingers interwoven tightly but palms open, begin to shrug your shoulders toward your ears. Try to not lock out your elbows. Begin to lift your elbows away from your back. Resist the urge to pull your shoulders together,

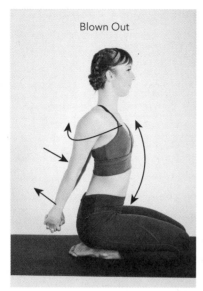

Blown Out

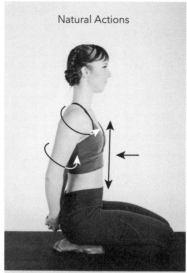

Natural Actions

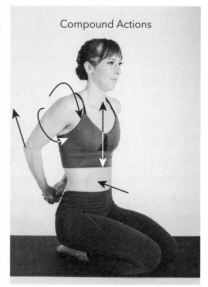

Compound Actions

It's tempting to lock out the elbows and allow that mechanical advantage to assist this movement, but that imposes too much shear force on the soft tissues of the shoulder. Instead, we need to move within the muscular bounds and natural compound movement of the shoulder, building strength and mobility over time.

and instead let them rise and tip forward. The bottom tips of the scapulae will pull away from the ribs, and your collarbones will lift up and away from the top ribs. Breathe into that new hollow at the base of your neck/top of your shoulders."

This rendition of this posture feels odd at first, but you'll find over time that it is profoundly freeing! Mechanical advantage is reduced, there is less tendency to lock out elbows, and it requires intentional muscular contraction. This is the natural way of movement in deep extension and builds strength to move into greater opening without the aid of gravity. When you do use gravity in forward-folded versions of this bind, you'll find you can access far more range than in the more traditional version with pinched scaps.

When practicing deeply rotated binds, as in Eagle or Cow Face, it's important to allow the scap to move naturally with the rotation. If too

much counteraction occurs, all that force gets concentrated into the soft tissues of the GH joint, and the strain will damage those tissues over time. There's really no need to memorize the compound movements for your own practice—you can feel the pull as the arm moves. I encourage you to play with these movements and notice how it actually feels to work against the natural flow of the rotation and abduction/adduction. When teaching these binds, it's good to have a clear understanding of how to cue the compound movements so there isn't too much counteraction. Your students will find more range than they expect when they access the movements of the scapulae.

Let's work with Cow Face to feel this fully. With right arm overhead and left behind the back, here are the cues for the compound actions needed to keep it safe.

"Right triceps rotates forward toward midline, encouraging the shoulder blade to wrap forward around the armpit.

Reach the elbow upward, letting scap rise up or shrug toward ear. Neck soft, head bobbly.

"Left triceps rotates forward, pulling shoulder blade with it slightly so that chest is engaged. You should feel a little space created between the forearm and back body, allowing you to slide elbow closer to side-waist, and room to bend the elbow deeper.

"Lift the chest, engaging upper back, but be careful not to force the shoulder blades together at the spine. You need those scapulae to be wrapping forward around the ribs, but a subtle counteraction at the back of the heart is appropriate."

All these cues are appropriate any time there is a bind behind the back, whether in a Bound Side Angle or Bird of Paradise, or in all the Marichi's Pose variations.

Arm Balances

The blueprint for all arm balances is Low Plank (Chaturanga Dandasana). We need to practice Low Plank very precisely for a time long enough to:

- Develop the forearm strength to use wrist/finger flexion effectively and maintain Hasta Bandha
- Become habituated to the alignment of the elbow over the wrist and not beyond it

- Integrate the scapula in good alignment and cohesion with the ribs
- Find continuity from the shoulder girdle into the back-spine, core, and lower extremity

While the physics of arm balances are rooted fundamentally in finding the "balance point," a feat that takes mental practice more than sheer strength, the dexterity and stamina we build in our hands and wrists will ensure we have adequate time to work on our deeper core strength and movements. The second point in the list is important because for all of our bent-elbow arm balances, we are strongest when we use the bony alignment to our advantage, without exploiting our joints or tendons. If we get used to aligning our elbow just over our wrist without hyperextending, we can use more bony support and shift our muscular awareness to our core, which is really where our arm balances activate from. So, points one and two work together to build adequate forearm strength to maintain proper flexion-action while deeply extended, and then we can be focused on the balance between the wrist and elbow. Points three and four effectively incorporate the shoulder girdle and the actions deep in the core to create buoyancy and lift, so we feel lighter through our torso, whether or not our feet remain on the mat.

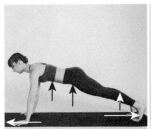 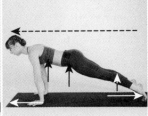 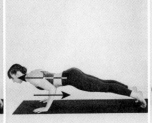 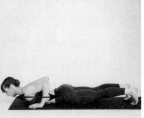

Cueing Practice

You'll start in a strong Plank. To achieve the most efficient architecture in Low Plank, you'll need to continually reinforce the alignment points of Plank while also moving through space in precise ways. If any part of the core/spine/lower body degenerates, your Low Plank will degenerate and overly stress the shoulder, elbow, and/or wrist.

> "Use the toes to press the whole body forward, taking the shoulders well past the wrist. Don't look down at your hips or feet, or at the front wall; keep back-neck long. On your exhale, begin to bend the elbows slowly, in a controlled fashion; stop before you reach 90 degrees. Pull elbows to ribs, shoulder blades toward spine, lift solar plexus. Elbow should align directly over the wrist, and shoulders should be beyond your fingertips. Maintain neutral spine, don't let hips drop or lift too high ... keep them level with the heart."

You'll notice the particular instruction to deliberately take the wrist into hyperextension. Although typically we want to avoid this, in this instance we are here for only a fraction of a breath as we set up the geometry necessary to find final alignment. We avoid hyperextension as much as possible intentionally so we can kind of "save up" for this pre–Low Plank moment. If we don't shift forward in preparation, the shoulder will be over our hands as we bend the elbow, instead of out in front, and this is not a strong position for anyone. By bringing the body forward first, we can pull the elbow back into alignment over the wrist as it bends, while the heart and crown continue to lengthen forward. This is the only way to make that nice, squarish angle in the arm while also keeping the core fully alert and the spine neutral.

If this forward movement is new to you, I highly recommend practicing simply shifting forward and back for a bit, without coming down into Low Plank. Once that feels comfortable, and you can do this without losing any lift in the belly and hips, then practice bringing the knees down before bending elbows. Make sure you keep the chest broad and don't come down too low. Ensure you are pulling the elbows back in order to lower the upper body, but only until they stack over the wrist.

THE VINYASA FLOW

The ubiquitous vinyasa flow! Now that we've learned to observe the spine, lower extremity, and upper extremity, we can put them all together to perform the full-body expression of the core movements of many vinyasa classes. While I myself don't teach this sequence as often as many vinyasa-style teachers, it remains the integrating factor for many teachers, which means that we should have a focused and detailed understanding of its mechanics and component poses.

The poses, however, aren't the only things we need to pay attention to. This is where emphasizing transitional acuity is integral to safe practice. If we merely stitch together the poses, we can miss out on the strength and integrity of each pose—and also disregard the nuance of the transitions themselves. That is setting us all up for potential injury, especially in the delicate tissues of the shoulder and wrist joints.

So for those who haven't already gotten the Kool-Aid that is "The Vinyasa," it's really a selection of postures pulled from Sun Salutations (Surya Namaskar A). Here is the outline:

- Forward Fold or Plank (sometimes stepping or jumping directly back to the next pose, or coming from someplace else, like Down Dog)

- Low Plank (or Plank all the way to the floor)

- Baby Cobra/Cobra/Up Dog

- Down Dog

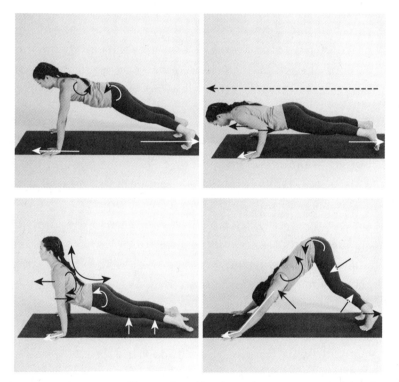

There is a constant sense of forward and backward momentums helping keep the entire body active and neutrality strong in the spine (except in the backbend).

This sequence is often used as a link between other short sequences of standing poses. Because it becomes so repetitive, many folks get really habituated to the way they do it, and they run the risk of just going through the motions or succumbing to movement patterns they aren't aware of. Once this happens, they will reinforce those bad habits and increase the risk of injury with every single pass through.

You'll likely see many bodies do a deep nose-dive style flow that begins in Down Dog, arching into a moving backbend as the face careens toward the floor between the hands, only to barely escape crashing into the earth before a quick dust-off up into the sky, throwing the head back at the peak of something in between a big, broken Cobra and some version of Up Dog. They won't actually BE in any of the postures in the model, and they're very likely to blow out their shoulders and low back in the process. The truth is, to remain safe AND actually have the opportunity to experience each posture in The Vinyasa, there is a geometric imperative to the transition between these poses.

What I'm about to describe will sound remarkably robotic, but I assure you, once this form is instilled, a beautifully dynamic flow thrums through the movements from beginning to end. When people witness it in action, they are often blown away by how strong and graceful it looks and feels. There isn't really a sacrifice of rhythm, but a natural reinforcement of each pose in deep relation to the next. The mechanics of the individual postures are outlined in the following section. Here we'll focus on the transitions.

The Flow

- The transition from either Down Dog or a standing pose at the front of the mat to the Plank/Low Plank requires that we maintain a neutral spine. The core must remain active and contained while the shoulder and hip make some pretty dynamic movements, especially if you choose the jump-back option. So, I strongly suggest that you omit the jump-back for now, or at least until you become familiar with how this new version will feel through each transition. In fact, it may serve you best to simply start in Plank, so you can suss out the finer details of this nuanced sequence.

- From Plank: Ensure that your hands are active with Hasta Bandha and your feet are alive with Pada Bandha. Don't allow the wrists to collapse down— you'll need to keep a full grip on the mat throughout the sequence. Now you'll need to shift forward, way forward, bringing the shoulders past the wrists and pushing onto the very tip-tippy-tips of the toes, even rolling over them completely, all without sacrificing the neutral spine or levity of the hips. (You are welcome to drop the knees as needed at this point. But make sure you always shift forward BEFORE bringing knees down.)

- Low Plank: Now you can begin to bend the elbows straight back, realigning them over the wrists so that the forearm is roughly upright (if looking at it from the side). There may be a slight tilt inward from wrist to elbow if your hands are wide with an adequate turn-out. Be aware that you may reach this alignment long before the elbow reaches a 90 degree bend, and that is A-OK. In my opinion 90 degrees is a rather arbitrary point to meet, so we don't care about getting there. What we do care about is building the strength you need to actually hold yourself in this flexed-elbow posture for more than a breath cycle. You need to do that without the chest collapsing, or the hips dropping out, or the spine dropping in the middle. If you cannot hold all of these at one time while also maintaining a fluid breath cycle, I highly recommend you practice very slowly descending all the way to the earth, or dropping the knees to build up your strength over time.

- Upward Facing Dog: In the previous steps, the chest has not dropped below the level of the elbows; it has merely hovered there or slightly above. The transition to Up Dog then will not have that diving quality, but instead it will feel a little like a rebound up and off a cushion of air beneath the chest. The arms engage backward, as if doing a pull-up, the chest opening toward the front wall, the scapulae adducting and retracting to create a "coiling" behind the heart. The hips still haven't dropped!! The legs engage downward and the thighs upward, tail pulling toward the heart to create a continuous arc instead of a deep break at the ribs or sacrum. You embody a long graceful Cobra pose that has been elevated off the mat by the stilts of your long, strong arms.

- Downward Facing Dog: Since your feet and legs are already pressing down, and the thighs already have lift in Up Dog, you merely need to increase the effort of those actions to make the transition back to Down Dog—at least that's how it appears from the outside. You're really continuing those actions while engaging the deep Uddiyana Bandha/upper belly actions of Cat pose, so the upper body is just as actively lifting as the lower body. There is backward momentum and upward lift though the hinge in the hips. The chest lands light and suspended between the shoulders, not jamming down toward the floor as the armpits collapse. The legs remain active even with softened knees, heels pull back instead of down. There is a sense of gathering toward the center hinge while pressing out through the hands and feet. These opposing forces contribute to the rising effect.

Practice Mechanics

For each of the following postures, I've listed fundamental alignment points for the upper extremity. For many of these, especially when we bear weight, we need to account for individual differences and make adjustments for each student accordingly. You'll notice pretty quickly that this is a practice in repetition. The key concepts here are that when you are reaching, you need to integrate with the core using counteractions between the core, scapulae, and arms; and when the hands bear weight, you need to use counteractions to stabilize the entire system from floor to core. The cues here are specific to the upper extremity, but you should always consider and cue the concurrent spinal activations.

Keep in mind that we are working within the confines of a system that is not built to do what we are asking it to do. That's not to say we shouldn't do these things (unless a particular body protests in earnest), but we certainly need to remain mindful as we make these movements. It's imperative that we consider the tissues—bones and squishy bits alike—and where they will be happiest as we execute each pose.

Standing Poses: Reaching

These are the postures that get the least amount of attention because we make so many assumptions about our range of motion. It will serve you and your students to constantly reinforce the range-of-motion rule: only 30 degrees in any direction will actually come from the GH. You MUST move the shoulder girdle to achieve safe alignment and movement while reaching. Also remember that EXTERNAL ROTATION is the name of the GH game. This simple action will change how your arms, shoulders, and upper back engage and work together forevermore.

Upward Facing Hands (Urdhva Hastasana)

Upward Facing Hands pose—we do it so many times during a typical class that it certainly becomes one of the postures we are mostly thoughtless about. We are also probably conditioned to automatically drop the shoulders as we reach up. This is one of the bad habits we must endeavor to break. Your students may resist at first, but I assure you, if you explain what's really happening at the shoulder in these movements, they will change their habits. Often a "before and after" practice of both positions will offer perspective on what feels restricted and what feels truly free.

- Neutral spinal curves, active belly, stable rib cage.
- External rotation of the arm at the shoulder joint.
- Abduction of the scapula, shoulder blades wrapping forward around the armpits.
- Upward rotation of the scapula, allowing acromion to rise even as medial borders drop slightly.

- Let hands remain shoulder-width when overhead, at least until the new shoulder position becomes more familiar.

- Arms may be forward of head at first, instead of alongside the ears. Allow this to maintain integrity in spine and shoulder girdle to avoid compensations for short lats and shoulder muscles.

- Maintain active Uddiyana Bandha.

Warrior II (Virabhadrasana II) Family of Postures

- Neutral spinal curves—do not tuck tail—stable rib cage.

- Heart rotation while leaving hips to their individual "open" alignments.

- External rotation of the arm at the shoulder joint.

- Neutral scapula—stabilization actions without compensation or overwork.

  - Retraction/Uddiyana Bandha

  - Abduction/adduction

- Arms align over top of thighs—avoid back arm cranking back to force/fake a deeper twist.

- Hands raise to shoulder height, reaching out from the anchor of the shoulders/heart, through the fingers into space.

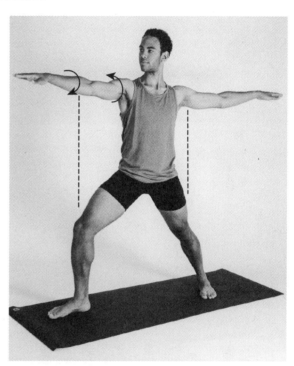

Backbends

There can be some counterintuitive actions in the upper extremity as part our backbending practice. Because of the compound actions that need to occur between the shoulder joint and shoulder girdle, we need to be pretty precise as to how we cue the minute details of these postures. There is also a huge difference between the backbends that integrate flexion in the shoulder versus extension ... as you can imagine.

Remember this: the primary directive of the shoulder girdle in every backbend is to create a support structure for the rib cage and heart. How does the shoulder girdle assist in extension of the thoracic spine? This is the question you need to answer through your alignment.

Cobra or Upward Facing Dog (Bhujangasana or Urdhva Mukha Svanasana)

These are the backbends that will incorporate the neutral/extension actions of the shoulder. The arm will be just at neutral or slightly extended, using the friction of the floor to entice the engagement of the lats and serratus, stabilizing the shoulder girdle so the back-spine muscles can fully extend the spine.

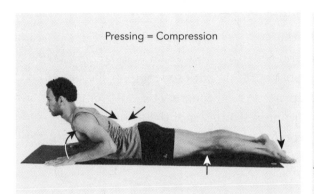

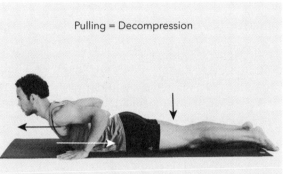

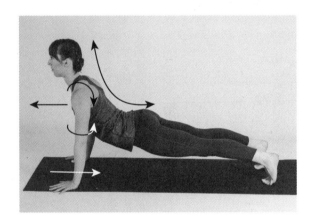

- Active abdominal core coupled with lumbar lordosis; avoid breaking at T10.

- Elbows align under shoulder joint; hands find appropriate width and turnout.

- Adduction at scapulae without total back-heart collapse.

- Retraction at scapulae, anchoring to back ribs without depressing down. Avoid overstretch of neck muscles.

- Adduction and external rotation to neutral of the arm; elbows will point straight back without locking. Remain engaged muscularly at each joint.

- Pull-back of hands and upper arms to engage lats and create forward momentum of chest and heart.
- Knees press down to fire hip flexors (in Cobra); or for Up Dog, press feet into the earth with fully engaged and stabilized leg, no locking of knees, focusing effort into hip flexors to keep hips lifted and spine actively extending.

Upward Facing Bow (Wheel) (Urdhva Dhanurasana)

Upward Facing Bow and its counterparts utilize the flexion actions of the upper extremity. It's very easy to compensate for short lats, chest, and shoulder muscles by breaking in the spine. It's integral that you maintain the abdominal stabilizers AND work to lengthen the lats/chest/shoulder AND align the shoulder girdle properly to create the necessary support for the ribs and heart. Though Bridge is generally lumped into this group in terms of the spine, it doesn't fit in here—its upper extremity actions are a bit of a hybrid between the previous Cobra points and the upcoming Camel points.

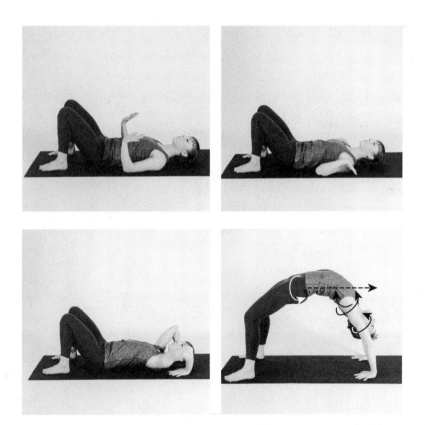

Using her carrying angle as her blueprint throughout the process, Jessica can find her best hand placement then engage external rotation, scapular abduction, and retraction all at once.

- Active abdominal core coupled with lumbar lordosis; avoid breaking at T10.

- Hands appropriate width and turn-out. (Photos illustrate this process.)

- External rotation of the arm at the shoulder, the elbows will wrap in (adduction); or at least activate in adduction, even if no movement is available.

- Abduction of the scapulae as the compound action of the external rotation of the humerus.

- Upward rotation of the scapulae. You are reaching overhead, so this principle still stands and is integral to the safety of the GH.

- Elevation of the scapulae; slight shrugging of the shoulders. Since you're upside down, this cue can feel confusing. It needs to be balanced with the external rotation, neither overpowering the other.

- Retraction of the scapulae, anchoring through the ribs to encourage the extension specifically in the thoracic spine.

Camel (Ustrasana)

The Camel family of backbends asks us to extend the arm fully, at least until we work up to a full drop-back, in which case we have to revert to the prior Upward Bow instructions. (I know ... the opportunity for confusion is high.)

- Active abdominal core coupled with lumbar lordosis; avoid breaking at T10.

- Extension of the arm. Hands may find a perch on the sacrum or back-thighs, or they might reach back in space to eventually find the heels or blocks aligned with the heels.

- Internal rotation of the arm at shoulder joint (some variations remain supinated in forearm).

- Protraction of the scapulae to support and facilitate the full extension of the arm.

- Abduction of the scapulae just enough to stabilize the protraction and support the expansion of the chest and extension of the thoracic spine. (Really tempting to squeeze scaps together here, but by pressing them side-on the ribs they seem to tuck under your armpits a little, which stabilizes gently and helps give lift to the chest.)

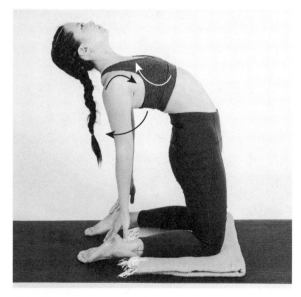

Shoulder extension requires scapular protraction, but Elena can still lift her heart up with spinal extension and Uddiyana activation.

Twists and Binds

Keep in mind that twists require us to use the upper extremity for information instead of as cranks, and in binds we want to use our muscles and not just bony mechanical advantages. This group of alignment points requires many small, refining actions instead of gross movements alone. Remain aware of what the "core" of the posture is asking on the inside and how the upper extremity can support it—not how fancy-shmancy the arms make the pose appear from the outside.

Simple Bind (and Jackrabbit/Sasangasana)

The following instructions offered seem specific to the Child's Pose variation, but the rules of the upper extremity remain the same if you are seated or standing: you must allow/encourage the scapulae to protract to achieve full extension, and therefore you must make extra space by elevating as well.

- From a Child's Pose, fingers interwoven at low back to bind hands, but palms remain wide.
- Extension of the arms at the shoulder; do not lock out elbows.
- If hands cannot move much, release bind and use a strap to enable wider hands.
- Protraction of the scapulae, allow shoulders to descend toward Earth as hands lift away from sacrum.
- Elevation of the scapulae, creating space between clavicles and ribs (make more room for increased extension/protraction). (Shrug!)
- Adduction of the scapulae; this is very subtle and acts as a soft counteraction, not so much as to override the protraction.

Lord of the Fishes (Matsyendrasana) (no bind)

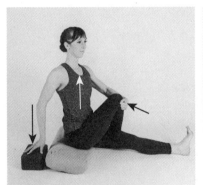 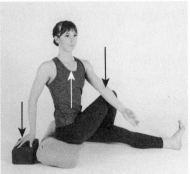 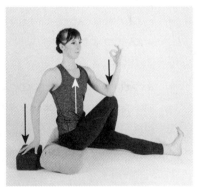

Jessica uses her arms to encourage height in her spine, not to crank in to deeper rotation.

This twist is often accompanied by a bind, but many bodies who do this find themselves off their spinal axis and collapsing. Here we offer the arms as a support to the core revolution first ... the bind may come after this, once stability is already achieved. Whether the base leg is bent or straight, the core must remain upright, and the arms act to inform the center, not pull you off center. For the following cueing, consider this a left twist, left foot crossed over right thigh. Left arm will be the "supporting" arm while right crosses the leg.

- Neutral scapulae; avoid depressing the shoulder blades onto the ribs.

- Extended left arm acts as a stabilizer, not a crank.

- Left hand should be wider than shoulders before the twist begins. Remain high on finger-tips to avoid axis collapse.

- Firm frame in abducted right arm (crossing arm); elbow at shoulder height to avoid ribs dropping on that side.

- Crossing hand pulls straight back through bent leg, no cranking. I like to use a fist to meet the leg to avoid gripping the knee/shin and inadvertently pulling it across my midline.

Cow Face (Gomukhasana)

Common cues associated with this posture run contrary to what we now know are the proper biomechanical compound movements of the shoulder girdle and shoulder joint. In the alignment points that follow, we specifically support the abduction of the scapulae to accommodate the deep rotations being asked of the shoulder joints. This can feel confusing since one arm is internally rotating and one is externally rotating, but because of the flexion or extension in each arm, these rotations will both pull the shoulder blades away from the spine. It really helps to feel this in your body, and to become familiar with what it looks like in others, instead of trying to memorize it. I swear it makes sense when you do it!!

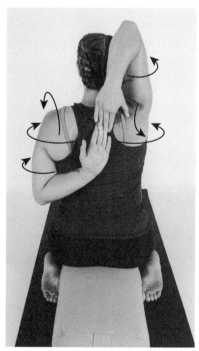

Upper Arm:

- Flexion of arm at shoulder, to maximum reach without pinching or compensating in spine.

- External rotation of arm at shoulder to make space in shoulder joint.

- Abduction of scapula as the compound action to achieve full external rotation of arm. Eventually the biceps points directly behind you.

- Elevation of scapula to allow plenty of room under collarbone. The previous action will ensure elevation cannot be overdone.

- Deep flexion at elbow; fingers will tap the back of the neck, or the center of spine, or the same-side shoulder blade, depending on available shoulder rotation.

- Neutral forearm rotation.

Lower Arm:

- Internal rotation of arm at shoulder joint, to maximum, without dropping shoulder or compensating in spine.

- Abduction of scapula, necessary for complete internal rotation at shoulder joint.

- Extension + adduction of arm, bringing extended arm in toward core-body, toward the spine.

- Deep flexion at elbow, bringing forearm into alignment with spine if possible, fingers pointing up toward heart.

- Internal rotation of forearm; back of hand rests on back-spine, palm open and exposed.

- Avoid binding hands together until both arms can be held steady with muscular actions alone.

Eagle (Garudasana)

This posture is integral for yogis to practice because it can help open up and strengthen the posterior rotator cuff muscles that tend to get so fascially bound up. The key, however, is to practice by actually using your muscles instead of relying on the mechanical advantage of the bind itself. I often make students practice without the bind for a while, keeping the forearms parallel instead of crossing, with elbows at shoulder-height to build upper back resilience. They don't always like me for it, but they get open and strong in the long run, so eventually they see it my way.

- Flexion of the arms at the shoulder, keeping elbows at shoulder-height if possible.

- Abduction of scapulae to allow the next step.

- Adduction of the arms, crossing arms above the elbow if possible. This will make for a deeper, more intrinsic bind.

- Flexion at elbows. This is where I keep them to build stamina. (Subtle extension at elbows to stabilize once bound, pressing forearms away from face.)

- Forearms cross; deep external rotation at the shoulder achieves this. Watch the biceps roll open as forearms cross.

- Internal rotation of forearms against each other (once bound) to create subtle internal resistance to help provide levity to the whole system.

- Subtle adduction of scapulae to stabilize once bound; do not overdo!!

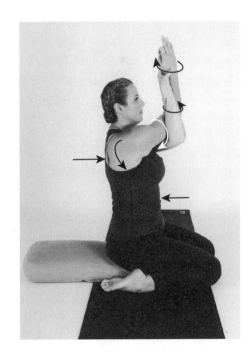

Inversions

Inversions by nature ask us to do things with the upper extremity that we aren't necessarily designed to do. Therefore, precision is of utmost importance, and refinement should be practiced from the beginning, no just as an afterthought. Like the neck-spine in headstands, the shoulder is particularly vulnerable in weight bearing, so any momentum that gets employed to achieve your inversion posture should be minimized. Earn your strength with slow, deliberate movements that are supported on a strong and stable base, and avoid haphazard leaping and flailing about. That stable base ALWAYS begins and ends with a well-developed Hasta Bandha.

Downward Facing Dog (Adho Mukha Svanasana)

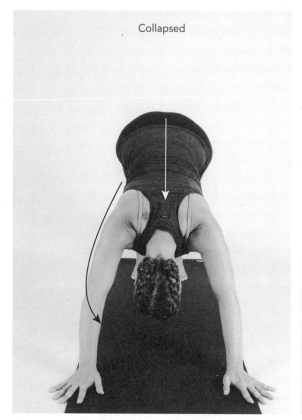 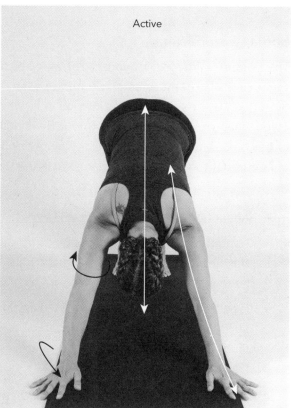

Collapsed

Active

It's counterintuitive, but Richelle shrugs her shoulders to create the space she needs to externally rotate her arms and reach back through her hips.

Although Downward Facing Dog is a quintessential posture, not many of us think of it as an inversion. We are in fact upside down, with our heart lower than our hips, even though some of our weight is still held in our lower body. In my eyes, then, this pose is the precursor and preparatory pose for all other inverted postures. Here, where we land at the end of each and every vinyasa, we learn to find a stable and neutrally curved spine while hinged deeply at the hip and bearing weight through our hands. It is here that we first experience the sense of lightness that can arise when we connect fully to the earth with Hasta Bandha and begin to lift up through the core bandhas. It is here that we earn the stamina of the upper back, shoulder girdle, and shoulder joint, learning to lengthen out of the upper extremity instead of collapsing into it.

- Hands wide enough with appropriate turnout; you should be able to access Hasta Bandha, index and middle fingers' knuckles rooted down and thumbs light.

- Soft elbows, no locking; subtle extension at shoulder as if pulling arms under you and heart forward.

- External rotation of arms; elbows should attempt to point straight back toward thighs, not out to the sides. More turn-out of hands may be needed to fully achieve this. (Play with that at will until you can achieve full Hasta Bandha while rotating elbows back.)

- Abduction of scapulae (the ribs should not collapse toward the floor); using active Uddiyana Bandha to get light in the core, ribs will press up slightly between shoulder blades.

- Retraction of scapula; avoid winging out from ribs. Fire serratus to help lift ribs to meet shoulder blades.

- Elevation of scapulae; subtle shrug in the shoulders while also externally rotating shoulder joint will result in arms lengthening up and back out, leaving plenty of room for the head to surrender.

Headstand (Sirsasana)

Headstand comes in many forms—and as far as I'm concerned, if your head is on the ground (or even in proximity to it) and your hips are in the air, *you are already there*. This pose is not dependent on the feet leaving the floor. Therefore, there is no reason whatsoever to try to get them off the floor by leaping or jumping or using any momentum of any sort. In fact, all those create so much risk that if you need them to get where you're going, you ought not to be practicing this posture at all; you should go back to getting your core strong enough that you can hold yourself in place indefinitely, even with your feet touching the ground.

In the following description, we will work through Supported Headstand (Sirsasana I), with the elbows on the mat and hands clasped, but the principles are the same for the tripod version—you'd just need to activate Hasta Bandha directly on the floor.

- Deep flexion of arms at the shoulder joint, elbows flexed and rooted to floor, hands clasped (loose or tight varies from person to person, though I prefer a loose basket).

- External rotation of arms at the shoulder; this action works against the friction of the floor but must remain constant.

- Abduction of scapulae; this is the compound action to achieving full external rotation in the shoulder joint.

- Elevation of scapulae (pressing elbows into mat); avoid collapse in the shoulder girdle—do not let head take full weight; the majority of your weight should be borne through the arms, not the neck.

- Extension at elbow (pressing wrist/hand into mat to stabilize); you should feel the entire forearm anchor into the ground, not just the elbows, or your head will be too heavy.

- Retraction of shoulder blades countered by Cat pose effort through the chest/solar plexus; gather the ribs and press them against the scapulae while scapulae hug into ribs. This counteraction gives you lift and supports the lightness of the head and neck.

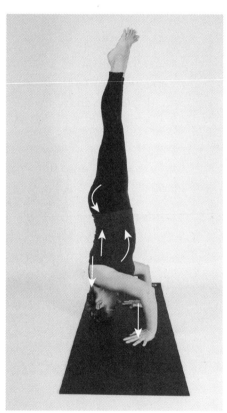

Again, Richelle shrugs shoulder slightly to help lift the ribs and take weight off the head.

Forearm Stand (Pincha Mayurasana)

In this inversion, strength in the shoulder girdle is paramount in order to avoid collapse and a not-so-graceful face-plant. But for many people, balance is really at the heart of the pose. Finding the perfect center of gravity and employing the central core in a balanced fashion will mean never needing to use the arms to overpower the rest of the posture. You do not need the upper body strength of a power lifter to manage this pose if you come at it with solid, healthy alignment and a profound awareness in the core.

Forearm Stand is notorious for looking really curvy and bendy, but this should only be the case if you intend to do a Scorpion variation. The fundamental posture should be straight upright and strong through the belly and back channels. Do not allow the back-spine to collapse; this is not a backbend!!

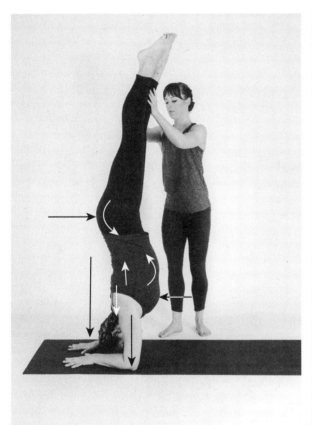 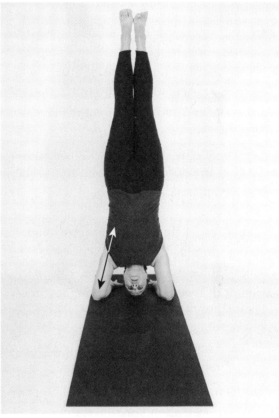

The entire elbow, wrist, and hand line must press down evenly to create an even base and help find the center of gravity. Do not rely on only one point.

- Flexion of arm to maximum at shoulder joint. (You can do this pose if full flexion isn't available, but it requires more inherent strength in triceps and deltoids.)

- External rotation of arms at the shoulder; this action is against the friction of the mat but must be maintained constantly to avoid splaying out and collapsing.

- Internal rotation of forearms so that hands root firmly and evenly to the floor.

- Extension at elbows (press forearm/wrist/hand into mat to stabilize); this action keeps you aloft, so press press press! Your center of gravity will end up slightly forward of the elbow, so the arm will be a significant part of your base.

- Uddiyana Bandha; do not allow the back-spine to collapse. Cat pose is the definitive action of the core in order to maintain neutral spinal curves.

Handstand (Urdhva Mukha Vrksasana)

Handstand is a posture that, much like Forearm Stand, requires a deep sense of balance and counteraction rather than brute strength alone. If you endeavor to hold this pose without the assistance of a wall, your awareness of your core is the most important component. You do not want to succumb to the back-spine collapse that is seen in many handstands. Front body and back body must find an equilibrium, a deep and fundamental counteraction that supports uplift and buoyancy.

Don't forget that your upper extremity is an integrated part of that central core. The strength and stamina needed to engage this upper core independently from your lower body, building a solid base on which to lift and stack the legs, require a deep sense of slow engagement. This is the opposite of momentum. If you only ever teach yourself to leap up wildly to reach the wall, the shoulders and deep core will miss out on the opportunity to build strength at every position in the transition from forward fold to inversion. You will always need the wall to catch you.

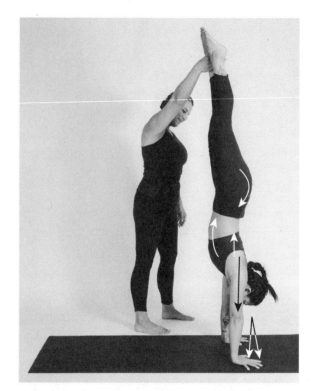

Allowing natural hand turnout makes more space in the shoulders to achieve this weight-bearing posture without crushing the soft tissues. Shoulder shrugging is also key to lifting the ribs toward the sky.

Be mindful as well that you have a much smaller "footprint" on which to build this pose. Your two hands are very compact compared to the full length of the forearm and hand in postures like Headstand and Forearm Stand. This means you'll need to engage your Hasta Bandha more fully and use the fingers' full length to assist in maintaining balance.

- Hands wide enough with appropriate turn-out; you need to be able to engage Hasta Bandha and not collapse into thumbs and wrists.

- Full flexion of arm at shoulder. If full flexion is not available in this pose, collapse in the back-spine is more likely.

- Soft elbows; no locking. For some people who lack upper body strength, a slight lock occurs in order to get up to Handstand, but once up, effort should be made to find a micro-bend in order to build up counteractive strength and stamina.

- External rotation of arms at the shoulder joint. You're reaching overhead!! This rule still applies, especially since you're bearing weight.

- Abduction of scapulae; this is the compound action needed to achieve full external rotation.

- Elevation of scapulae, necessary to prevent collapse in shoulder girdle. This is how you'll work to feel light in the shoulder joints.

- Retraction of scapulae; press the shoulder blades "through" the ribs.

- Uddiyana Bandha to stabilize against the retraction of the scapulae. The counteraction provides lift to the entire rib cage, lengthening the whole body, and helps you feel buoyant and integrated.

Planks and Arm Balances

Plank is the blueprint for pretty much all our hands-grounded poses, and it sets us up for Low Plank, which becomes the blueprint for all other arm balances. This means that establishing a powerfully supportive Plank will translate into strong arms and a solid connection to the central-core actions required to float and fly. Your Hasta Bandha is an integral building block of all these postures, and it should be emphasized repeatedly throughout every pose. Your wrists will work harder in these postures than anywhere else, so if your turn-out isn't appropriate and precise, then you're going to feel cramped and jammed pretty quickly. In hyperextension, which some of these postures require, it is very difficult to maintain Hasta Bandha, so it's important to build up your strength over time in more neutral poses like Plank and Low Plank, in order to be able to handle the more extreme extension of the other arm balances.

Plank (Phalakasana)

Since Plank is the blueprint for all our upper extremity weight-bearing postures, getting the hand placement dialed in properly is key. You need to make clear assessments of the natural width of your hands, making sure to accommodate the reality of your own personal carrying angles and torsions. In some bodies this may mean that the fingers point more out to the sides than straight ahead. Variation is vast in the arms, so taking the time to find your personal alignment, and then observing and adjusting your students', will make a huge impact on the strength and stability of all your weight-bearing poses.

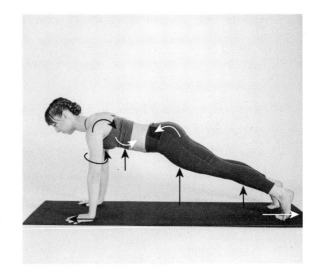

Keep in mind that the lower body will be very important in many of these postures, but for now we're leaving out the cues for that. See the Lower Extremity chapters for those actions.

- Hands wide enough with appropriate turnout.

- Shoulder joint aligned *behind* the crease of the wrist (avoiding hyperextension); doesn't need to be much. Consider a 95 degree bend in the wrist instead of a 90 degree crease.

- Hasta Bandha!! Press into middle/index knuckles; if this isn't possible, more turn-out may be needed, or there may be a strength differential in play. (Folks may need to earn this over time, learning to actively apply weight forward in the hand using muscles instead of just shifting forward.)

- Elbows point straight back (adduction + external rotation); this helps seat the scapulae on the ribs at neutral and align the head of the humerus safely in its socket.

- Neutral scapulae (abduction + adduction to stabilize); muscular counteraction in the upper back is needed to keep the scapulae in their neutral position; otherwise the chest is likely to take over and fully abduct them.

- Retraction of scapulae; similar to the prior step, serratus will need to contract to prevent protraction, but not overpower the adduction of the upper back between the shoulder blades (traps and rhomboids).

- Uddiyana Bandha!! This helps keep the ribs and spine aloft and prevent them from dropping into a collapsed backbend. This action is integral to maintaining a neutrally curved spine whenever we are prone.

Side Plank (Vasisthasana)

All the previous cues will be appropriate for the weight-bearing hand in Side Plank. Generally speaking, we want to keep a neutral spine in this posture, though there are variations that include an active side bend up and out of gravity. You'll see a cue at the very bottom that instructs how to integrate the upper extremity and the central core.

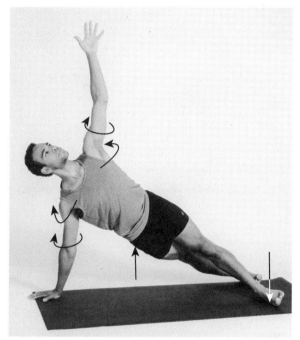
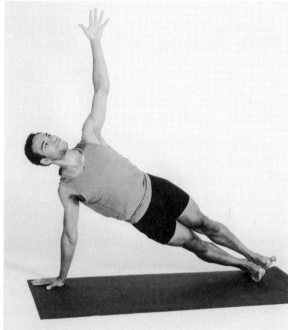

Bottom hand:

- Begin in Plank pose with your individual hand placement and turnout.

- Hand aligned just in front of shoulder (avoid wrist hyperextension); about 95 degree bend in the wrist.

- Hasta Bandha!! Press into middle- and index-finger knuckles to achieve slight lift in the center of palm. Ensure that the thumb remains light.

- Elbow points toward feet; do not lock out! Keep a slight bend in the joint and maintain muscular counteraction to stabilize.

- Slight abduction of scapula; press the earth away from you instead of sagging into the shoulder girdle. You should feel broad across the chest and lifted up off the ground.

- Retraction of scapula; the tendency is to protract and collapse into the chest. Wrapping elbow to point back toward thighs can help activate serratus in retraction.

- Uddiyana Bandha!! Ribs should press back into the shoulder blades, using this counteraction to feel lighter and more buoyant.

Top hand:

- Hand reaches up to sky actively (scapular abduction), aligned directly over center of heart. (Tendency to drop hand and arm back behind you with a collapsed shoulder girdle—avoid this!)

- External rotation of arm; biceps turning to face front wall to ensure plenty of bony space in the shoulder joint.

- Retraction of scapula; usually occurs naturally as you externally rotate the arm. Need to keep the shoulder blade anchored to the ribs.

- Slight internal rotation of forearm so hand faces side wall; counteraction keeps arm very active and straight, energetically lifting instead of falling into the ribs.

- Uddiyana Bandha!! Active solar plexus to prevent ribs blowing out.

- Slight horizontal abduction of the arm to stabilize between arm and solar plexus; press hand toward side wall while ribs pull back. Eliminates tendency to let hand fall behind you and completes the integration of upper extremity and central core. Creates extra length in spine and uplift off the base hand.

Low Plank (Chaturanga Dandasana)

This posture and its transitions account for more yoga-related injuries than you can imagine. There is a lot of precise geometry that accounts for a strong and stable Low Plank. We already covered the transition a bit earlier, describing the method for getting all your parts in place in order to remain strong and aloft. Here we'll assume you're already in the posture and describe all the active components needed to maintain healthy alignment in your shoulders—and hopefully prevent those injuries to the labrum and biceps tendon that are so ubiquitous here.

I highly recommend bringing knees to the ground for this pose, so you can gradually build up the strength in the upper back, belly, deltoids, triceps, and biceps that will be necessary to hold you up in the floating position. Many of us, whether we like to admit it or not, are simply not strong enough right out the gate to be able to achieve proper alignment throughout the movement. Many times it's not even a direct function of how strong you are, but it's a learning curve for recruiting the appropriate muscles in the correct order and timing. To avoid injury, modification is needed until that strength and proper recruitment are reached. I assure you, it will still be tough with your knees down. You will still need to work very hard. You are not in any way cheating by shortening the lower-body lever. You are simply doing the smartest thing for your tissues.

Be smart. I dare you.

- Hands wide enough with appropriate turn-out to take less weight directly into the thumb.

- Hasta Bandha!! It is far more difficult to achieve this action in this position, but your effort to press through the knuckles must be present to prevent collapse of the wrist.

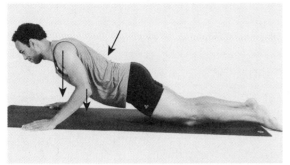
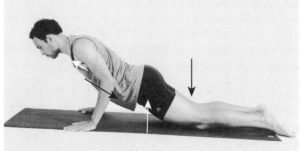
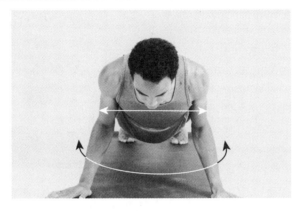

- Chest out in front of wrists (shift whole body forward prior to elbow flexion); active lengthening of sternum toward front wall throughout, neutral neck.

- Elbow directly over/behind wrist (no wrist hyperextension); forearm appears to stack over wrist and NOT over the hand.

- Elbow flexion larger than 90 degrees; in order to maintain the midrange of both biceps and triceps (one working primarily at shoulder, the other primarily at elbow), you should not bend the elbow beyond 90 degrees ... so why not err on the side of a little extra, just to make sure you're not overtaxing those tendons??

- Adduction of arms; elbows pull in toward ribs, just until the elbows point back, no need to squeeze the ribs completely. This helps keep the head of the humerus seated in the center of its socket and prevents some compound compensations.

- Equal abduction and adduction of scapulae; just like Plank, you need to achieve balanced counteraction in the chest and upper back to maintain neutrality in the shoulder blades.

- Uddiyana Bandha!! The solar plexus activates firmly to help lift the ribs up to meet the scapulae, creating more lightness and helping maintain a neutrally curved spine. No backbends!!

Crow/Crane (Bakasana)

After Low Plank, Crow or Crane pose is usually the next arm balance that yogis learn to execute. In a sense, it is a Cat pose balanced on the arms of Low Plank. Advanced versions of Crow have you straightening out the arms completely, but only attempt this after your core and shoulder girdle gain the acuity to help make the body feel lighter and offer more central uplift. Fundamentally, Crow pose is developed from your center; it is far less about muscling it out in the arms and more about finding the precise balance point on the hands, while using the shoulder girdle, central core, and pelvis to activate the rebounding effect off the ground.

As you move on to other arm balances, you'll find that there is always a sense of counteraction between the front and back channels, a sense of finding the actions of both Cat and Cow at the same time. Each form will find a slightly different equilibrium, but there always needs to be a deep lift of the solar plexus or you will definitely collapse.

One hazard in learning this pose is lifting the hips instead of the central core. There are many lower-body actions that contribute to this posture, and I'll note a couple at

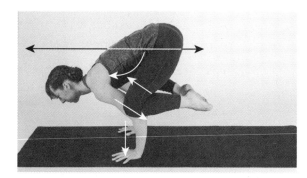

The goal is to get long and light, not to get the hips high in the air.

the end so you can feel how the lower, central, and upper core sections end up totally integrated in the flying family of arm balances. But, and this is very important, don't just lift the hips and wonder why your head feels so heavy. Lifting the hips only makes you front-load and leaves you top-heavy. The rising action must come from the ribs and belly if you intend to build into other, more extended arm balance postures.

- Hands wide enough with appropriate turn-out.

- Hasta Bandha!! This will be difficult to maintain, but don't let the thumb-side or wrist take the brunt of your weight; rebound through the entire palm is essential.

- Chest out in front of wrists (shift whole body forward prior to elbow flexion); if chest aligns between the hands, there is no hope of stacking your forearm upright and you will certainly collapse.

- Elbow directly over/behind wrist (no wrist hyperextension); you won't be able to fire those wrist flexors if you hyperextend, which leaves your tendons and ligaments to hold you up. If you do hyperextend, it's nearly impossible to rest into the balance point, and you won't have the energy to access the heart/chest required to integrate to the central core.

- Elbow flexion larger than 90 degrees (advanced version = straight arms). It's even more important here than in Low Plank; you can't allow the chest to drop below the elbows or you will face-plant for sure.

- Adduction of arms; downward forces will attempt to push the elbows out and you will fall down. You've gotta wrap those upper arms in toward the midline to maintain your foundational framework.

- Abduction of scapulae; Cat pose!! Press the ribs up between the shoulder blades, round the back body.

- Uddiyana Bandha!! Cat pose!! The belly needs to gather up the organs and lift the mid-low back.

- Mula Bandha!! The lower extremity works in a few ways:

  - Pada Bandha! Make sure feet are active even once they leave the floor. Dangling feet mean no energy feeding the root.

  - Shins press down actively on arms; slight extension action in the flexed knee, but not so much that hips lift higher than heart.

  - Adduction of thighs at hip joints; squeezing the thighs into the midline creates lift and stability in the lower body, while contributing to the Mula Bandha.

  - Flexion in hips; this translates to added lift in the low back.

  - Contraction of rectus abdominis; this is one place you really do want to pull your pubic bone toward your sternum to assist in the Cat-flexion of the spine, and to amp up the connection between Mula Bandha and Uddiyana Bandha.

Practice Teaching
Adjustments

As discussed throughout the manual, the existence of individual differences in the upper extremity means we are certain to need to make many personal adjustments. That said, there are many ubiquitous cues that we already know we need to throw out and replace with more relevant instruction. Perhaps more in the upper extremity than anywhere else, we will need to change up our words and make more hands-on adjustments, if for no other reason than people are perplexed by the definite contradictions we are making with respect to their former training.

Take care to acknowledge that some of these cues are new, that they are an evolution in how we think about the tissues of the body, and that they are in agreement with our internal engineering. Also be prepared for some active resistance. It is not your job to change the minds and bodies of every student before you, but it is your responsibility to present the most accurate and relevant information to them so they can make better decisions in their practice. Tell them that they are tailoring their practice to their own actual body, drawing a new blueprint that is individual to their frame and their appropriate alignment. That is how you can stand strong in your integrity.

Reaching

When reaching out or overhead, our highest regard must be for the soft tissues of the shoulder joint. Because so many students have heard repeatedly to pull their shoulders down, you have a big hurdle to leap in retraining them to make space. Begin by offering the external rotation. You'll want to mime this repeatedly yourself.

When reaching out to the sides, even when just coming up to shoulder-height, that rotation is imperative:

> "Make sure hands rotate open to the side walls. As you reach out, biceps need to face the sky, regardless of what the hands end up doing."

Then you'll likely need to offer hands-on instruction to some individuals. For most people, a light touch is effective and offers a tactile cue to move in association with the words "external rotation."

With one hand on the arm and the other on the scapula, use a light touch to show how external rotation brings the biceps away from

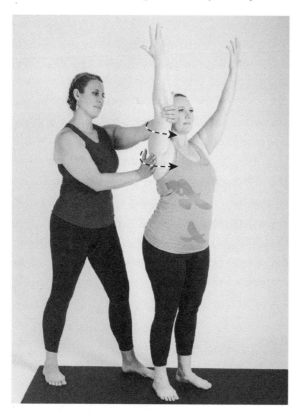

the face (when overhead). The scapular hand can help guide the adduction that is necessary in the shoulder girdle as the compound action to external rotation.

> "See how this rotation pulls the shoulder blade around the ribs? It kind of hollows out the armpit a bit. This is very important to the health of the shoulder tissues and will help seat the scapulae at their optimal height. It's really important to reinforce this movement here in upward reaching, so that we are familiar with it once we start weight bearing in Downward Facing Dog."

In this way you can bring attention to the fact that this is not an arbitrary stylistic choice but one rooted in the safe alignment principles you are trying to ingrain. This is particularly true when eliminating the "draw down" cue. So many students are going to do this without being told because it is already habituated. You'll need to verbally encourage over-shrugging the shoulders, you'll need to explain that it's safe, you'll need to prove it by showing them in their own body. You'll need to go into some detail at times as to why this cue is being replaced ... you may need to ask them to feel the difference in the two versions, paying deliberate attention to the shoulder joint itself. Once you show them this and give them permission, maybe even insist at first that they try it, realization will dawn.

For some, you'll need to give them time to make the change. For others, they may simply insist that they know better than you. In this case, I suggest backing off and focusing instead on those in the room who are receptive to your guidance—they are your actual students, and your attention will be much more appreciated there.

Downward Facing Dog

Since Down Dog is so ubiquitous and places gravitational force on those overhead arms, we need to be clear about this rotational adjustment. For most folks, rotation will be very difficult with hard or locked elbows. First, a softening of the elbows, perhaps a soft thumb in the "eye" of the elbow to encourage a bend. Then, using that soft touch, guide the elbows to point back instead of outward. Trace your fingers over the scapulae to show how they will widen and shrug slightly. Lastly, a light touch at the solar plexus or front ribs to encourage the lifting of the ribs up into the space created by the spreading shoulder blades.

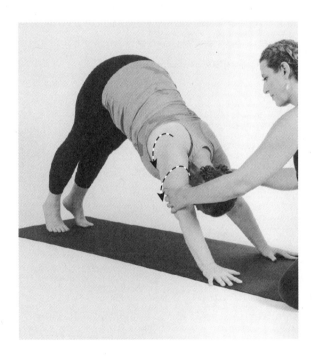

Weight Bearing

Weight-bearing postures are everywhere, and most people aren't doing them right for their personal bony frame. My own adjustments once the hands are on the ground consist of pointing and miming, since it's tough to pick up someone else's hand when they have it rooted to the floor. Again, it will be helpful to offer the entire class a general instruction to get their hands wider than they are, then offer more personal alignment suggestions.

Carrying Angles

It's likely that your students are unaware of their carrying angles, and they have been told to align their hands under their shoulders since they first stepped on the mat. In fact, many teacher trainings explicitly instruct this alignment, so this is not going to be an easy habit to break, but it's an important one. This is perhaps the one cue I give most consistently over time, repeating it to the same students for years ... "make sure your hands are wide enough." Your students will find more strength and stability when their bones land where they're built to go. This is our opportunity to help them tune in to the shape of their own body and become more aware of how they are built to move. Keep in mind that the health of the shoulder and wrist are our priority, so even if postures end up looking vastly different than a *Yoga Journal* photo, as long as you can see healthy positioning of the GH and the wrist crease, you're on the right track.

I always give the general cues to the entire class, including steps to find their shoulders behind the wrist, then encourage each person who needs it to take a turn-out or even wider stance than they have. Consider all the ways that you can approach individual or hands-on adjustments—using their name, pointing to where you want them to go, miming the turn-out motion, etc. You can also show them how wide their elbows need to be and see where the hands land from there.

Have the whole class look at their carrying angles. Sitting back on their heels (Rock pose) with arms reaching out in front of them:

> "Reach toward front wall. Now align your elbow directly in front of the shoulder joint. Acknowledge that the shoulder joint is just outside the crease of the armpit."

You'll very likely need to go around and make tactile adjustments here. It's admittedly a little tough to see our own width in a realistic way; there are some optical illusions at play here.

> "Now notice your hands. Are they wider than your elbows? Probably. If yours are not wider, well, you're the odd one out! This carrying angle is a natural part of our design, and to ignore it is to build all of our weight-bearing postures on a faulty foundation."

Once aligned, you maybe offer a moment to compare and contrast to their neighbors. I wouldn't do this in every class, but you can choose one class every so often where this particular trait is highlighted. Remind them that keeping their wrists and shoulders healthy will help them continue to practice for decades to come.

> "Hinge at your hips and bring your hands to the ground exactly as they are. Resist the urge to bring them toward midline, don't worry if they land wider than your mat. Yoga mats aren't wide enough for most people. It's likely that some of us will only have the index and middle fingers directly on the mat, and that's okay, since that's where we want to bear most of our weight."

Make gestures directly in front of students who have come back in toward midline, encouraging them to challenge the edge of the mat. Make it personal.

Don't be surprised if a student who has a profound carrying angle needs to turn out their hands to a great degree in order to achieve their optimal Hasta Bandha activation. I've seen students who, based on the shape of their bones and the healthiest alignment for their shoulders, end up with their fingers pointing nearly straight out to the sides. It seems crazy, but when you consider that the health of the shoulder and wrist joints is our highest priority, then you just follow what the bones tell you. It always pays to question the extremes of alignment, but be open to the idea that sometimes the extremes may be appropriate for a particular individual.

Hasta Bandha

For many students, their hand turn-out is fundamental to their ability to activate a healthy Hasta Bandha. They will need to find the softened elbows pointing back first, then assess how the hand has responded to that rotational force. Getting the index- and middle-finger knuckles to press down evenly is the key to achieving appropriate counteraction through the arm and forearm. If you can't root down there, you won't be able to fully access the upper extremity/core integration.

Adjustments here are subtle and, besides miming the turn-out action, are mostly intended to reinforce the anchor of the knuckles and lightness of the wrist.

Make sure that the hands are wide enough. Then instruct the turn-out, miming as needed. You may mention specifically that their fingers may not point forward at all, and that it's fine. It's more than fine. Why should their fingers point forward? Who says? What good does it do? If they don't have an answer, well, they're more likely to listen to you and try a new way!

"Notice that once you rotate the hand outward, you can root with more ease through the knuckles and less in the wrist. It will take some time to adjust to this, and more time to build the strength needed to make the wrist feel truly light, but at least now you can begin to access this strength."

Once they make the adjustment, press down gently on those root knuckles. This tactile cue reinforces the place you are referring to so they can feel it. This will make it a little easier to activate it once they really start working.

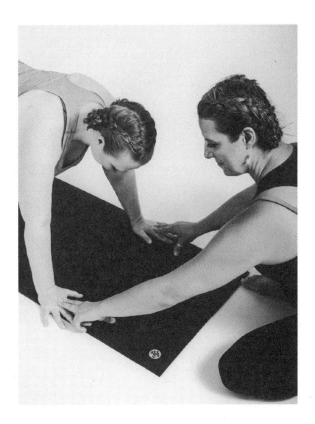

Since this alignment and action serve to make the link between the earth and the heart, it can be very helpful to cue the connection; describe the work of both the arm (in its counteractive rotations) with the counteractions of the shoulder blades (adducting and abducting to stabilize on the ribs) and the active lifting of the solar plexus and Uddiyana Bandha. Often students aren't aware of these integrations until you point them out ... even if they are actively engaging them.

Binds

Most of my adjustments in binds are done verbally instead of hands-on, because of the tender nature of the shoulder joint and the relatively pervasive condition of very stuck shoulder blades. To force these parts to move in any direction risks some serious injury to the shoulder joint tissues, and frankly, no one needs extra risk associated with this area.

There is one exception, and that is in a simple bind in extension. For postures such as Jackrabbit (Sasangasana) or the "C" position in Wide-Legged Forward Fold, students are likely to need some extra instruction in the shrug + protraction maneuver. They have been told for ages to pull the shoulders down and together in this move, so even though our version will help them achieve deeper and safer movement overall, they are likely to ignore the cue in favor of forcing movement into the shoulder joint.

First, it can be helpful to ease them out of their current level of extension with a soft hand on their bound fingers. Then ask them to shrug the scapulae toward their ears just a bit. Then instruct the pressing of the "tips" of the shoulders forward toward the ground or the heart (depending on the pose they're in).

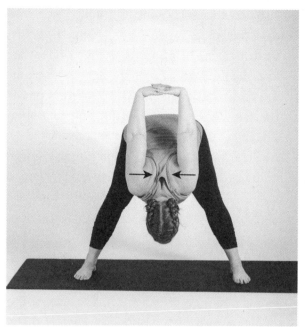
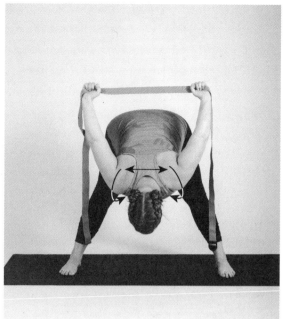

The strap allows Ka Shawna ample space in the posterior shoulder to find more movement. Otherwise, the joints get jammed up on the back side.

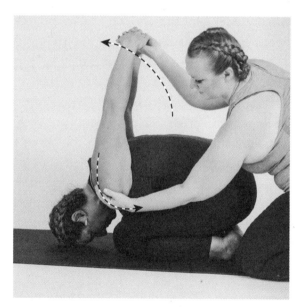

Encourage movement to originate at the shoulder girdle, not just cranking the hands higher.

I use soft touch and tracing motions on their shoulder blades to encourage these motions. Sometimes I'll place hands on so my thumbs rest on their shoulder blades while my fingers reach under to the collarbones or around the lateral edges of the scapulae and create the subtle rocking action that is protraction. I will often comment on the space and/or resistance between the collarbones and ribs that this motion will cause, and what a great achievement that space is!!

Verbal reinforcement of these altered alignments is key to long-term adoption. When students can feel the difference between two versions, and they are given permission to do what feels more natural, they are more likely to keep it up. They will begin to hear your voice in their head, even when other teachers offer more-traditional options.

The most difficult part of relearning how to cue and adjust binds is that we have to consider and articulate the compound actions that the shoulder girdle and shoulder joint require for healthy functioning. It's hard to straight-up memorize those things, unless that's your superpower—in which case, please, be my guest—but it does make sense when you feel it in your body. What is the natural progression of the shoulder blade when internally or externally rotating the arm? Do it, feel it, then instruct it.

Modifications

Modifications take many forms and may be needed for a number of reasons. As students arrive to class, they come through the door with a lifetime of impacts on their body. In the upper extremity these may be as simple and common as a lack of strength. In many cases the neck, shoulder, or wrist may have suffered an injury that limits range of motion, strength, or contractility. Since most folks aren't using their body correctly in life, and in yoga are asked to do some pretty crazy things we aren't designed to do, I am perhaps a bit more conservative in my teaching of the upper extremity. I try to instruct hard work but allow for more breaks. I am even more aware of misalignments and pretty emphatic about props. Blocks for standing postures, straps for binding poses. More space will usually equal more safe movement.

Bear in mind that some folks will try to push through pain because they think they are just weak, or that it's supposed to feel crummy until they do it enough times. Other students will back off at the slightest impression of discomfort. It is our job to try to tease out who is who and encourage their internal conversation to figure out whether they are experiencing the discomfort of growth or the pain of injury. We need to teach endurance where it is appropriate but also know how to modify postures to keep these tender bits safe and healthy.

This is not always a clear-cut situation. We need to ask specific questions and be able to make some interpretations without trying to make diagnoses. Remember, it is always okay to acknowledge that you aren't a physician, and that your student would be smart to have their condition assessed by a medical professional. Armed with proper diagnoses, you'll be able to offer more tailored adjustments and modifications.

Shoulder Injuries and Conditions

Keep in mind that many people, especially women, lack strength in their upper body. They need to do work in these muscles to change that, but we need to design work that is safe for them and not push them to overdo it. Too much too soon will lead to strain, and that's not good. Considering this, oftentimes we need to modify how much weight is being borne, which means a modification of the lower body instead of the arms. Assuming that you've already gotten them into their best alignment, they'll just need to bring knees to the ground for better leverage until they build up their acuity between the upper, central, and lower bodies.

Neck and Shoulder Girdle Spasticity or Tension

For most students who feel pain or tension in the shoulder/neck area, it is a condition of those muscles being overstretched ... the shoulders and arms hanging heavy in gravity, leaving the traps et al. to just hang on for dear life. They lack good circulation through this region and therefore need to contract these muscles. They need strength and blood flow and movement of the fascia—not stretching.

So instead of doing movements that drop the scapulae and laterally flexing the neck (as may be advised in a more traditional yoga class), we will instruct our students to reach out and overhead. We will insist that they practice shrugging their shoulders. We will challenge those muscles to hold the shoulder girdle up in gravity and get them toned up again over time.

So this is a generalized modification for your sequencing: Anyone who says "my neck and shoulder are super tight from sitting at a computer, reaching for a steering wheel, stooped over a kitchen counter, etc." is actually asking you to include really active Upward Facing Hands (Urdhva Hastasana), Chair (Utkatasana), Plank, and Down Dog. They need to work those shoulders, so you're gonna give them the opportunity, and you're gonna teach them how to do it all with integrity and great alignment.

Nerve Compression and Thoracic Outlet Syndrome

Make sure your student has a solid diagnosis for these conditions before making any assumptions. If they feel nervy sensations, it's possible that muscle spasm, not a bony impingement, is the culprit. If they are experiencing shooting pain up or down the neck or arm, they probably ought not to be in class that day.

If, however, they have a diagnosis for either of these conditions, freeing up the shoulder girdle will always be good medicine. As earlier, they need to contract their upper shoulders,

they need to lift the collarbones off the ribs, they likely need to open their chest and rotator cuffs and strengthen the upper back. They DO NOT need to stretch their neck. If they stretch spastic muscles that are stuck to the neurofascia, they will just irritate the nerve root more.

So again, encourage lifting, reaching, extending, and simple binding in the arms and shoulders.

Labrum/Rotator Cuff

Most times a "rotator cuff tear" is the official diagnosis given to a patient. Unfortunately, this reference is pretty vague. Ask the following questions:

- Did you get imaging? (MRI is the only way to be totally definitive.)

- Did they say whether it was a labrum tear or mention the word "slap"? (A SLAP tear is a specific diagnosis for a kind of labrum injury.)

- Did they tell you if there was a muscle strain? (Since the rotator cuff is really a set of muscles in our definition, it's important to tell whether their injury is a muscle or tendon injury there.)

- Did they talk about their biceps tendon? (Since this tendon is often knitted into or through the labrum, this could be a big deal. It's also possible that they have an isolated biceps strain [stretch or tear].)

Having a clearer idea about what is really going on in the very complicated shoulder system may inform how you modify. The following are some modification guidelines when reaching:

- When reaching, overly emphasize the external rotation to ensure maximum room for the squishy bits.

- Shrugging is imperative, as is a bit of scapular abduction.

- They may not bring their arms all the way up to shoulder height when reaching out to the sides.

- A deep bend in the elbows when reaching out to sides will offer slack in the fascia and will adjust the leverage so the shoulder doesn't have to work as hard.

- When flexing at the shoulder, arms need not go all the way overhead in line with the ears. Some will be fine with arms just in front of the face, while others will need to keep arms out in front of them, just below shoulder height.

Weight bearing presents some additional issues with rotator cuff injuries, because we're not really built to do that under the best circumstances. This is one area where I really try to not push them hard. Grinding, pinching, shooting, popping, and snapping are all NOT GOOD in these tissues. With or without pain, these are indications that more damage is likely, so I would advise they opt out completely until they can mitigate the signs through more specific therapies.

That said, here are some modifications that can offer some relief if they really want to go for it.

- Some people will feel more stable on their elbows in weight-bearing postures, because it changes the arm-lever and their shoulder/arm rotation is a bit more fixed.

- Even on the elbows, students may not feel stable in full flexion, so they may do postures like Downward Facing Dog with shoulders stacked over or just behind the elbows, instead of arms alongside the ears.

- In Side Plank, if they can do it at all, these students need to pay extra attention to keeping the scapula retracted; rotating the elbow to point back toward thighs will achieve external rotation in the shoulder joint and encourage that scapular stabilization.

Arm-Length Differences

If you observe students with profound arm-length differences, you may need to stagger their hands on the mat a bit, especially for postures like Downward Facing Dog. I myself need to do this. If I don't, my spine compensates and I end up in a side bend; my hips go all off-kilter, and a funky rotational compensation presents in my ribs. It's also very difficult for me to access my deep core effectively, leaving me to collapse a bit through my chest. If I slide my short-side hand back just a bit, all of those misalignments resolve themselves.

This is mostly true for those with bony differences, not functional ones. If, however, a student has significant scapular adhesion or shoulder joint soft tissue restrictions, and it's obvious that repetitive actions are not going to improve this situation, staggering of their hands may be warranted.

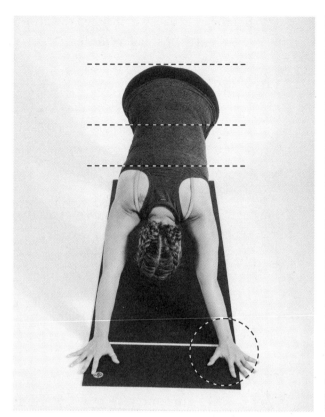
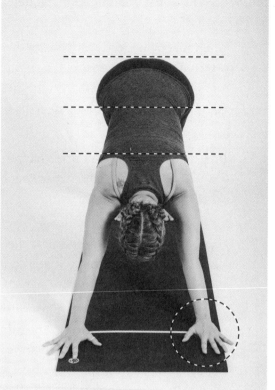

Because Richelle has one arm that's significantly shorter than the other, if her hands are on the same line her whole body is thrown off-center. By adjusting her hand back, her shoulders, hips, and spine no longer compensate.

Wrist Injuries

For those who come to class with wrist conditions or limitations, make sure to offer extra props like wedges, extra padding, blankets, hand weights, etc. Sometimes just extra padding helps, so folding the front edge of their mat, or adding layers under their mat, is sufficient. Some other folks need to significantly change the wrist angle, so wedges will offer the best results. For those with chronic issues in the hands and wrists, insist that they keep knees on the ground, reducing the total weight-bearing and giving them more direct access to the lower body connections and contractions. This will take some burden off the hands.

Some conditions may be aided by using fists instead of flat palms, but this is not a fix-all. If the wrists are weak, this isn't likely to be a much more supportive feeling. Also, the knuckles themselves will want extra padding, like a double mat layer. Using fists also requires some transition from Table/Plank to Downward Facing Dog. You can't use your fists for this pose—you need to transition to flat palms or forearms instead.

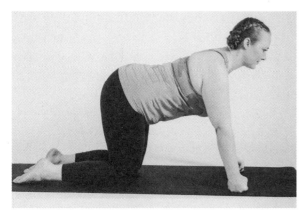

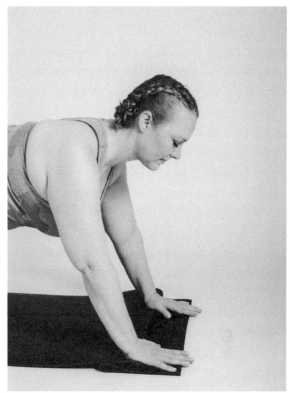

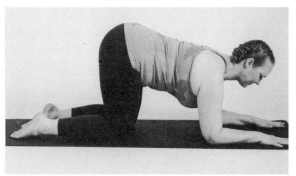

Tendinitis

Since tendinitis is the inflammation of tendons, and many tendons travel through the wrist, most flare-ups are going to be initiated by the stretching, the contracting, and the direct pressure on those tissues in weight-bearing postures. Therefore, it's important that you be clear with your students that if this is their diagnosis, it is in their best interest to REALLY rest their parts. They can still engage in a yoga practice, but they should mindfully opt out of the weight-bearing postures.

This is an instance when taking it down to the elbows is appropriate. Fists are an option, but because those tendons still have to work to stabilize the wrist, it can be irritating. Provide extra padding for their knuckles if they choose this option, and remind them that their transitions are likely to feel clunky ... they'll need to maintain their core stability as they move from fists to elbows in vinyasa, so they don't inadvertently tweak their low back or SI through compensatory movements.

Carpal Tunnel Syndrome

It's important to note that people with an existing carpal tunnel dysfunction diagnosis have a whole set of issues that need to be addressed at the individual level. I am usually a proponent of using the hands as properly as possible to help build strength over time, and in some mild cases this might actually help alleviate some of the symptoms. But if the carpal tunnel has already fully collapsed, if there is already significant nerve damage, or if there is a profound lack of strength/circulation, then there is an unmitigated need for props or alignment that help take the pressure off the wrist.

Fists are an option for Cat/Cow or Plank/Low Plank but are not ideal for Downward Facing Dog or Upward Facing Dog. Wedges or folded mats under the wrist can relieve some pressure for these postures. If you have a client with severe carpal tunnel syndrome, it may be best to find them some dumbbell blocks. The gripping action may not work for everyone, but it can be a major help to those for whom it does work.

If a student has a diagnosis of carpal tunnel syndrome, it may be relevant to ask the following:

- Have you had surgery on the affected hand?

- Do you know if the condition was due to a bony collapse or to overly inflamed tendons with not enough space through the canal?

- Are there any clearly aggravating actions you've identified?

While you cannot make any diagnoses yourself, it can be helpful to know these things so you can provide better or more appropriate modifications. If they have already had surgery, building strength may be their best approach, but wedges may be needed at first. If there is bony collapse, they need strength but also extra padding to cushion the soft tissues that they can't lift completely with Hasta Bandha. Any actions that currently aggravate their symptoms may give you specific insights to whether or not they should bear weight at all.

Experiential Learning

When you teach postures of the upper extremity, it's important to be very clear about small movements. Both in reaching and in binds, relating the complementary movements of the arm and shoulder blade is very important. Most students haven't heard these cues in this context. As we know, it's likely they've heard the exact opposite. It's now our job to slowly unwind those old beliefs and behaviors, so take your time, use your words, and don't be shy about explaining how and why these changes are needed.

Practice teaching the basics: Upward Facing Hands, Plank, Simple Bind. Consider the gross movement of the arm, the supporting action of the scapulae, the fine-tuning of the forearms and hands. If you practice covering these repeatedly, you'll be prepared for most other postures.

For Teachers

Practice observing the energetic lines from the ground, up the arms, and into the core-body. Consider making adjustments for individual differences in carrying angle and muscle tone. Consider offering modifications for strength and core integration, like dropping the knees. Pay close attention to how these changes affect the way energy flows from one point to another. How does the heart change? How do the neck and head change? Do these adjustments make for a more integrated posture? If so, make sure to say these things out loud to help encourage your students to be thoughtful about these changes for future practices.

For Students

This is a distinct opportunity to learn things about your own body and alignment that may have been mysteries before. While your work here is definitely about helping your peers learn how to use their voice and knowledge effectively, this may offer some distinct take-aways for you personally. Do exactly as you are told, but also communicate what you feel along the way. Do you notice more power from Hasta Bandha? Have you turned too far out with the hands? Do you have your own strengthening work to do in your forearm flexors? Are there differences in your abdominal core as you make these upper body adjustments? Share these experiences in real time with your student-teacher. Both of you can benefit from this experience of give and take.

Once you have taught the most basic postures for the upper extremity, and repeated them enough to feel comfortable with the primary cues, you can expand to teaching transitions. I think the movements of the basic vinyasa are next in line, as these are so ubiquitous in the current culture. Shifting from Plank to Down Dog, and then to Up Dog and back to Down Dog—focusing on the actions of the arm and shoulder girdle specifically—will help you develop the skills over time to teach fluidly in class, without having to overthink the process.

13

Unifying the Practice

Now that you've come to the final chapter, I ask you to look back at your former perspectives on alignment, personal practice, risk, and mitigation. How has the experience of the Yoga Engineer changed those? Have you been compelled to work in a different way?

I also ask you to reflect on how observing and experiencing your asana practice in this precise manner has affected the other limbs of your yoga practice. Are there tools that you have gained through the process that can be applied to the study of the deeper layers of your body and life?

Asana is practiced, in part, to teach you how to observe, to become a witness to both your outer and inner worlds. It is not an escape from the harried daily activities and pressures, it is the opposite: the path into truly experiencing those activities and examining what creates the pressure. Yoga practice asks us to look at the frightening, feel the discomfort, hold the bitterness on our tongue, all to determine a way to actively make change and find a

path through. If escape is your plan, then you are doing it wrong.

That is not to say that all practice must be uncomfortable, but when it is, we must be willing and able to enter into the internal conversation of why there is discomfort. "Is this the discomfort of growth or the pain of injury?" "Am I feeling a physical resistance or a psycho-emotional one?" "Why do I feel panicky in this position and at ease in another, similar one?" These are some of the questions that our yoga practice trains us to ask in order that we may become more self-aware off the mat as well.

My intention in teaching you the Yoga Engineering principles of asana practice is to provide a looking glass into your first layer of physical practice. It insists that you apply Ahimsa, the first Yama, to the world—outside yourself and within. By observing yourself as a sacred body, and endeavoring to protect it from harm while also asking it to work hard on your own behalf, you are abiding in a way that propels an intention of non-harming into the world with better, more informed context.

Though *The Yoga Engineer's Manual* focuses on the physical body, it provides a roadmap of sorts. The practice of becoming more aware of your placement, more studied in your movement, builds the internal tools necessary to turn your gaze deeper, to apply those observation skills to your breath, to your thought, to your emotion, and ultimately to how and why you respond to those things in the manner you do. You cannot ever change something you do not know is there. The *Manual* provides tools to become more interested in the minutiae, to begin to question old paradigms and develop more informed views. Your asana practice occurs on your mat, but the effects of this approach move with you into your daily life.

In this modern world, it can be difficult to reconcile our needs with our wants, our privilege with others' suffering. Our yoga practice gives us a path to growing into better, more observant, and compassionate people. But we must still do the work. The tapas is real—it burns through the haze of our wrong-thinking and brightens our perspective with Truth—but only through the struggle can we find a rhythm. It does not just happen; it is called "Practice" for a reason.

Thank you for opening this book, for walking down this path. Thank you for your curiosity and your willingness to question, your pursuit of growth. I appreciate you for all those reasons and more. *The Yoga Engineer's Manual* is a study in changing perspective and changing action, my own included. The yoga practice breeds curiosity, and my own curiosity is only more piqued by the process of writing this book. I hope that yours is by reading it.

When we are curious about the nature of anything, we seek out new voices, new resources to inform us in one direction or another, and that process breeds more questioning. I love that! I hope that as time goes on, your curiosity leads you down unknown paths of discovery, that you realize interests you didn't know were there, that you continue to question and ponder and relate to the world in new ways. It's my intention to do the same.

This book is a compendium of decades of observation, practice, study, questioning, more practice, and an ever-evolving view. This will continue in my own practice, and I look forward to sharing with you the fruits of those labors. Since our practice is a living thing, changing over time, I hope that you'll keep me informed of your progress and your questing. This book is the beginning of a conversation, not just an instruction manual. YogaEngineer.com will continue to evolve to offer you the answers you seek. I'll be adding video and visual references from the book, as well as some discussion videos to the Readers' Access page as time goes on, so check back often. There are podcast episodes and full-class videos already up and running for the public, so avail yourself of those and let us know what you think.

Until we meet again, I pray that we may all walk with the intentions of Clarity, Compassion, Grace, and Devotion.

Namaste.

Artwork Attributions

All original artwork provided by commission. The remainder of the illustrations are public-domain images from *Anatomy of the Human Body* (Henry Vandyke Carter and Henry Gray, 1918) and *Atlas and Text-Book of Human Anatomy* (Johannes Sobotta, 1914). Digital editing and annotating to remove outmoded labels and add those relevant to the current content were done by Kathryn Stevens and the author.

Illustrations on the following pages are original works by Rachel Schneider with digital annotation by Kathryn Stevens and the author: 14, 15, 25, 27 (lower image), 28, 29, 32, 33, 35, 38, 62, 78, 159, and 162. Copyrights reserved.

All photography is the original work of Kathryn Stevens. Editing, labeling, and annotations were completed by Kathryn Stevens and the author. Copyrights reserved.

Models for this book are Javan Mngrezzo, Elena Cheung, Jessica McCarthy, Ka Shawna Bell, and the author. The ladies are all wearing signature styles from Oiselle, and Javan is outfitted in prAna.

Contributors

KATHRYN STEVENS

Kathryn Denelle Stevens contributed her talents as a photographer to this book. When Kathryn isn't photographing (mostly) people, she is thinking about how to remain IN her body ... she has been practicing specific embodiment practices for two+ decades, with names like yoga, meditation, Qi Gong being given to all these practices. Kathryn is a newly trained yoga teacher who is building skills around teaching various embodiment techniques from her home in Portland, Oregon. Her embodiment practice fuels her creative endeavors and vice versa. It's all cyclical, and Kathryn enjoys watching the illumination dance play out before her, as she braids her way among the vines and weeds of life ... She also makes a mean margarita. Please reach out to see about how to connect!

hello@kathryndenellestevens.com
IG: kathryndenellestevens
kathryndenellestevens.com

RACHEL SCHNEIDER

Rachel Schneider drew the illustrations for this book. She is a painter/illustrator/mixed media artist currently residing in Albuquerque, New Mexico, with her partner Matt and her cat Oscar. Rachel has a BFA in painting and drawing from the Pacific Northwest College of Art in Portland, Oregon.

SALLY BERGESEN

Sally Bergesen is the reason the models in this book are wearing clothes. She is the owner and founder of Oiselle, a Seattle-based women's athletic apparel company (www.oiselle.com/pages/our-story). Sally is a marketing genius, a social activist, a dance fiend, and a total badass who has the most amazing laugh. Her company provided the women's wardrobe for the book's photos, but she has been outfitting Richelle for teaching yoga and living life since 2015.

Acknowledgments

This list is far from complete. I am a person who collects people—friends, colleagues, neighbors—and they become family pretty quickly. There aren't enough pages to include all the people who have helped make me the woman I am, or have helped me do the things I am able to do. I take nothing for granted (or at least I try not to) and am grateful each day for this astounding life I get to live. I marvel at my privilege and the grace I've been granted. If I have been in class with you, or worked with you, or had you on my table; if I have shared coffee or cocktails and talked about books or breathing or Spirit or food; if you are my family or my friend; if you are not mentioned below specifically, you are still acknowledged by me here. I would not be writing these words if not for your love, support, laughter, tears, heavy-lifting, spell-binding, and hugs. Thank you for being a part of me.

These are in no particular order ... except for one!

JAMES

First and foremost, it would not have been possible to undertake the actual writing of this book without the motivation and the opportunity of Time afforded to me by my best friend and Partner For Life, James Stevens. You trusted my passion and my knowledge. You trusted me to sit and do the work. You trusted that I would be able to create something worthwhile while you went to a job each day. You trusted that I had something to say, and maybe even something to believe in. For you, I am grateful. For your trust in me, I am grateful. For your motivating spirit and your leading by example, I am grateful. It is an honor and a privilege to be loved and supported by you, you remarkable human being. I am a writer because you knew I could be and convinced me of the same. All the way(s).

THE DONORS

To the students and fans and bandwagoners who trusted this project enough to front some money so I could commission and compile the artwork: I could not have done this without you. Through your support of the GoFundMe campaign, you made it possible to meet my deadlines (one of them, anyway) and honor the work of some remarkable artists at the same time. Your generosity of spirit and support for this book has humbled me to the core. Some of you are students of mine, some of you have trusted the rumor that this book would be a thing for years, some of you have never even met me, but trust your friends who have. Each of you is a gift to me in this life and beyond: Richard and Patti Ricard, Helen McConkey, Gina Colorossi, Syrinda Sharpe, Randi Riesenberg, Clare McCahill, Shari Larsen, Rosa Mercer, John Sindelar and Kristi Coulter, Emily Crocker, Raina Rose, Robyn Brezinski, Ciara Tice, Janelle O'Bannon, Amy Gaskill, James Stevens, Lizzie Van Brocklin, Sara Proctor, Debra Del Castillo, Sarah Akhtar, Katie Chatwood, Elena Cheung, Rachel Stern, Ka Shawna Bell, Karlyn Nourse, Chris Eddy, Jolynn Jensen, Stephanie Martin, Suzanne Smith, Pat McCotter, Jeni Martinez, Erin Taylor, Jenni O'Brien, Jennifer Kuduk, Amanda Mitchell-Norrgard, Thao Ly Snider, Chelsea Hanson, Candice Morrow, Megan Gallant, Kim Tull-Esterbrook, Claudine Pedersen, Brittany Paris, Kristen Larsen, Mark Butler, Lori Snow, Grace Parker, Ali Clark, Lynn Long, Diana Viney, and Stu McDonald.

JENNIFER + FRAN + CATHERINE + LIZ

If not for these women, my yoga practice would have been a different beast. You are my first teachers, my deepest teachers. You helped me find my feet on the mat and my voice in front of class. Your guidance initiated me into the dance, the flow, the beat, the seat, and the challenges of the evolving culture of practicing and teaching yoga. I have been equally humbled and inspired by you. You have trusted me to step into the realm of "peer" and I still am not sure I live up to it well enough. I will spend my whole life working toward that. To you, I bow: Jennifer Isaacson, Fran Kao, Catherine Munro, and Liz Doyle.

RACHEL + SUSAN

When I arrived in a yoga classroom in Vancouver, BC, I was very new at teaching teachers-to-be,

and totally overwrought to have to teach to some professionals who had been doing this much longer than I. I needn't have feared, though, because these two women embraced me and my anatomical perspectives from the get-go and proved to be some of my most powerful allies along this path. Thank you, ladies, for being my friends first, my colleagues next, and my advocates always. I am grateful to have you in my life, even when far away. Please know what an inspiration you have both been, and continue to be, as I move into new realms of this profession.

PAULA + KIRK

When I was only twenty years old, I stepped into my massage therapy training and into my future. I said out loud, "I wanna be like Paula when I grow up ... especially that gray hair." My most beloved teachers, Paula Pelletier-Butler and Kirk Butler helped set me firmly in the seat of anatomist and physiologist, as well as healer. With their tutelage, I had the confidence to begin teaching with an authentic voice. Their support in my early career was unparalleled. Thank you both for being such an integral part of my evolution from student to practitioner to teacher. You are and will always be family to me. I have the gray hair, but I'm not sure I'll ever be quite as Magical as you!

WANYE + LIS + ALISON + KEITH + TRISHA + MATTHEW + EMMA

If it were not for my generous clients Wayne and Lisbeth, this particular relationship with North Atlantic Books may not have manifested as it has. Thank you both for your trust in me and this message, and for stepping into the role of magic-makers and getting my proposal into

Alison Knowles's hands. I am still in wonder at the way this opportunity was bestowed upon me through you two. Thank you, Alison, for believing in my project and going to bat for me over and over. I hope the final project lives up to our hopes. To Keith, who has kept my spirits up when things were hardest, and who held my hand through the circuitous process of publishing for the first time, my deep and abiding gratitude. Your respect for this project and for my process is wondrous—and for someone who didn't know me already, your ability to know just what to say to talk me off the ledge is profound. Trisha, you helped me recognize that I really am an author and that this complex book is worth the efforts. Thank you for trusting my gut alongside me and allowing the space for improvements even when it got complicated. Matthew, this is a much better book because you are absolutely brilliant at doing what you do. To Emma and the whole design team: you move mountains. I appreciate you turning that remarkable mass of data into such a stunning presentation.

THE SCHOOLS + JEAN + JULIE + JENI + KAREN + SUZY + BETH + SALLY G + RACHEL + COMMUNITY

When I started teaching weekly yoga classes, I was on my own for a while, renting space from Soma Yoga and Dance, an independent home for teachers who didn't work so well into the mainstream fabric—Jean Hindle still owns this sweet space, and I am eternally grateful for the beginning I was offered there, the place where I could develop my voice and my passion, my style and direction. I did find a home in established studios later, and through various teacher trainings I found a new voice—Yoga Works and Semperviva in Seattle and Vancouver—thank you for the chance to put my ideas into action and to begin the journey toward being the Anatomy Girl. To the many Seattle teachers and program managers who invited me into your own yoga sanctuaries and trusted me with your beloved student body—special thanks to Jamie Silverstein, who not only asked me to teach in her first YTT but also offered me a new yoga home in Portland.

To Julie at Aditi, I cannot believe my fortune in our paths crossing at such potent times. Thank you for hearing my voice and trusting that we would work so closely in the future, for not letting time or space keep us apart in Spirit. My most abiding love and thanks to Jeni, Karen, and Suzy at Three Trees Yoga—and to Jennifer B. for connecting us. You have been a particularly special tribe for me. Your graciousness as I upended all the traditional alignments and rewrote the rules is unparalleled. It's been an honor to be a part of your team for each and every training. And finally, to the crew at The People's Yoga—Beth and Sally for giving me the chance to enter into your astounding family of teachers, and most importantly, Rachel Stern. In just a single class you renewed my hope and joy in my own practice and reaffirmed that there is a healthy swath of folks who want what we offer. Thank you, Rachel, for sharing with me your devoted students and turning to me as your sub—it is an honor and a privilege to work with you and your loving following of yogis. It has made my transition to Portland a magical experience.

STEPHANIE

For her vision of a sustainable asana practice, I salute Stephanie Adams and company. By imagining that yoga asana could be practiced with the life-long health of the body in mind, you have changed the potential of the practice for so many. I am honored to be a part of the advisory board for the Sustainable Asana Yoga Foundation (SAYFyoga.com). Since I met you all those years ago at your beloved yoga festival, I have trusted that we were kindreds and would connect again. I'm so lucky to be so much closer to you now! Thank you for trusting in my perspective and offering me a chance to be part of your team of innovators. I hope this book can add to the standard in some small part.

ELENA + AMANDA

My friends, protégés, and Certified Bad-asses, Elena Cheung and Amanda Mitchell-Norrgard—damn. You've been by my side for so long it's hard to think of you as my students. Your love and support and help and devotion to growth in your teaching are beyond compare. You both inspire me to get off my ass and get stuff done, and somehow never make me feel guilty when I'm slacking. You help me stay organized and keep me on track, except when you don't, which just means a lot of fun being had. Thank you for being the rookies, the beta-testers, the editors and collaborators—your hours and hours of assistance have allowed this project (and so many more) to come to fruition. Thanks for trusting me when you have questions, thanks for offering me your wisdom and perspective, thanks for having answers too. Thank you most for thinking of me as Teacher—because you do, I can.

THE MODELS

Yes, you get an extra nod here! There were many hours of prep and time and toil to get the thousands of photos done for this book. Your energy, humor, and enthusiasm made it almost seem like not-work for eighteen hours. Kathryn Stevens brought out the best in all of us, and Alina made us all look like professionals. Elena, you braved traffic and Gresham to be there all weekend—you are a true friend. And of course, our mascot, Inky ... thanks, doll, for keeping it real ... your headshots will be on the website even though they were cut from the print.

THE FAERIE-WRITERS

A few friends had words when I had none. Thanks to the inspiration of these ladies, there is both a beginning and a graceful ending to this book. Hannah darling, who even when very far away still manages to whisper wisdom into my ears, your perspective gave rise to a preface I could have confidence in. Your words convinced me all over again why what I have to share has meaning. To Annie, my dear friend, thank you for the inspiration for the closing chapter of this book (and for so many other magics!). What seemed obvious to you was like a dawning light for me. Thank you for reminding me of what I do when I'm not overthinking.

SHASTA

I have a name, a brand, a color scheme, a product, and a website because one woman did all the real work. Shasta Brewer is a magician herself in all the technical bits that keep my machine running, and looking good to boot. You made it possible to think I could manifest this book, even if I never found a publisher, and were ready to help make it happen if it came to that. Thank you for always being there for me when I panic, when I have silly ideas, when I have confusion, when I need to get grounded and seek sanctuary ... You are a brilliant creator and I appreciate your patience with me all of these years.

ERIN

Erin Taylor, self-described Driver of My Bandwagon, was there at the very outset of this anatomy adventure, and still she remains. Thank you for your moral support, all the talks about writing and publishing, trusting me with your own work and writing, and being a great friend and inspiration. You don't know what a comfort it is to have an ally who's been through it all before! Your generosity is overwhelming, in all the ways. And of course, you are the faery who connected me to the magic of Oiselle ... Whew. That's a biggie.

SALLY + LESKO + LAUREN

The team at Oiselle—my favorite company for women's workout apparel, a huge relationship in any yoga teacher's life—has been with me long before I set these words to paper. Through the magic networking of Erin Taylor, I was introduced to this tribe of women who Run The World from their headquarters in Seattle. Sally Bergesen, Sarah Lesko, and all of my other teammates at HQ (past and present), along with Lauren Fleshman and the current and former members of Little Wing and the Haute Volee—you goddesses make my day. Between the active support of my bodywork career, our ongoing professional relationships and personal friendships, and the all-out effort to outfit the models for the photos in this book, I can honestly say, "I am here because of you!" Sally, Lesko, and Lauren, my heart swells with gratitude for trusting me with your bodies and those of your cherished athletes. Thank you for the opportunity to be such a huge part of some very special events and for keeping me in the community after all these years. Special thanks to Sally for the photoshoot wardrobe, and to Josephine and Stephanie at the flagship store for coming through in a pinch (or two).

THE CIRCLE

There is a Circle of friends who sit in sacredness and have held me in their hearts and minds and hands at my most vulnerable. This group has fostered my knowledge and growth and curiosity in magical ways, always available with love and support at a moment's notice. Your collective and individual Grace has helped me to trust my own magic and be more generous in sharing it with the world. Thank you for your guidance and your leadership. To you all, but particularly to the holders of the space, Cosetta Romani and Ivo Grossi. My teachers and friends, thank you for being present for this journey into understanding. Cosi, you told me my hands would begin different work ... and these pages prove that is true.

THE PACK

To the Wolf Babes—who reminded me that this book "isn't about me," who reminded me to get out of the way and let the book happen as it is meant to—thank you. I bow to each of you, your grace, your wisdom, your seeking of ways to find meaning and Truth. I am honored to be a member of the pack—Owwwwwoooooooowoowoowoo!

Index

elbow
    carrying angle. *See* carrying angle
    joint, 235-236
    limitations, 258-259, 262
    muscles, 254-255, *254*
elevation
    hips, in seated folds, 95
    shoulder, 237, *238*
ellipsoid joints, 41, *42*
endocrine system, 23-24
eversion, foot joint, 140
Equal Standing (Samasthiti), 90-91, *90*
erector spinae group, 77
eversion, ankle muscles, 157
experiential learning
    lower extremity, 158-159, 173-175,
        182-183, *174*
    practice-teaching, 124, 125
    spine and core, 78-79, 106-107
    upper extremity, 256-277, 322-323
Extended Hand to Big Toe (Utthita Hasta
    Padangusthasana), 191
Extended Triangle (Utthita Trikonasana), 203, *203*
extensibility/elasticity, muscles, 33
extension, 16, 67, *67, 81*
    ball and socket joints, 138
    elbow, 242, *242*
    hip muscles, 147-149, *148*, 162
    knee joint, 139
    knee muscles, 154-155, *154*
    shoulder, 238, *239*, 240, *240*
extensor digitorum, *156*, 157
extensors, wrist/hand/fingers, *255*, 256
external, 14
external obliques, 75, *76*
external rotation
    ball and socket joints, 139
    hips, 152-154, *152*, 162-163
    knee muscles, 155, *155*
    seated postures, 211-212, *211*
    shoulders, 238, 240, *239, 240*
    upper extremity, 267

F

Facebook, 11, 125
facet joints, 41, *58*, 60, 62-63, *63*
facets, 59
Facing Hands (Urdhva Hastasana), 292-293, 318
FAI (femoroacetabular impingement), 165
fascia, *27, 28, 29*
    deep fascia, 28-29
    integumentary system, 27-29
    muscle bellies, 29, *29*

feet. *See also* lower extremity
    bones, 130-131, *131*
    common conditions, 169
    flexing to protect knee, 194-197, *194, 196, 197*
    heel to knee to hip alignment, 180-181, *180*
    Pada Bandha (Foot Container), 157-158
    range of motion, 140-141
    relation to gait, 141-142
    soft tissue limitations, 164
    talus, 130, *131*
    talus notch, 160, *160*
    joints, 135, *135*
femoroacetabular impingement (FAI), 165
femur, 129-130, *130*
    angle of femoral neck, 159, *159*
    dysplasia, 171
    torsions, *159*, 160
fibrinogen, 31
fibula, 130, *130*
fingers
    bones, 230, *230*
    muscles, 255-256
    thumb, 259, *279*
Fire Log (Agnistambhasana), 195
    modifications, 224
    practice mechanics, 211-212, *211*
flexing foot to protect knee, 194-197, *194,
    196, 197*
flexion movement, 16
    ball and socket joints, 138
    elbow, 242, *242*
    hip muscles, 143-145, *143*
    hips, 162
    knee joint, 139
    knee muscles, 154, *154*
    shoulders, 238, *239*, 240, *240*
    spine and core, 67
    wrists/hands/fingers, 242-243, *242, 243*
flexors, wrist/hand/fingers, 256
foot. *See* feet
forearm, 229
    bones, *229, 230*
Forearm Stand (Pincha Mayurasana), 303-304, *303*
form follows function, 14, 26, 39
forward folds
    adjustments, 120-122, *121*
    cueing practice, 92-94
    forward momentum, 122
    practice mechanics, 110, *110*, 206-211
    spinal risk factors, 84
    spine and core, 110, *110*, 120-122, *121*
Frog pose (Bhekasana), 108
frontal (coronal) plane, 15-16, *15*
functional anatomy, 2-3

L

L5/S1, 70 *83*
    backbends, 81, 212
    glutes, 100
    lumbar/low back, 83–84
    neck, 81
    twists, 83–84, 103
labrum, 41
    lower extremity, 129, *133*, 165
    modifications, 318–319
    tears, 44, 170–171, 263
    upper extremity, 230, *231*
language, 8–10, 13. *See also* terminology; vocabulary
    babies, 5
lateral, 14, *14*
lateral collateral ligament (LCL), 133
lateral flexion, 67, *67*
lateral longitudinal arch, 135, *135*
latissimus dorsi, *245*, 249–250, *249, 251*
Law of Compensation, 17–18, 78, 80
    pelvis-spine relationship, 171
LCL (lateral collateral ligament), 133
legs. *See also* lower extremity
    ankle across thigh poses, 195
    bones, 129–130, *130*
    compartment syndrome, 168
    shin splints, 168
levator scapula, 246
leverage, 36
levers and torsion, 192
lifting kneecap, 191, *191*
ligamentous joints, 40
ligaments, *30*, 40
    common conditions, 165–169
    foot, *135*
    hip, *132*
    injury risk factors, 43, 44
    integumentary system, 27, 30
    knee joint, 133–135, *134*
    SI joint, *131*
    spine, 63, 79
    sprains, 85
    upper extremity, 231
Light on Yoga (Iyengar), 200
limitations
    lower extremity, 159–165
    spine, 79–86
    upper extremity, 257–262
linea aspera, 150
Locust, 108
longissimus, *76*
Lord of the Fishes (Matsyendrasana), 204, *205*, 224
    adjustments, 220
    practice mechanics, 297, *297*

lordotic curve, cervical spine. *See* lumbar lordosis
Lotus (Padmasana), 139, 147, 211
    knee protection, 195
    modifications after knee surgery, 164
Low Plank (Chaturanga Dandasana)
    arm as lever, 245
    cueing, 55, 287–288, *287*
    practice mechanics, 308–309, *309*
    serratus anterior, 247
    using fists, 322
    vinyasa flow, *289,* 291
lower appendicular skeleton, 38
lower extremity, 127–128
    bones, 128–131
    bony limitations, 159–161
    common conditions, 165–170
    cueing, 185–199
    exercises, 225–226
    experiential learning, 158–159, 173–175, *174,* 182–183
    foot, relation to gait, 141–142
    hip-width, 182
    integration with upper extremity, 283–285, *283, 284*
    joints and connective tissue, 131–137
    muscles, 142–158
    observation skills, 178–181
    practice exercise, 225–226
    practice mechanics, 199–214
    practice teaching, 215–225
    principles of teaching, 177
    range of motion, 137–142
    relationship to spine, 171–173, *172, 173*
    risks, 170–171
    skeleton, *38*
    soft tissue limitations, 162–165
    students, 225–226
    teachers, 225
    vocabulary, 183–184
lumbar, *59*, 60
    backbend support, 97
    forward folds, 84–85
    rotation, *69*, 70
    supine twists, *105*
    twists, 83
lumbar lordosis, *59*, 60–61, 65, 80, 97–98, 108–110, 186, 206, 294, 296
Lunge, 225–226
lunge-based (asymmetrical) backbending
    postures, 109
lunges
    cueing, 187, *187*
    experiential learning, 174–175, *174*
    heelkneehip plane, *178,* 179
    knee conditions, 167
    momentum, 185

About the Author

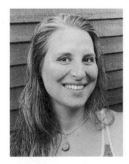

Richelle Ricard is an educator, bodyworker, and movement specialist whose work across the Pacific Northwest and beyond has earned her notoriety as the "Anatomy Girl." She has been teaching yoga teachers about anatomy, kinesiology, and preventing injury in asana practice since 2008. Her own twenty-year asana practice has shown her the value of critical thought regarding alignment and execution, and it brought her deeper into understanding of the How and Why we practice yoga. She has written curricula for teacher trainings worldwide and hopes that, together, the yoga teachers of the world can shift out of a practice of rhetoric and regurgitation and into a closely observational style of teaching that honors the individual as well as the deeper energetics of asana practice.

Richelle is currently devoted to designing online support courses for *The Yoga Engineer's Manual* and her other teacher training programs, as well as continuing to teach yoga and provide clinical bodywork to her community. Her favorite escapes from her various realities are beaches, mountains, novels, and a long hot bath. Really good tequila also helps.

About North Atlantic Books

North Atlantic Books (NAB) is a 501(c)(3) nonprofit publisher committed to a bold exploration of the relationships between mind, body, spirit, culture, and nature. Founded in 1974, NAB aims to nurture a holistic view of the arts, sciences, humanities, and healing. To make a donation or to learn more about our books, authors, events, and newsletter, please visit www.northatlanticbooks.com.